Allergic Skin Diseases of Dogs and Cats

Second Edition

Allergic Skin Diseases of Dogs and Cats

Second Edition

Lloyd M. Reedy DVM
Animal Dermatology Referral Clinic
Dallas, Texas
USA

William H. Miller Jr VMD
New York State College of Veterinary Medicine
Cornell University, New York
USA

Ton Willemse DVM, PhD
Faculty of Veterinary Medicine
University of Utrecht
The Netherlands

W.B. Saunders Company Ltd
LONDON PHILADELPHIA TORONTO SYDNEY TOKYO

W.B. Saunders Company Ltd 24–28 Oval Road
London NW1 7DX

The Curtis Center
Independence Square West
Philadelphia, PA 19106-3399, USA

Harcourt Brace & Company
55 Horner Avenue
Toronto, Ontario M8Z 4X6, Canada

Harcourt Brace & Company, Australia
30–52 Smidmore Street
Marrickville, NSW 2204, Australia

Harcourt Brace & Company, Japan
Ichibancho Central Building, 22-1 Ichibancho
Chiyoda-ku, Tokyo 102, Japan

First edition published in 1989 by W.B. Saunders Company, Philadelphia

This book is printed on acid-free paper

A catalogue record for this book is available from the British Library

ISBN 0-7020-1974-7

Typeset by Saxon Graphics Ltd, Derby
Printed in Great Britain by The University Press, Cambridge

Contents

List of Color Plates

Preface

We (Drs Reedy and Miller) were immensely pleased with the reception given to the first edition of *Allergic Skin Diseases of Dogs and Cats*; so much so, in fact, that we forgot the pain involved and agreed to produce a second edition. In order to improve upon the first edition and to make the book more international in scope, we asked Dr Ton Willemse, a well-known and respected teacher and scientist from Utrecht, to be the third author. We were delighted when Dr Willemse agreed. All three of us were honored as well as humbled at the enormous and enlightening task.

Each and every chapter has been completely re-written, updated, and referenced to include not only the latest scientific information but the viewpoints from all three authors. We also feel that the addition of selected color photographs and larger print will enhance the value of the text for the readers. We hope that the result will be a useful, practical guide to the allergic skin disorders which plague dogs and cats.

The authors would like to thank all the researchers and clinical investigators whose works we quoted. We would also like to thank W.B. Saunders Company Limited for their assistance and expertise in this undertaking. In closing we would also like to give our personal thanks to our respective wives, Juanita, Kathy, and Marlies for their encouragement, patience, and understanding.

Lloyd M. Reedy, DVM

William H. Miller Jr VMD

Ton Willemse, DVM, PhD

1
Introduction to Allergy

Introduction

Allergy is an altered state of immune reactivity. A basic function of the immune system is to protect by distinguishing self from nonself, and by the elimination of the latter. If the normal controls fail, the immune system may not clear noxious substances and may attack harmless materials such as pollens or even self. Allergy is a specific hypersensitivity that triggers complex biochemical and inflammatory sequences that are harmful to the tissues or disrupt the physiology of the host. The symptoms depend on the degree of responsiveness of the effector cells and interactions with other biochemical agents. Thus, it would not be too simplistic to suggest that allergy is immunity gone awry.

With increased understanding of the pathogenesis of allergic disease, we have developed renewed appreciation for the complexity of the allergic response and of the immune system. The immune system is extremely complex and new information about its function and regulation is added daily. Much of the recent information on the pathogenesis of allergic disease arose from more clearly defining the intricate interplay between cells of the immune system and the plethora of chemical substances (inflammatory mediators and cytokines) that these cells are capable of elaborating. Allergic sensitization can affect virtually any tissue in the body and cause a multitude of clinical diseases, which vary in their pathogenesis, immunology, and pathology. Consequently, there is hardly any area in veterinary medicine where a knowledge of allergy and allergic reactions is not important. The correct diagnosis and management of allergic diseases requires a thorough knowledge of basic immunologic principles. This first chapter will present some background and the vocabulary necessary to understand the chapters that follow. A brief outline of the immune response and how it applies in allergy is also included. Only very basic information is provided here and the reader is referred to immunology texts and the references for a more complete discussion.

History of Allergy

Much of our present knowledge of allergy (Coca and Cooke, 1925) is based on early fundamental observations relating to experimental anaphylaxis in animals. In 1902, Richet (see Richet, 1913) demonstrated that repeated injections of toxic extracts of sea anemone (*Actinaria*) provoked progressively more severe reactions in dogs rather than protection as expected. They coined the word *anaphylaxis* ('without protection') and theorized that the first injection destroyed any natural resistance the animal might have had against the toxin. Thus they produced an increased susceptibility rather than immunity. Similar reactions occurred after repeated injections of relatively harmless products such as milk. Anaphylaxis could also be transferred to normal animals by the injection of serum from a sensitized animal, clearly indicating that some circulating factor conferred specific anaphylactic sensitivity. Since this was artificially induced, there was some doubt that animals other than man spontaneously developed allergies. The erroneous assumption that hay fever in man was caused by pollen 'toxins' prompted early workers to attempt to induce protection by immunization. Clinical improvement indicated efficacy of this mode of treatment (Noon, 1911). The discovery of 'blocking antibodies' in the serum of these patients added further support to the usefulness of immunization. Prausnitz and Küstner (1921) demonstrated the presence of skin sensitizing antibody (reagin) in the serum of allergic humans by passively transferring it by injection to normal individuals. This important discovery, the Prausnitz–Küstner (P–K) test, laid the groundwork for the eventual identification of IgE as reagin or the allergic antibody.

History of Allergy in Small Animals

As in man, the first published case reports of canine allergies, although anecdotal, were to foods (Burns, 1933; Pomeroy, 1934). In 1941, Wittich reported on a dog with recurrent seasonal pruritus that coincided with the ragweed season. Skin tests and P–K tests were positive for ragweed and other fall pollens and the dog was successfully hyposensitized to these pollens. The association of IgE antibodies with canine mast cells was demonstrated in 1973 by Halliwell.

Man and dogs are not the only species of animal capable of developing spontaneous allergy to aeroallergens. Clinical allergic diseases have been demonstrated in cats, horses, sheep, cows, and a variety of laboratory animals (Halliwell *et al.*, 1979; Halliwell and Gorman 1989). No doubt, allergies exist in all species of animals.

Definitions

Adhesion molecules: Cell surface molecules that regulate cell-to-cell or cell-to-extracellular matrix adhesion.

Adjuvant: A substance that nonspecifically enhances the immune response to an antigen.

Allergen: An antigen that induces an allergic reaction.

Allergenicity: The property of a substance that makes it capable of inducing an immune response.

Anamnestic: The faculty of memory.

Anaphylactoid reactions: Mimic anaphylactic reactions, clinically but not immunologically mediated.

Anaphylaxis: An immediate hypersensitivity reaction resulting from the degranulation of sensitized mast cells following re-exposure to an allergen. It is typically thought of as a systemic hypersensitivity leading to a shock-like state, but it can be localized to one specific organ system such as the gastrointestinal tract, nasal mucosa, or skin.

Anergy: No response to an injection of antigen; anti-anaphylaxis.

Antibody: A complex protein produced in response to an antigen that has the ability to combine specifically with the antigen that induced its formation. The term immunoglobulin is also used.

Antigen: A molecule that induces the formation of antibody.

Antigen presentation: The process by which certain cells in the body – antigen-presenting cells (APCs) – express antigen on their cell surface in a form recognizable by lymphocytes.

Antigen-presenting cells (APCs): Cells – usually monocytes, macrophages, or dendritic cells – that process and present antigen within an antigen-binding cleft of their major histocompatibility complex (MHC) molecules.

Antigen processing: The conversion of an antigen into a form in which it can be recognized by lymphocytes.

Atopy: A genetically determined immunologic reactivity in which IgE (or IgGd) antibody is readily produced in response to ordinary exposure to common allergens in the subject's environment. In man, atopy consists of hay fever, asthma, and atopic dermatitis, while in animals the term is applied to allergic dermatitis.

Autoimmunity: A state in which tolerance to self is lost.

Chemokines: Molecules that regulate leukocyte trafficking and migration.

Cluster designation (CD) markers: Cell surface molecules of leukocytes and platelets that are distinguishable with monoclonal antibodies and may be used to differentiate different cell populations.

Cross-reaction: The reaction of an antibody with an antigen other than the one that induced its formation. Cross-reacting antigens share some common determinant groups. Some grass pollens have similar determinant groups so an individual allergic to one grass may react to certain other grass pollens.

Cytokines: A generic term for soluble molecules that mediate interaction between cells.

Cytotropic antibody: An antibody that can attach to or sensitize cells. Homocytotropic antibodies are those that will fix to tissues of animals within the same species while heterocytotropic antibodies will fix to tissues of different species.

Determinant groups: Individual chemical structures on the antigen that determine antigenic specificity. The number, type, and nature of the determinant groups determines the immunologic uniqueness of an antigen. Two or more antigenic determinants are necessary to stimulate an immune response. Antigens that share common determinant groups immunologically can be viewed as similar and may cross-react.

Epitope: A single antigen determinant. Functionally it is the portion of an antigen that combines with the antibody paratope.

Hapten: A small molecule that by itself is incapable of eliciting an antibody response, but can act as an epitope. For a hapten to induce an immune response, it must be coupled to a larger carrier molecule, which in itself need not be antigenic.

Immunogenicity: The property of a substance that makes it capable of inducing an immune response. The immunogenicity of an antigen is dependent upon the molecular size, solubility, shape, electric charge, and accessibility of its determinant groups.

Immunotherapy: The process of preventing or diminishing allergic symptoms by modulating the immune response. This process was previously called desensitization or hyposensitization.

Interleukins: A group of molecules involved in signalling between cells of the immune system.

Intolerance: An exaggerated nonimmunologic physiologic response to a substance. The term is used to distinguish symptoms caused by an idiosyncrasy or an irritation to a substance from those caused by allergy. Erythromycin-induced vomiting is an example of drug intolerance.

Major histocompatibility complex (MHC): A genetic region found in all mammals that functions in signalling between lymphocytes and cells expressing antigen. Originally identified in transplant rejection, it is now recognized that proteins encoded in this region are involved in many aspects of immunologic recognition, including interaction between different lymphoid cells as well as between lymphocytes and APCs.

Paratope: The part of an antibody molecule that makes contact with the antigenic determinant (epitope).

Receptor: Cell surface molecule where antibody, cytokines, etc. bind to initiate some cellular event. The affinity of receptor molecules can vary from cell to cell.

The Skin Immune System

In the not too distant past, the protective functions of the skin and the immune system were thought to work independently. The skin mechanically blocked the entrance of foreign antigens into the body and the immune system dealt with those that got through. Today, it is well known that the skin is an active immunologic organ that participates in immunologic surveillance and reactivity. In recognition of these roles, the skin has been joined to the immune system in the well accepted concept of the skin immune system (Bos, 1989).

Traditionally, the immune system has been divided into three separate arms: namely the humoral, the cellular, and the nonspecific systems. The four types of hypersensitivity reactions described by Gell and Coombs were defined with this segregation in mind (See general immunology texts – Halliwell and Gorman, 1989; Roitt *et al.*, 1989; Tizard, 1996). These concepts are, however, far too simplistic. It is not possible to consider cell-mediated and antibody-mediated responses separately. Cells involved in the initiation of an antibody response and the resultant antibody act as an essential link in some cell-mediated reactions. Moreover, no cell-mediated response is likely to occur in the total absence of antibody. Inflammation, the heart of hypersensitivity reactions, is a complex process involving elements of nonspecific and specific cellular and humoral immunity and a growing network of interlocking soluble mediators, the cytokines and interleukins. The following discussion breaks down the skin immune system into individual components, but due to the complex interactions in the immune system, this separation is artificial. The reader is also reminded that what follows is intended to be a brief overview to allow a more complete understanding of the material that follows. Current immunology textbooks should be consulted for more complete details.

Cellular components of the immune system

All of the cells of the immune system and the ancillary networks that work in concert with the immune system's cells arise from pluripotential stem (PPS) cells in the bone marrow. This PPS cell gives rise to lymphoid and myeloid stem cells (Shearer and Huston, 1993). The lymphoid population differentiates into three cell types: the T lymphocyte, the B lymphocyte, and the non-T non-B large granular lymphocyte. The myeloid stem cell population gives rise to megakaryocytes, erythrocytes, neutrophils, mast cells, basophils, eosinophils, monocytes, and macrophages. Differentiation and development of all these various cell lines is critically dependent upon an array of cytokines and cell-to-cell interactions.

All cells of the skin immune system express many different molecules on their surface. Some of these appear for short periods at a specific stage of cell differentiation or activation while others persist. Molecules that can be used to distinguish cell populations are called cell markers and many of them can be identified by specific monoclonal antibodies. A systematic nomenclature has been developed for these surface markers and the term cluster designation (CD) has been adopted. The markers are numbered CD1, CD2, etc. and over 130 markers have been assigned so far (Tizard, 1996).

Antigen-presenting cells
Allergens are large proteins or glycoproteins, which in most instances must be phagocytized, metabolized, and broken down into smaller subunits before an immunologic reaction can occur (Figure 1.1). Traditional APCs of the immune system include mononuclear phagocytes (monocytes, macrophages), dendritic cells, and B lymphocytes (Bos, 1989; Nickoloff, 1993; Tizard, 1996). Although details of antigen processing can differ with the type of APC in question, the basic process is similar. The allergen is internalized and digested into its peptide fragments and these interact with the major histocompatibility complex (MHC) class II. The peptide–MHC complex migrates to the surface of the APC where it interacts with T cells. The trimolecular interaction of the APC, peptide–MHC II complex, and T cell triggers a specific immunologic reaction to the allergen in question. The type of reaction, humoral or cell-mediated, depends upon the cytokines present. Cell-mediated processes result from the production of interleukin (IL)-2, interferon (IFN)-γ,

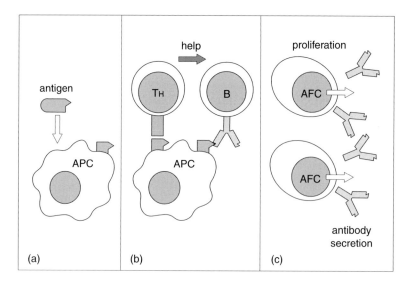

Figure 1.1   *Simplified overview of the immune response.*
(a) Antigen encountering the immune system is processed by antigen-presenting cells (APCs) which retain fragments of the antigen on their surfaces. (b) T-helper cells (TH) recognize the antigen via their surface receptors and provide help to B cells (B) which also recognize antigen by their surface receptors (immunoglobulin). (c) The B cells are stimulated to proliferate and divide into antibody-forming cells (AFCs) which secrete antibody. (From Roitt et al., 1989, with permission.)

and tumor necrosis factor (TNF)-β. A humoral response is encouraged by the production of IL-6, IL-7, IL-10, IL-11, IL-14, and transforming growth factor (TGF)-β (Fishman *et al.*, 1996).

Keratinocytes can also express the MHC class II (MHC II) of APCs, but their role in antigen presentation is uncertain. Since keratinocytes produce a variety of cytokines (IL-1, IL-3, IL-6, IL-8, and TNF-α, and colony stimulating factors, and express adhesion molecules, they no doubt play a pivotal role in allergic reactions (Bos, 1989; Suter, 1995).

The dendritic cell population of the skin is composed of Langerhans' cells and dermal dendrocytes. The Langerhans' cells are best known and are derived from cells of bone marrow origin and migrate to the suprabasal epidermis during the sixth week of gestation (Hogan and Burks, 1995) where they make up 3–4% of the epidermal cell population, but can also be found in the dermis, lymph nodes, thymus, and mucosal surfaces. The classical ultrastructural feature of the Langerhans' cell is the Birbeck granule, a rod-shaped body with central striations and, occasionally, a saccular terminus. The function of the Birbeck granule is unknown, but it probably represents endocytosis of receptor–ligand complexes. Birbeck granules have been identified in dendritic cells of the cow, horse, goat, and sheep, but are usually absent in the dog (Goodell *et al.*, 1985; Schroeder *et al.*, 1994). The immunohistochemical marker considered best for the Langerhans' cell is CD1a. Langerhans' cells express the MHC II complex of APCs as well as receptors for complement (C3b) and the Fc region of IgG and IgE. Their major function is antigen processing and presentation. IgE and Langerhans' cells are found in increased numbers in lesional skin of atopic dogs, suggesting that transdermal allergen exposure might be important for both sensitization and clinical disease in animals (Olivry *et al.*, 1995).

Other dendritic cells are found in the dermis and elsewhere in the body (Anttila *et al.*, 1994; Nickoloff, 1993). Immunohistochemical studies have shown that these cells are not antigenically related to Langerhans' cells. Despite differences in surface markers, all immunocompetent dendritic cells probably act in a similar fashion, with antigen processing and presentation a primary function.

The monocyte–macrophage

The monocyte develops from bone marrow precursors, but most of its functional development occurs outside the bone marrow. The cells migrate into the tissues where they develop into longlived macrophages. These mononuclear cells have an important phagocytic function and as phagocytes, macrophages act as scavengers of cellular debris and inorganic material as well as being capable of ingesting infectious agents. Their function as phagocytes is similar to that of neutrophils, but unlike neutrophils, macrophages can synthesize new enzymes on demand and thus sustain the phagocytic response (Reedy and Miller, 1989).

Although an important phagocyte, the macrophage also plays a critical role in immune regulation via its antigen processing and cytokine production. Activated macrophages produce IL-1, which activates lymphocytes, is chemotactic for neutrophils and, in conjunction with IL-6 and TNF-α, induces the liver to produce complement components, clotting factors, protease inhibitors, metal-binding proteins, and acute-phase proteins – C-reactive protein (CRP), serum amyloid P (SAP), and serum amyloid A (SAA) (Tizard, 1996). Macrophages are also a source of IFN, can act as killer cells and may help regulate natural killer (NK) cells (Reedy and Miller, 1989).

Lymphocytes

Lymphocyte populations are the backbone of the immune system and are divided into B cells, T cells, and null cells. Null cells are killer cells with Fc receptors on their surface and are responsible for antibody-dependent cell-mediated cytotoxicity. Classes and subclasses of lymphocytes are defined on the basis of their surface markers, the cytokines they produce, and other characteristics. Both B and T cells are activated when they bind their specific antigen in the presence of accessory cells. Once activated, they produce cytokines and cell surface receptors for these and other cytokines. These cytokines drive the cells through the cell cycle into currently active effector cells and memory cells. The memory cells are longlived, antigen-specific amplifier cells, which function in secondary or anamnestic responses. At the very first exposure to an antigen, only a few B cells can recognize and respond to the antigen. During the generation of active effector cells, multiple memory cells are also produced. With subsequent re-exposure to the antigen, these cells are activated and result in a more rapid and more intense response to the antigen.

The B cell is the antibody-secreting cell of the immune system and produces the immunoglobulins of the IgG, IgA, IgM, and IgE classes (Reedy and Miller, 1989). A fifth class of immunoglobulin, IgD, is also produced as a cell surface molecule. B cells mature in the bone marrow or partially in the fetal liver. There is supposedly a specific clone of B cells capable of recognizing each unique antigen. B cells have cell surface receptors for immunoglobulins, complement, cytokines, and for the specific antigen they recognize. The antigen receptor is termed the BCR and 200 000–500 000 are found per cell (Tizard, 1996). These receptors are immunoglobulins that can bind to intact allergen, whereas antigens that initiate a T cell response must first be processed by APCs.

For most antigens, a humoral response requires an intercurrent T cell interaction. When the B cell binds antigen, it activates helper T (TH) cells so that the B cell's surface IgD molecule is lost and is replaced with an antigen-specific IgM molecule. As proliferation and activation continue, memory cells and antibody-producing plasma cells are generated. The cytokines produced determine the nature of the plasma cell response. In allergic disorders, antibody production switches from IgM to IgE and the IgE production is regulated primarily by IL-4, IL-13, and IFN-γ (Fishman *et al.*, 1996; Kapsenberg *et al.*, 1996). Il-4 and IL-13 are up-regulators and result in IgE production. Co-stimulation with IL-2, IL-5, IL-6, and IL-14 results in a more marked IgE response. IFN-γ inhibits the development of IgE cell surface receptors and IgE production and promotes IgG production. The initial source of IL-4 triggering the switch to IgE production is unknown, but may arise from null cells (Tizard, 1996).

T cells comprise most (60–80%) of the mononuclear cells in the peripheral circulation and over 90% of the lymphocytes in the lymph channels (Tizard, 1996). They develop from stem cells, which enter the thymus gland where they develop into mature T cells with a distinct genome, surface antigens, and functional characteristics (Shearer and Huston, 1993). As with B cells, there is one T cell clone for each unique antigen. All peripheral T cells bear the T cell antigen receptor (TCR) complex, and thus CD3 serves as a pan T cell marker. In addition, T cells have specific cell surface receptors for histamine, immunoglobulins, cytokines, MHC, and complement. Traditionally, T cell subpopulations have been categorized into those that help or upregulate (TH), those that suppress or downregulate (Ts), or those that kill (Tc). Currently, the existence of the suppressor group is being debated. Convincing evidence exists that downregulation is accomplished by inhibitor interactions of the TH populations (Tizard, 1996).

Th cells (CD4$^+$) are necessary to initiate and perpetuate most immunologic reactions. Three subsets (TH0, TH1, and TH2) have been characterized by their surface markers and cytokine repertoire. TH1 cells appear to interact best with antigen processed by B cells while TH2 cells deal with antigen processed by macrophages and Langerhan's cells, etc. (Tizard, 1996). TH1 cells produce IL-2, IFN-γ, and TNF-β while TH2 cells produce IL-4, IL-5, IL-10, and IL-13 (Fishman *et al.*, 1996; Tizard, 1996). TH0 cells secrete a mixture of cytokines from both TH1 and TH2 cells and may represent precursors of TH1 or TH2 cells or be a transition phase where a TH1 cell is converting to a TH2 cell or vice versa.

The CD8$^+$ T cells are referred to as Ts cells, which modulate or downregulate an immunologic reaction and also function as effector cells in delayed hypersensitivity reactions, graft-versus-host reactions, and the direct killing of cells. As mentioned previously, suppressor influences attributed to these cells may be due to the interplay of the cytokines produced by the TH1 and TH2 cells. As killers or modulators of delayed hypersensitivity reactions, Tc cells can be activated by IL-2 produced by TH1 cells or by direct interaction with the processed antigen at the MHC II receptor.

NK cells

NK cells are mononuclear cells of uncertain origin that can cause spontaneous cyto-toxicity (Reedy and Miller, 1989). Killing is antibody independent and does not require previous sensitization. Virus-infected or tumor cells are typically the targets of NK cells. NK cells are upregulated by IFN-γ.

Polymorphonuclear leukocytes

Neutrophil. The neutrophil is a bone marrow-derived cell that migrates into the tissues where it plays a central role in the host's defense against infection, especially by rapidly dividing organisms such as *Staphylococcus* spp., but it is also important in other immunologic reactions. Neutrophil migration is influenced by a variety of chemoattractant factors, which include:

- histamine, eosinophilic chemotactic factor of anaphylaxis (ECF-A), neutrophil chemotactic factor (NCF), platelet-activating factor (PAF), and lipid chemotactic factors (e.g. leukotriene (LT) B4) from mast cells;
- prostaglandins (PGs) and LTs from a variety of cells;
- C3a, C5a, and C567 from the complement cascade;
- kallikrein from the kinin system;
- plasminogen activator, fibrinopeptides, and fibrin-derived products from the coagulation system;
- lymphokines;
- bacterial products;
- immune complexes (Reedy and Miller, 1989).

Neutrophils have complement and IgG receptors on their surfaces and these medi-ate the binding of opsonized (antibody- and/or complement-coated) particles to the cell membrane. Phagocytosis of small particles or surface adherence activates the cell to produce or release reactive oxygen products, LTs, PGs, and various enzymes. If an activated neutrophil is damaged or a particle is adhered to the cell's surface, these agents are released into the surrounding fluid space where they will damage tissues, activate other cells, and suppress some humoral and cell-mediated processes.

Eosinophil. The eosinophil is another phagocytic granulocyte and has an important role in allergic and parasitic conditions (Martin *et al.*, 1996). Eosinophils have receptors for complement, histamine (H_1 and H_2), and IgG on their surface and contain gran-ules, which contain toxic cationic proteins – major basic protein (MBP), eosinophilic cationic protein (ECP) – lipid mediators (LTC4, LTD4, PAF), oxygen metabolites, and various enzymes such as eosinophilic peroxidase (EPO), histaminase, and kinase. Degranulation is regulated by numerous factors including immunoglobulins (IgG, IgA), lipid mediators, cytokines (IL-5), and adhesion molecules.

Although the eosinophil is a phagocytic cell (immune complexes, immunoglobu-lins, etc.), its primary role in allergic disorders is to modulate the allergic reaction. The eosinophil is capable of both downregulating and upregulating the reaction. It produces IL-3, IL-5, and granulocyte-monocyte colony-stimulating factor (GM-CSF), which are necessary for activation, differentiation, and survival of eosinophils

(Martin *et al.*, 1996). Destruction of histamine, kinins, and PAF by histaminase, kinase, and phospholipase, respectively, damp allergic inflammation. The inflammation is prolonged or intensified by the release of LTs and PGs by eosinophils.

Basophil.   Both mast cells and basophils are derived from hematopoietic precursors and both have surface receptors for IgE and IgG molecules (Sainte-Laudy and Prost, 1996). The affinity of the IgGd receptors in the dog appears to be low. As with mast cells, bridging of two adjacent antibody molecules can result in basophil degranulation with the release of various chemotactic factors and vasoactive substances. At one time basophils were thought of as circulating mast cells or precursors of tissue mast cells, but recent studies indicate that basophils and mast cells have quite distinct function (Schroeder *et al.*, 1995). Basophils appear to be more reactive then mast cells (Schroeder *et al.*, 1994). They are upregulated by more cytokines and chemokines and generate more proinflammatory cytokines than mast cells. As discussed previously, IL-4 is important in the production of IgE and the basophil is an important source of this cytokine. Lymphocytes generate only about 10–20% as much IL-4 as basophils. Basophils infiltrate tissues many hours after the immediate reaction to administered antigen and cause mediator release in the late-phase response (LPR), a clinically relevant model of chronic allergic inflammation, and are also important in some delayed hypersensitivity reactions and basophil hypersensitivity.

The mast cell
Mast cells are oval-to-spindle-shaped cells with numerous large intracytoplasmic basophilic metachromatic granules and are repositories for or synthesizers of numerous inflammatory substances (Figure 1.2). Under the influence of IL-3, a growth factor from T lymphocytes, pluripotential stem cells grow and differentiate into mast cells (Siraganian, 1993). Although mast cells are thought of primarily in the context of allergic disorders, they have also been implicated in biologic responses as diverse as angiogenesis, wound healing, bone remodeling, reactions to neoplasms, and many chronic inflammatory conditions (Galli, 1993). They are widely distributed in connective tissues and are prominent around dermal blood vessels in the skin. Mast cells in different anatomical sites, and even in a single site, can be substantially different in terms of mediator content, sensitivity to agents that induce activation and mediator release, and response to pharmacologic agents (Galli, 1993). Such heterogeneity is regulated by many factors, but especially cytokines, which influence the cell's stage of maturation, differentiation, proliferation, and other characteristics.

Two types of mast cells, types I and II, can be identified and both are found in dog skin (Scott *et al.*, 1995). In the dog, 4–12 mast cells/high power field (hpf) is considered normal while up to 20/hpf can be found in normal cats. Although the number of mast cells in the dog's skin is 20% less than in human skin, dogs' mast cells are calculated to contain 50% more histamine (DeBoer, 1994).

Mast cells have a variety of surface receptors including receptors for immunoglobulin (IgE or IgGd), histamine (H_2), cytokines, complement, and eosinophilic MBP and can be activated in an immunologic or nonimmunologic fashion (Figure 1.2). The former is most important in the allergic patient. When antigen cross-links two IgE (or IgGd) molecules bound to the mast cell's surface receptors

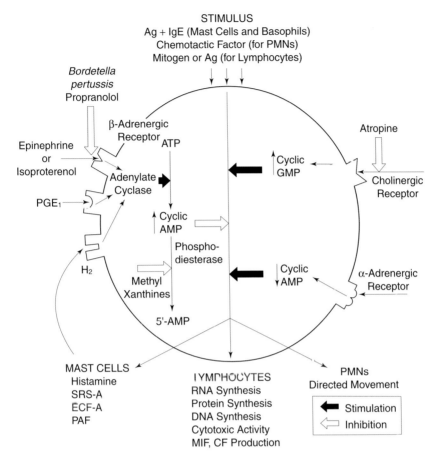

Figure 1.2 *Diagrammatic representation of pathways by which pharmacologic mediators might act on mast cell, lymphocyte, and polymorphonuclear (PMN) leukocyte membrane receptors to alter intracellular cyclic nucleotides, which in turn may either enhance or inhibit the function of those cells. Ag = Antigen; PGE_1 = prostaglandin E_1; SRS-A = slow-reacting substance of anaphylaxis; ECF-A = eosinophil chemotactic factor of anaphylaxis; PAF = platelet-activating factor; MIF = migration inhibition factor; CF = chemotactic factor. (From Hanifin and Lobitz, 1977, with permission.)*

the cell undergoes a characteristic pattern of biochemical and morphologic changes, which are collectively designated anaphylactic degranulation, and result in the release of a panel of biologically active mediators. After stimulation, adenylate cyclase is activated and several proteins are phosphorylated (Reedy and Miller, 1989). A transient calcium flux occurs across the membrane, causing the cytoplasmic granules to swell and move towards the cell membrane. The granules push the cell membrane from the inside and produce multiple bulges from the cell surface. The perigranular membrane fuses with the cell membrane and the granule is discharged into the extracellular space. Mediator is released very rapidly after activation and histamine can be found in the extracellular space within 15 seconds (Reedy and Miller, 1989). At activation, phospholipases, especially phospholipase A_2, are activated and liberate free arachidonic acid, resulting in the formation of various lipid mediators. At activation, mast cells also produce multiple cytokines and chemokines, including IL-3, IL-4, IL-5, IL-6, IL-13, ECF-A, NCF, GM-CSF, and TNF-α (Burd *et al.*, 1995; Tizard, 1996).

Mast cells modulate allergic reactions through their cytokines and preformed, granule-derived, or newly-formed membrane-derived mediators. Granule-derived mediators include histamine, heparin, chondroitin sulfate, and various proteases. Newly-formed mediators include PAF and the PGs, thromboxanes, LTs, hydroperoxyeicosatetraenoic acids (HPETEs), and hydroxyeicosatetraenoic acids (HETEs). Histamine is the primary vasoactive mediator and its effects are exerted through interactions with H_1 or H_2 receptors. In the skin, H_1 activation:

- causes the induction and augmentation of the wheal and flair reaction;
- increases vascular permeability by causing venular endothelial disconnections;
- stimulates the production of PGs;
- stimulates directed and random migration of neutrophils and eosinophils;
- mediates pruritus (Reedy and Miller, 1989)

Stimulation of H_2 receptors downregulates allergic reactions by:

- inhibition of lymphocytotoxicity, random and directed migration of granulocytes, and vasoactivity;
- stimulation of suppressor activities of regulatory T cells;
- inhibition of further mast cell degranulation (Reedy and Miller, 1989).

The impact of the lipid mediators is discussed under eicosanoids.

Chemical components of the immune system

Antibodies

Antibodies or immunoglobulins are protein (primarily glycoprotein) molecules synthesized by lymphocytes. Five major classes, namely IgG, IgM, IgA, IgE, and IgD, are recognized. IgD is a noncirculating antibody found in large quantities on many B cell membranes and although its precise biologic function is unknown, it may play a role in antigen-triggered lymphocyte differentiation (Roitt *et al.*, 1989). The remaining classes enter the tissues or circulation. Plasma cells produce the circulating antibody, which has the same antigenic specificity as that found on the original B cell initiating the immune response. Plasma cells are prolific antibody producers, with estimates that each cell can produce 10^6 molecules of immunoglobulin/hour (Tizard, 1996).

All immunoglobulins have the same basic four polypeptide chain structure consisting of two light and two heavy chains (see Figure 1.3). Each of these chains has a constant and variable region where the amino acid sequence is either constant or variable. The amino acid sequence in the constant region of the heavy chain determines the class of the antibody. For example, IgG has two γ heavy chains while IgE has two ϵ heavy chains. In nature, these chains are folded so that the molecule appears to have six globular units.

Immunoglobulin molecules are divided into the Fab region where antigen binding

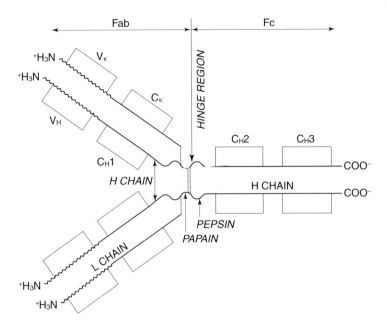

Figure 1.3 *A simplified model for an IgG1 (k) human antibody molecule showing the four-chain basic structure and domains. V indicates variable region; C, the constant region; and the vertical arrow, the hinge region. Thick lines represent H and L chains; thin lines represent disulfide bonds. (From Goodman and Wang, 1987, with permission.)*

occurs and the Fc region where cell binding occurs. The Fc region of the IgE molecule has a special segment that facilitates binding to mast cells (Reedy and Miller, 1989). IgG and IgM also bind complement in the Fc region. Antigen binding occurs in the variable zone of the Fab region. Although the heavy and light chains each have some individual binding activity, the natural binding site for an antigen involves both chains. With two Fab units per molecule, the immunoglobulin can bind to two antigens.

Antibodies have a unique amino acid sequence in the variable region that enables them to recognize a specific antigen or an antigen that is very similar to it (cross-reaction). Plasma cells can produce one class of antibody or switch from the production of IgM to IgG, IgA, or IgE with the same antigenic specificity. Switching is under genetic control. Genes coding for the amino acid sequence in the variable region remain unchanged while those coding for the constant region of the heavy chain are replaced (Reedy and Miller, 1989). The signal(s) inducing the switching are not completely understood, but cytokines have a critical role. In switching to IgE production, IL-4, IL-13, and IFN-γ are most important (Fishman *et al.*, 1996). IFN-γ inhibits the allergic response while IL-4 and IL-13 promote it.

IgG is the basic workhorse of the immune system and comprises 70–75% of the total immunoglobulin pool. Four subclasses have been characterized in the dog and one, IgG4 or IgGd, is cytotropic and can participate in immediate hypersensitivity reactions (Tizard, 1996). Three subclasses of IgG have been identified in the cat and a fourth probably exists. The role of a subclass of IgG in allergic diseases of the cat is unknown.

IgA is considered to be a barrier antibody as it is the predominant protective immunoglobulin in seromucous secretions such as saliva, colostrum, milk, tracheo-bronchial and genitourinary secretions. IgA is also found in the skin, and dogs with selective IgA deficiency can develop recurrent pyodermas (Scott *et al.*, 1995). Although serum IgA levels can be normal in some atopic dogs, atopic dogs tend to have lower mean serum levels then normal dogs (Hall and Campbell, 1993; Hill *et al.*, 1993). The significance of this IgA deficiency remains unclear. Since environmental allergens gain access to the body through the skin and respiratory tract, IgA deficiency may play a central role in atopic sensitization. It is one author's (WHM) view that IgA-deficient atopic dogs have more severe clinical signs then atopic dogs with normal serum IgA levels. Whether this relates specifically to the IgA deficiency or a more basic abnormality in immunoregulation is unknown.

IgE is the antibody generated in response to parasitic infections or allergens. As discussed previously, the switching of B cells to IgE production in allergic patients is upregulated by IL-4 and IL-13 and downregulated by IFN-γ. All immunologically normal individuals can produce IgE and titers increase or decrease with antigen exposure. In nonallergic individuals, antibody production stops with antigen withdrawal and titers drop to unmeasurable levels, typically within 60 days (Miller *et al.*, 1992), but because of various genetic factors, atopic individuals continue to produce antibody after allergen withdrawal (Miller *et al.*, 1992: Blumenthal and Blumenthal, 1996). How these genetic factors influence the allergic individual's immune system is incompletely understood, but an IgE-augmented persistent activation of APCs via their IgE receptors is postulated (Mudde *et al.*, 1996).

IgE is a homocytotropic antibody with a molecular weight of approximately 190 000 and a sedimentation coefficient of 8s. IgE is found in the fast γ region of protein electrophoresis and is heat and acid labile. Heating of IgE to 56°C for 4–6 hours (Sainte-Laudy and Prost, 1996) alters the Fc portion of the molecule and destroys its reactivity. The two Fc antigenic determinants on canine IgE have a different degree of heat lability (Reedy and Miller, 1989): one is very labile and can be destroyed within 30 minutes, while extended heating is required to destroy the other. Canine and human IgE share some heavy chain antigenic determinants, and antibodies from the dog will bind to human basophils and mast cells (Sainte-Laudy and Prost, 1996). Feline IgE no doubt exists, but its characterization is not complete.

Of the immunoglobulins in man, IgE has the lowest serum concentration due to its highest turnover rate, shortest half-life, and lowest rate of synthesis. Metabolic turnover studies in man have shown that IgE has a total body pool of 0.01 mg/kg [1030 for IgG]; a synthesis rate of 0.004 mg/kg/day [36 for IgG]; a plasma half-life of 2.7 days [21 for IgG] and a fractional turnover rate of 94.3%/day [6.9 for IgG]. The serum IgE levels in dogs are much higher than they are in humans, but IgE is still the least prevalent immunoglobulin. Halliwell has shown that there is a poor correlation between serum and cell-bound levels of IgE (Halliwell, 1973). Metabolic turnover studies for IgE in dogs have not been reported, but because P–K reactivity in man and dogs is similar, the trends shown in man probably apply in the dog.

Cytokines and chemokines

Cytokines are low molecular weight glycoproteins that act as intercellular messengers to regulate their own production as well as the activity of other cells in the immediate area (Table 1.1). Although textbooks assign specific actions to the various cytokines, knowledge of their actions is far from complete since the response the cytokine can evoke depends upon the species being studied, the cell type and its location, the developmental state of the target cell, and the other cytokines present in the local milieu (Fishman *et al.*, 1996). Chemokines are chemotactic cytokines. Most histamine-releasing factors (HRF) are chemokines (Alan and Grant, 1995).

Arachidonic acid cascade

Essential fatty acids, long carbon chain molecules of the Ω-6 (N-6) and Ω-3 (N-3) groups, are necessary for skin to function normally. Dogs and cats require a dietary source of linoleic (18:2N-6) and linolenic (18:3N-3) acids and the cat has an additional requirement for arachidonic (20:4N-6) acid (Scott *et al.*, 1995). Other acids (see Figure 1.4) can be produced from the essential acids through the actions of various elongases and desaturases. Both the Ω-3 and Ω-6 acids use the same enzyme systems for their metabolism. The accumulation or depletion of substrate at one point in the metabolism of either the Ω-3 or Ω-6 acids will impact the metabolism of the other series since enzyme system activity will be altered. This modulation of metabolism by supplying specific fatty acids is the basis for the clinical responses seen with fatty acid supplementation (see Chapter 6).

The most important fatty acid is arachidonic acid, and its metabolites have wide ranging impacts on immunoregulation and inflammation. Arachidonic acid metabolites have been found in all cell types involved in hypersensitivity reactions. Arachidonic acid is stored in an esterified state in the cell membrane where it is unavailable for metabolism. With cellular activation, phospholipases, especially phospholipase A_2, release arachidonic acid from the cell membrane. This release results in the production of PAF and the prostanoids and LTs, collectively called eicosanoids (Campbell, 1993; Horrobin, 1993; Triggiani *et al.*, 1995; Scott *et al.*, 1995). The prostanoids, the thromboxanes and PGs, are produced under the action of cyclooxygenase enzymes, while the LTs and lipoxins are generated by lipoxygenase

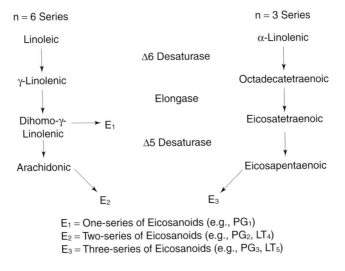

E_1 = One-series of Eicosanoids (e.g., PG_1)
E_2 = Two-series of Eicosanoids (e.g., PG_2, LT_4)
E_3 = Three-series of Eicosanoids (e.g., PG_3, LT_5)

Figure 1.4 *Schematic of fatty acid metabolism.*

Table 1.1 *Immunological properties of cytokines.*

Cytokine	Principal cell sources	Primary type of activity	Predominant effects
IL-1	Macrophages and others	Immunoaugmentation; promotes B cell activation	Inflammatory and hematopoietic
IL-2	T lymphocytes	T & B cell growth	Activates T and NK cells; promotes B cell growth and Ig production
IL-3	T lymphocytes	Hematopoietic growth	Promotes growth of early myeloid progenitor cells, eosinophils, mast cells and basophils
IL-4	T lymphocytes	B and T cell growth; promotes IgE switch; mast cell growth cofactor*	Promotes B cell activation and IgE switch; promotes T cell growth; synergizes with IL-3 for mast cell growth*
IL-5	T lymphocytes	Eosinophil growth; B cell growth*; T cell growth*	Promotes eosinophil growth; terminal differentiation factor for B cell Ig production*; costimulant of T cell proliferation*
IL-6	Fibroblasts and others	Hybridoma growth; augments inflammation	Terminal differentiation factor for B cells & polyclonal Ig production; enhances IL-4 induced IgE production
IL-7	Stromal cells	Lymphopoietin	Promotes growth of pre-B and pre-T cells
IL-8	Macrophages and others	Chemoattractant for neutrophils and T lymphocytes	Regulates lymphocyte homing and neutrophil infiltration
IL-9	T lymphocytes	Erythroid precursor; T cell tumor; macrophage and mast cell growth	Maturation of erythroid progenitors; T cell tumor growth; synergizes with IL-3 for mast cell growth
IL-10	B lymphocytes T lymphocytes	Thymocyte proliferation; CTL differentiation; B cell growth and differentiation	Synergizes with IL-2 and IL-4 for thymocyte growth; increases CTL precursor frequency and CTL effector function; enhances B cell proliferation and Ig production

Cytokine	Source	Function	Effects
IL-11	Stromal cells	Megakaryocyte and plasma cell growth	Enhances IL-3 effect for megakaryocytes; mitogenic for plasma cells
IL-12	B lymphocytes	Cytotoxic lymphocyte maturation	Synergizes with IL-2 for generation of CTL and LAK
G-CSF	Monocytes and others	Neutrophil growth	Neutrophil proliferation
M-CSF	Monocytes and others	Monocyte growth	Macrophage proliferation
GM-CSF	T lymphocytes and others	Monomyelocytic growth	Myelopoiesis
IFN-α	Leukocytes	Antiviral; antiproliferative; immunomodulating	Inhibits viral replication; stimulates macrophages and NK cells
IFN-β	Fibroblasts	Antiviral; antiproliferative; immunomodulating	Inhibits viral replication; stimulates macrophages and NK cells
IFN-γ	T lymphocytes and LGL	Immunomodulating; antiproliferatve; antiviral	Induces cell membrane antigens (e.g., MHC, FcR); enhances IL-2 effects; antagonizes IL-4 effects; enhances macrophage, CTL, and LGL effector function
TNF-α	Macrophages and others	Inflammatory, immunoenhancing, and tumoricidal	Vascular thromboses and tumor necrosis
TNF-β	T lymphocytes	Inflammatory, immunoenhancing, and tumoricidal	Vascular thromboses and tumor necrosis
TGF-$\beta_{1,2,3}$	T & B lymphocytes, macrophages, platelets, and others	Fibroplasia and immunosuppression	Wound healing and remodeling; broadly immunosuppressive but increases IgA production

Modified from Oppenheim JJ, et al: Cytokines, basic and clinical immunology, ed 7. Stites DP, Terr AI, editors, Norwalk, CT, 1991, Appleton and Lange, pp 78–100 with permission.
*Not shown for human cells.

enzymes. The LT group includes 15-HPETEs, 12-HETEs, 15-HETEs, and five LTs, namely LTA_4, LTB_4, LTC_4, LTD_4, and LTE_4. LTA_4 is an unstable compound and is hydrolyzed to LTB_4 or conjugated with glutathione to form LTC_4, LTD_4, and LTE_4, previously known as SRS-A. The lipoxins, L_{XA} and L_{XB}, are formed through the actions of the 5- and 15-lipoxygenases and their actions await characterization.

As a group, the two-series of PGs (e.g. PGE_2):

- alter vascular permeability;
- stimulate cell proliferation;
- suppress leukocyte function;
- potentiate the sensations of pain and itch (Campbell, 1993; Horrobin, 1993).

The four-series of LTs, especially LTB_4, have significant pro-inflammatory effects. LTC_4, LTD_4, and LTE_4 (SRS-A) increase vascular permeability and enhance PG production. LTB_4:

- is an important chemotactant for eosinophils and neutrophils;
- upregulates endothelial adhesion molecules;
- induces DNA synthesis;
- causes pain.

PAF is produced by all cell types participating in allergic reactions and has wide ranging impacts well beyond wound healing (Triggiani *et al.*, 1995). PAF:

- promotes its own generation by upregulating arachidonic acid metabolism;
- is a complete stimulus for the chemotaxis and activation of platelets, neutrophils, and eosinophils;
- induces histamine and LTC_4 release from basophils;
- induces cytokine (IL-1, IL-4, and TNF-α production by monocytes and macrophages;
- regulates immunoglobulin synthesis.

PGs and LTs derived from fatty acids other then arachidonic acid either have minimal inflammatory effects or are anti-inflammatory. Fatty acid supplementation to control inflammatory disorders has its basis here. For example, when fatty acid metabolism is overloaded with dietary eicosapentaenoic acid, the lipoxygenases produce the five-series of LTs and 15-HETE, which among other actions, inhibit the production of LTB_4 (Campbell, 1993).

Humoral amplification systems
Four separate but integrated serum protein systems – namely complement, coagulation, kinin, and fibrinolytic – affect the immunologic responsiveness of an animal. Each is composed of proteins, substrates, inhibitors, and enzymes, which produce a specific response. Products from one system can activate or modulate another system. These systems are dynamic and proteins must be activated in an orderly sequential fashion, and undamped activation is prevented by a variety of inhibitors.

The complement system.   The complement cascade is composed of at least 20 chemically and immunologically distinct proteins, which interact with each other, with antibody, and with cell membranes. The complement cascade is the primary humoral mediator of antigen–antibody reactions and results in the formation of products which:

- increase vascular permeability;
- induce histamine release from mast cells and basophils;
- are chemotactic for granulocytes;
- are cytotoxic (Reedy and Miller, 1989).

The cascade can be activated by the classical or alternative pathway. The alternative pathway joins the classical pathway at the C5 level. Immunologic activation of the classical pathway occurs when C1 binds to the Fc region of IgG or IgM molecules found in immune complexes or aggregations of immunoglobulins. Alternative pathway activation is typically antibody independent and stimuli include microbial polysaccharides, lipopolysaccharides and certain cell membranes. During complement activation, anaphylatoxins (C3a, C5a, and possibly C4a) are generated and influence immune regulation and mast cell and basophil degranulation.

The coagulation system.   Blood clotting involves the formation of a platelet plug and the activation of the clotting cascade. The clotting cascade consists of a series of factors, which are activated sequentially by either an intrinsic or extrinsic method. The activated cascade not only produces various factors required for hemostasis, but also results in the generation of kinins. Activated factor X produces thrombin, which among other actions can cleave C3 to C3a and activate C5 (Reedy and Miller, 1989). Platelet aggregation and activation is regulated by products of the cyclooxygenase metabolism of arachidonic acid generated in the endothelial cells of the vessel walls. PAF and thromboxanes (TXA_2) cause strong aggregation while prostacyclins (PGI_2) inhibit it (Reedy and Miller, 1989). TXA_2 and PGI_2 also have opposite affects on the local blood vessels: TXA_2 is vasoconstrictive while PGI_2 is vasodilatory.

The kinin system.   Kinins (e.g. bradykinin) are basic polypeptides produced from serum kininogens cleaved by kallikreins. They cause vasodilation, increase vascular permeability, and are chemotactic for granulocytes (Reedy and Miller, 1989). The kallikreins are produced by mast cells, basophils, or platelets (Tizard, 1996).

The fibrinolytic system.   The fibrinolytic system is designed to dissolve the fibrin in a hemostatic plug so that tissue repair can take place. Plasmin generation, an essential step in fibrinolysis, can be triggered during the complement, clotting, and kinin cascades, or by the production of tissue plasminogen activators from lymphocytes, macrophages, or basophils (Reedy and Miller, 1989). Beyond its effect on clot dissolution, plasmin can influence inflammatory reactions by its impact on the complement cascade where it activates C1 and cleaves C3 and C5.

Adhesion Molecules

Since cytokines and other cellular products only operate in the area immediately around the cell that produced them, leukocytes must be drawn into an area in order for the inflammation to continue. Chemotactic factors (e.g. LTB_4) and adhesion molecules play key roles in this trafficking. There are three families of adhesion molecules, namely integrins, immunoglobulin superfamily, and selectins, which have wide-ranging impacts on the immunologic reaction. These molecules play a pivotal role in the control of the migration and accumulation of leukocytes, but also influence cellular activation, cell-mediated cytotoxicity, antigen presentation, and antibody production (Schroth, 1996). Integrins are expressed on lymphocytes, eosinophils, basophils, and various other cells and mediate cell-to-extracellular matrix adhesion as well as cell-to-cell adhesion. The immunoglobulin superfamily consists of intracellular adhesion molecule-1 (ICAM-1), ICAM-2, and vascular cell adhesion molecule-1 (VCAM-1). ICAM-1 is important in trafficking neutrophils, eosinophils, lymphocytes, and monocytes into areas of inflammation. VCAM-1 has similar actions, but is not expressed on neutrophils so has no influence on these cells. The role of ICAM-2 is uncertain. Three families of selectins have been identified and these molecules work in conjunction with the intregrins and immunoglobulin superfamily.

Control mechanisms for the expression of adhesion molecules are complex and influenced by the type of immunologic reaction in question. For example, IL-4, the cytokine that influences IgE production, upregulates the expression of VCAM-1, allowing basophils and eosinophils to enter and concentrate in the area.

Hypersensitivity Reactions

In 1963, Gell and Coombs defined four types of hypersensitivity reactions to aid in the understanding of the immunology of allergy (Types I and IV) and immune-mediated disease (Types II and III) (Coombs and Gell, 1963). With the advances in immunology in the 30 plus years since, their list could be enlarged and refined considerably. Since their initial description of Type I and IV reactions is still the basis for our understanding of most allergic disorders, these types of reactions will be described (Figure 1.5). The reader is referred to immunology textbooks to learn about type II and III reactions.

Type I: anaphylactic reactions

Type I reactions are mediated by antigen-specific IgE (or IgGd) molecules bound to high affinity receptors on mast cells. When the sensitized mast cell comes in contact with allergen, the mast cell is activated, degranulates, and releases or produces various inflammatory mediators, which cause an acute-onset but short-lived hypersensitivity reaction. The resultant clinical lesions may be visible (e.g. urticaria) or microscopic (e.g. canine atopy).

Late-phase reactions can be considered to be a subtype of Type I reactions and have been shown to be important in atopic dermatitis, asthma, and allergic rhinitis in man (Massey, 1993; Charlesworth, 1995). Late-phase reactions occur as a sequel to immunologic or nonimmunologic mast cell degranulation and peak 8–12 hours after allergen challenge, can occur in the absence of allergen, and are not mediated by mast cells. During the initial mast cell degranulation, LTC_4, PAF, and various

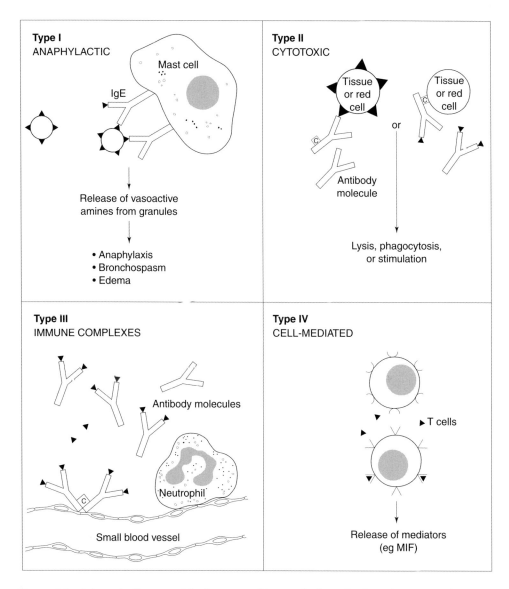

Figure 1.5 *Schematic diagrams of the four types of immunologic mechanisms that may produce tissue damage. C = Complement; ▲ = antigen; U and V = specific receptors for antigens. (Reproduced from Wells, 1980, with permission.)*

cytokines generated upregulate adhesion molecules and attract lymphocytes, especially CD4+ cells, eosinophils, neutrophils, and basophils into the area. During the initial reaction, monocytes, B cells, T cells, platelets, and neutrophils produce various chemokines such as monocyte chemotactic protein-1 (MCP-1), which are HRFs (Alan and Grant, 1995). These HRF molecules cause degranulation of IgE-coated basophils (and to a much lesser degree, mast cells) with the subsequent release of histamine and various other mediators. Although the late-phase reaction has been reported in the dog (Scott *et al.*, 1995), its role in the immunology and clinical symptomatology of the allergic skin diseases of animals is unknown. However, since clinical symptoms are longlasting and there is a preferential increase in CD4+ cells in lesional atopic skin from the dog and cat (Roosje *et al.*, 1996; Sinke and Thepen, 1996), the late phase may be important.

Type IV: cell-mediated

In the initial Gell and Coombs' description, Type IV reactions were strictly mediated by lymphocytes, which eliminated the offending antigen by secreting various lymphokines or by direct cytotoxicity. In the skin, Type IV reactions play a central role in allergic contact dermatitis. Although lymphocytes do play a central role in Type IV reactions, some components (e.g. IgE, basophils, and mast cells) of Type I reactions are active here, suggesting that there is great overlap in all allergic reactions (Tizard, 1996). In Type IV reactions, foreign antigen is presented by the APC network to Th1 cells, which drain to a regional lymph node. After sensitization in the node, γ/δ T cells migrate to the area of antigen deposition and secrete various cytokines and chemokines, which attract killer T cells and other cell types, including the basophil, to the area. When the basophils degranulate with antigen exposure or under the influence of HRF, the histamine causes more inflammation, resulting in even greater cellular infiltration. It has been estimated that no more then 5% of lymphocytes in the area are specific for the antigen that induces the response (Tizard, 1996). Since γ/δ T cells are rare in normal dog skin, but are increased in atopy, Type IV reactions may be more important in veterinary medicine then previously recognized (Cannon *et al.*, 1996).

References

Alan R, Grant A. The chemokines and histamine-releasing factors: Modulation of function of basophils, mast cells, and eosinophils. *Chem. Immunol.* **61:** 148, 1995.

Anttila M, Smith C, Suter M. Dermal dendrocytes and T cells in inflammatory dermatoses in dogs and cats. *Proc. Annu. Memb. Meet. Am. Acad. Vet. Dermatol. Am. Coll. Vet. Dermatol.* **10:** 43, 1994.

Blumenthal JB, Blumenthal MN. Immunogenetics of allergy and asthma. *Immunol. Allergy. Clin. N. Am.* **16:** 517, 1996.

Bos JD. *Skin Immune System.* Boca Raton: CRC Press, 1989.

Burd PR, Thompson WC, Max EE, *et al.* Activated mast cells produce interleukin 13. *J. Exp. Med.* **181:** 1373, 1995.

Burns PW. Allergic reactions in dogs. *J. Am. Vet. Med. Assoc.* **83:** 627, 1933.

Campbell KL. Clinical use of fatty acid supplements in dogs. *Vet. Dermatol.* **4:** 167, 1993.

Cannon AG, Olivry T, Ihrke PJ, *et al.* Gamma/delta T-cells in normal and diseased canine skin. *Proc. Third World Congress Vet. Dermatol.*, Edinburgh, 1996, p. 20.

Charlesworth EN. Role of basophils and mast cells in acute and late reactions in the skin. *Chem. Immunol.* **62:** 84, 1995.

Coca AF, Cooke RA. On the classification of phenomenon of hypersensitivities. *J. Immunol.* **8:** 163, 1925.

Coombs RRA, Gell PGH. Classification of allergic reactions. In Gell PGH, Coombs RRA (eds) *Clinical Aspects of Immunology*. 2nd edition. Blackwell Scientific Publications Ltd, Oxford, 1963.

DeBoer DJ. Enzymatically dispersed canine cutaneous mast cells characterization and response to secretagogues. *Proc. Am. Acad. Vet. Dermatol./Am. Coll. Vet. Dermatol.* **10:** 10, *1994.*

Fishman S, Hobbs K, Borish L. Molecular biology of cytokines in allergic diseases and asthma. *Immunol. Allergy. Clin. N. Am.* **16:** 613, 1996

Galli SJ. New concepts about the mast cell. *N. Engl. J. Med.* **328 (4):**257–265, 1993.

Goodell EM, Blummenstock DA, Bower WE. Canine dendritic cells from peripheral blood and lymph nodes. *Vet. Immunol. Immunopathol.* **8:** 301, 1985.

Goodman JW, Wang A. *Immunoglobulins: structure, diversity and genetics.* In Stites DP, Stobo JD, Wells JV (eds) *Basic and Clinical Immunology*, 6th edition. Appletion & Lange, 1987, p. 28.

Hall IA, Campbell KL. Serum immunoglobulins in normal dogs and dogs with skin disease. *Proc. Annu. Memb. Meet. Am. Acad. Vet. Dermatol. Am. Coll. Vet. Dermatol.* **9:** 45, 1993.

Halliwell REW. The localization of IgE in canine skin: An immunofluorescent study. *J. Immunol.* **110:** 422–430, 1973.

Halliwell REW, Fleischman JB, Mackay-Smith, *et al.* The role of allergy in chronic pulmonary disease in horses. *J. Am. Vet. Med. Assoc.* **174:** 277–281, 1979.

Halliwell REW, Gorman NT. *Veterinary Clinical Immunology.* W.B. Saunders Co, Philadelphia, 1989.

Hanifin JM, Lobitz WC. Newer concepts of atopic dermatitis. *Arch Dermatol.* **113:** 663, 1977.

Hill, PB, DeBoer DJ, Moriello KA. Levels of total serum IgE, IgA, and IgG in atopic, normal, and parasitized dogs. *Proc. Annu. Memb. Meet. Am. Acad. Vet. Dermatol. Am. Coll. Vet. Dermatol.* **9:** 32, 1993.

Hogan AD, Burks AW. Epidermal Langerhans' cells and their function in the skin immune system. *Ann. Allergy, Asthma Immunol.* **75:** 5–10, 1995.

Horrobin, DF. Medical uses of essential fatty acids (EFAs). *Vet. Dermatol.* **4:** 161, 1993.

Kapsenberg, ML, Hilkens CMU, Jansen HM, *et al.* Production and modulation of T-cell cytokines in atopic allergy. *Int. Arch. Allergy Immunol.* **110:** 107, 1996.

Martin LB, Kita H, Leiferman KM, *et al.* Eosinophils in allergy: role in disease, degranulation, and cytokines. *Int. Arch. Allergy Immunol.* **109:** 207, 1996.

Massey, WA. Pathogenesis and pharmacologic modulation of the cutaneous late-phase reaction. *Ann. Allergy* **71:** 578, 1993.

Miller WH Jr, Scott DW, Cayatte SM, *et al.* The influence of oral corticosteroids or declining allergen exposure on serologic allergy test results. *Vet. Dermatol.* **3:** 237, 1992.

Mudde GC, Reishi IG, Corraia N, *et al.* Antigen presentation in allergic sensitization. *Immunol. Cell Biol.* **74:** 167, 1996.

Nickoloff, BJ. *Dermal Immune System.* Boca Raton, CRC Press, 1993.

Noon L. Prophylactic inoculation against hay fever. *Lancet* **1:** 1572, 1911.

Olivry T, Moore PF, Affolter VK, *et al.* Langerhans' cell hyperplasia and surface IgE expression in canine atopic dermatitis. *Proc. Annu. Memb. Meet. Am. Acad. Vet. Dermatol. Am. Coll. Vet. Dermatol.* **11:** 36, 1995.

Pomeroy BS. Allergy and allergic skin reactions in the dog. *Cornell Vet* **24:** 335, 1934.

Prausnitz C, Kustner N. *Studien uber die Ueberempfindlichkeit Zbl. Bakt.* **68:** 160, 1921.

Reedy LM, Miller WH Jr. *Allergic Skin Diseases of Dogs and Cats.* W.B. Saunders Co., Philadelphia, 1989.

Richet C. *Anaphylaxis.* Translated by JM Bligh. Constable, London, Liverpool University Press, 1913.

Roitt I, Brostoff J, Male D. *Immunology,* 2nd edition. CV Mosby Co., St Louis, 1989.

Roosje PJ, Whitaker-Menezes D, Goldschmidt M, *et al.* MHC Class II+ and CD1a+ cells in lesional skin of cats with allergic dermatitis. *Proc. Third World Congress Vet. Dermatol.* Edinburgh, 1996, p. 59.

Sainte-Laudy J, Prost C. Binding of canine anaphylactic antibodies on human basophils: application to canine allergy diagnosis. *Vet. Dermatol.* 7: 185, 1996.

Schroeder JT, Kagey-Sabotka A, MacGlashan DW. The interaction of cytokines with human basophils and mast cells. *Int. Arch. Allergy Immunol.* 107: 79–81, 1994.

Schroeder JT, Kagey-Sabotka A, Lichtenstein LM. *The role of the basophil in allergic inflammation.* Allergy 50: 463–472, 1995.

Schroth MK. Adhesion molecules in asthma and allergy. *Immunol. Allergy Clin. N. Am.* 16: 643, 1996.

Scott DW, Miller WH, Griffin CE. *Muller and Kirk's Small Animal Dermatology,* 5th edition. W.B. Saunders Co., Philadelphia, 1995, p. 59.

Shearer WT, Huston DP. The immune system: An overview. In Middleton E Jr, Reed CE, Ellis EF (ed.) *Allergy: Principles and Practice,* 4th edition. Mosby, St. Louis, 1993, pp. 3–21.

Sinke JD, Thepen T. Immunophenotyping of skin-infiltrating T-cell subsets in dogs with atopic dermatitis. *Proc. Third World Congress Vet. Dermatol.* Edinburgh, 1996, p. 46.

Siraganian RP. Mechanisms of IgE-mediated hypersensitivity. In Middleton E Jr, Reed CE, Ellis EF (ed.) *Allergy: Principles and Practice,* 4th edition. Mosby, St. Louis, 1993, pp. 105–34.

Suter, MM. The skin as an immunologic organ. *Proc. Eur. Soc. Vet. Dermatol.* 12: 70, 1995.

Tizard I. *Veterinary Immunology,* 5th edition. W. B. Saunders, Co., Philadelphia, 1996.

Triggiani M, Oriente, A, Crescenzo G, *et al.* Metabolism of lipid mediators in human basophils and mast cells. *Chem. Immunol.* 61: 135, 1995.

Wells JV. Immune mechanisms in tissue damage. In Fundenberg HH, Stites DP, Caldwell JL, Wells JV (ed.) *Basic and Clinical Immunology,* 3rd edition. Large Medical Publictions, Los Altos, 1980, p. 193.

Wittich FW. Spontaneous allergy (atopy) in the lower animal: Seasonal hay fever (fall type) in a dog. *J. Allergy* 12: 247–251, 1941.

2
Urticaria, Angioedema, and Atopy

Introduction

Type I hypersensitivity disorders are characterized by a tissue reaction where anaphylactic antibodies are formed after exposure to antigens, and where as a consequence enzymatic reactions are initiated on mast cell and basophil surfaces, resulting in the release of various inflammatory mediators. Anaphylactoid reactions are clinically indistinguishable from anaphylactic reactions, but have no immunologic basis for the cellular degranulation. Anaphylactic reactions can occur locally or in a generalized fashion. In animals, urticaria, angioedema, anaphylaxis, and atopy are examples of Type I hypersensitivity disorders. Food hypersensitivity and flea bite hypersensitivity may involve Type I reactions, but other immunologic mechanisms may also occur so these are discussed separately.

Pathomechanism

Atopy – atopic dermatitis (AD), allergic inhalant dermatitis – in dogs shares many characteristics with its counterpart in man, such as a familial occurrence, early age of onset, chronic pruritus, skin lesions typically located at flexor and extensor sites of the extremities, and the presence of immediate skin test reactivity (Helton Rhodes *et al.*, 1987; Rhodes *et al.*, 1987). In both man (Van der Heyden *et al.*, 1991; Zachary *et al.*, 1995) and dogs (Nimmo Wilkie *et al.*, 1991, 1992) changes in cell-mediated immunity have been observed in atopic patients. Additionally, serum concentrations of allergen-specific IgE and some types of IgG are increased in dogs (Willemse *et al.*, 1985b; Kleinbeck *et al.*, 1989) as well as in man (Parish, 1981; Uehara, 1986). In man, IgE synthesis is mainly regulated by two cytokines produced by T-helper (TH) cells. Interleukin-4 (IL-4) induces (in conjunction with IL-2) synthesis of IgE, and interferon (IFN) γ suppresses IL-4-mediated production (Pène *et al.*, 1988). The majority of skin-infiltrating lymphocytes and allergen-specific peripheral blood lymphocytes from atopic patients exhibit the cytokine profile typical of the TH2 subclass. Upon stimulation these T cells release IL-4 and tumor necrosis factor (TNF) α, but are deficient in IFN-γ. In human AD patients a definite relationship has been observed between these cytokines: allergen-specific T lymphocyte clones from peripheral blood of atopic donors produce mainly IL-4, but no IFN-γ. In contrast, nonallergen-specific T lymphocyte clones from the same donors and allergen-specific T lymphocyte clones from nonatopic control donors produce IFN-γ, but little or no IL-4 (Wierenga *et al.*, 1990).

In human AD patients the skin contains an infiltrate of predominantly CD4$^+$ T cells (TH cells), and lesser numbers of CD8$^+$ T cells, which are thought to have mainly cytotoxic and suppressor effects (Leung *et al.*, 1981; Lever *et al.*, 1987). Over the last few years, information has become available about antigen-presenting cells (APCs) and the presence of IgE surface receptors, and skin-infiltrating T cells and the cytokines they produce in atopic dogs. The development of monoclonal antibodies specific for antigens expressed by canine T cells has been a major step forward for investigations in this field (Moore *et al.*, 1992). APCs have been characterized as CD1a$^+$/major histocompatibility complex (MHC) class II$^+$ cells with low-affinity IgE receptors (CD23) on their surface (Olivry *et al.*, 1995a). These cells may play a role in antigen presentation if the antigen penetrates the skin (Bruijnzeel-Koomen *et al.*, 1988; Bruijnzeel-Koomen *et al.*, 1991; Mudde *et al.*, 1995). Investigators have also found that the cutaneous infiltrate from dogs with atopy is composed chiefly of mast cells, dendritic APCs of probable Langerhans' cell lineage, and memory TH lymphocytes. Eosinophils and free eosinophilic granules were identified only in the epidermis of lesional atopic skin. Finally T lymphocytes expressing the γδ T-cell receptor were observed in the epidermis and dermis of all atopic dogs, but rarely in healthy animals (Olivry *et al.*, 1995b). This observation is in contrast to findings in man, where a decreased number of these T cells has been observed in peripheral blood. As γδ T cells secrete IFN-γ, a decrease may potentiate IgE production. Sinke *et al.* (1996) reported a preferential increase of CD4$^+$ T cells in lesional atopic epidermis. In nonlesional atopic skin, there was an infiltration with both CD4$^+$ and CD8$^+$ T cells within the epidermis, without preference for CD4$^+$ T cells. In the dermis, only CD8$^+$ T cells were increased, when compared with the numbers in healthy dog skin. It was concluded that CD8$^+$ T cells may be important regulatory cells in AD of dogs.

IgE is the classical reaginic antibody, but as discussed later, other immunoglobulins may also be important. All immunologically normal individuals can produce IgE antibodies, but allergic individuals have an exaggerated tendency to do so to substances that are normally innocuous. In man, there is a tendency for allergic patients to have a high serum IgE concentration while nonallergic individuals have a low concentration, which can be explained by the decreased allergen-specific γδ T cell activity in atopic patients.

In normal dogs, the serum IgE concentration varies from 30–350 μg/ml (mean 198 μg/ml) (Rockey and Schwartzman, 1967; Schwartzman *et al.*, 1971). Vriesendorp *et al.* (1975) found a mean serum IgE concentration of 198.8 μg/ml in normal dogs compared to a concentration of 180.4 μg/ml in atopic dogs. Schwartzman (1984) and Schwartzman *et al.* (1971) studied the IgE concentrations in 70 dogs born to atopic parents and found a mean concentration of 125.4 μg/ml in affected dogs, 130.0 μg/ml in skin-test positive but clinically normal dogs, and 100.6 μg/ml in skin-test negative, clinically normal dogs. IgE concentrations decreased with age, which supports the finding of Halliwell (1975) that the number of IgE-producing cells can decrease with age.

The most probable explanation why normal dogs have high IgE concentrations is the high incidence of external or gastrointestinal parasitism. In the atopic dog, parasite-induced elevations of IgE would mask rises caused by environmental allergens and thus the measurement of total serum IgE is of little diagnostic significance. Measurement of antigen-specific IgE levels may be useful and is the basis for the radioallergosorbent test (RAST) and enzyme-linked immunosorbent assay (ELISA) testing (see Chapter 4).

In the dog's skin, IgE binds firmly to mast cells and with low affinity to Langerhans' cells (Olivry *et al.*, 1995a). The binding of IgE to the cell surface receptors is reversible and in man the affinity constant is very high such that IgE tends to remain bound to the cell. Because of the high affinity constant, the half-life of IgE in the skin of man is 8–14 days compared to a serum half-life of 2.7 days. Prausnitz–Küstner (P–K) testing in dogs supports a high affinity constant in this species as well (Rockey and Schwartzman, 1967).

IgE molecules bind to mast cells that have surface receptors for the Fc portion of the molecule. In man, it has been estimated that 100 000–500 000 molecules of IgE can bind to one cell. For optimum mediator release it appears that a threshold number of antigen-specific IgE molecules must be bound to a cell. In man, the binding of at least 2500 molecules of antigen-specific IgE is thought to be necessary for optimum mediator release. No such data are available for the dog.

For mast cell degranulation to occur, bridging of IgE molecules is necessary. Accordingly, the allergen must be multivalent and have a stable antigenic configuration. Univalent allergens can bind to individual IgE molecules, but will not cause mast cell activation. Following the cross-linking of IgE molecules, the mast cell is very rapidly activated to release preformed mediators and to synthesize new compounds. The exact nature of the signal caused by the bridging of IgE molecules is unknown, but probably involves adenyl cyclase activation, augmentation of phospholipid metabolism, and phospholipid methylation.

The first report on the presence of non-IgE anaphylactic antibodies in dogs was from studies by Willemse *et al.* (1985a). They immunized dogs with eggs of *Toxocara canis* or *ortho*-dinitrochlorophenol-bovine serum albumin (o-DNCP-BSA) antigens, which induce considerable amounts of IgE in dogs (Rockey and Schwartzman, 1967; Schwartzman *et al.*, 1971). In all dogs, immediate skin test reactivity preceded or accompanied serum P–K and PCA reactivity. P–K and PCA reactivity was only observed after four hours of sensitization of recipient skin. In addition, heating of the sera at 56° C for two hours or reduction with 2-mercaptoethanol did not influence the P–K and PCA results. These measures would have destroyed any IgE activity. The induced non-IgE anaphylactic antibodies proved to be most likely IgGd, a subclass of immunoglobulin G. The reference values of serum IgGd in healthy dogs ranged from 1.6–17.8 mg/ml.

In dogs with clinical manifestations of atopy and immediate skin test reactivity, 89% had allergen-specific IgGd antibodies against one or more allergens. Antibodies were most frequently found against house dust, human dandruff, grass pollens, and spring tree pollens, and 55% of dogs with clinical signs of atopy but no immediate skin test reactivity also exhibited elevated IgGd titers (Willemse *et al.*, 1995b).

Subclasses of IgG are homocytotropic, but mast cells have fewer IgG receptors than IgE receptors. The affinity constant for the binding of IgG is very low so the antibody diffuses away fairly quickly. Sensitization persists for hours or days and not weeks as it does with IgE. Accordingly the IgG molecules have been termed short-term sensitizing antibodies. Short-term sensitizing antibodies have been found in some human patients with allergic diseases.

Other factors can affect the mast cell and make it more or less sensitive to immunologic stimulation. Szentivanyi (1968) proposed the β-adrenergic theory of asthma, which stated that the common factor responsible for the hyperreactivity of the airways of asthmatics might be a β-adrenergic receptor blockade. The autonomic nervous system is responsible for the visceral control of the body and is composed of the parasympathetic and the sympathetic or adrenergic systems. Adrenergically affected tissues include mast cells, lymphocytes, and polymorphonuclear leukocytes and they have α and β receptors on their cell surfaces. Although exceptions do occur, α receptors mediate cellular excitation while β receptors are inhibitory. These receptors work in concert with each other via a check and balance system. Decreased β reactivity or β blockade would cause a commensurate α hyperreactivity.

Cyclic nucleotides play a central role in cellular function. Reactions that increase the intracellular level of cAMP or decrease the intracellular level of cGMP will stabilize cells while actions that cause the reverse will have the opposite effect. Typically, α-receptors mediate decreases in cAMP while β-receptor stimulation causes an increase. Szentivanyi's theory was based on the observation that his experimental asthmatic animals showed a hypersensitivity to histamine and other vasoactive substances and a reduced response to β-adrenergic catecholamines.

A group of Basenji–greyhound crossbreed dogs have been studied because they were naturally allergic or could be sensitized to *Ascaris* antigen (Peters *et al.*, 1982; Butler *et al.*, 1983). These dogs show both nonspecific and allergen-specific airway hyperreactivity typical of asthma. Additionally, these dogs suffer from atopic-like dermatitis, which flairs after each allergen challenge and abates without treatment after antigen withdrawal. With antigen challenge, these dogs release histamine and leukotrienes (LTs) and show increased pulmonary resistance and decreased dynamic compliance. The pulmonary response to antigen challenge is potentiated by the administration of propranolol, which is a β-adrenergic antagonist. These dogs also show a blunted increase in intracellular cAMP when they are given isoproterenol, a β-adrenergic stimulant. All these facts indicate that the β-adrenergic response of these dogs is abnormal and that the β-adrenergic theory of Szentivanyi has some applicability in the atopic dog. It should be realized that there is considerable evidence in man that the β-adrenergic theory does not explain all aspects of atopy.

After mast cell degranulation is triggered, the vasoactive substances, chemotactic factors, and enzymes are released and the synthesis of reactive lipids – platelet activating factor (PAF), LTs, and prostaglandins (PGs) – proceeds (Thomsen *et al.*, 1993; Yager, 1993). The vasoactive substances cause immediate vasodilation and vascular leakage, which produces the clinical wheal. Depending on the sensitivity of the patient, the antigen load and the persistence of the allergen, the reaction may be terminated or may continue. The vasodilation and increased vascular permeability causes local tissue edema, which flushes the vasoactive substances away from the site. Histamine and PG binding to the mast cell receptors stabilizes the cell or adjacent cells and inhibits further mediator release. Eosinophils attracted to the area by eosinophilic chemotactic factor (ECF-A), LTs, histamine, bradykinin, and PAF block further tissue damage. In very sensitive patients or with a high persistent antigen load, the humoral amplification system may be activated. Neutrophils attracted by ECF-A, PAF, neutrophil chemotactic factor (NCF), and LTB 4 from mast cells and the chemotactic factors from the amplification system can cause tissue damage and continue the inflammatory response.

In cats reaginic hypersensitivity, presumably IgE, was demonstrated with passive cutaneous anaphylaxis testing in cats infested with *Otodectes cynotis* (Powell *et al.*, 1980). More recent publications show evidence for the existence of the putative feline IgE in cats experimentally infected with *Brugia pahangi* (Baldwin *et al.*, 1993; Foster *et al.*, 1994). DeBoer *et al.* (1993) showed cross-reactivity between monoclonal anticanine IgE and the putative feline IgE in serum of cats experimentally parasitized with *Toxocara canis*. Evidence for the existence of a heat-stable cytophilic antibody was found in cats with miliary dermatitis or eosinophilic plaques (Roosje and Willemse, 1995). Recently, increased numbers of CD1a[+]/MHC class II[+] Langerhans' cells were found in lesional skin of cats with AD (Roosje *et al.*, 1996). In addition, cats with AD have a significantly greater number of T cells in lesional skin than in the skin of healthy control animals. Healthy control cats have only a few CD4[+] cells and no CD8[+] cells. A mean ±SD CD4[+]/CD8[+] ratio of 3.9 ± 2.0 was found in lesional skin from ten cats with AD. The CD4[+]/CD8[+] cell ratio for healthy control cats could not be determined because of the absence of CD8[+] cells. The CD4[+]/CD8[+] ratio in the peripheral blood of the ten cats with AD was 1.9 ± 0.4, and did not differ significantly from that of the control animals (2.2 ± 0.4). The CD4[+]/CD8[+] cell ratio, predominance of CD4[+] T cells in lesional skin, and increase of absolute numbers of CD4[+] T cells in non-lesional skin of cats with AD are comparable to the findings in AD in man (Roosje *et al.*, 1995). Using immunohistochemical procedures, it has been shown that feline CD4[+] T cells in lesional skin can produce IL-4. Double staining indicated that all IL-4[+] cells expressed pan-T or CD4 markers. In addition, the combination of recombinant human IL-2 (rhIL-2) and recombinant human IL-4 (rhIL-4) induced more proliferation of peripheral blood lymphocytes (PBL) than rhIL-2 or rhIL-4 alone (Roosje *et al.*, 1995b). Although these T cells could be TH0 or TH2, there is abundant evidence that the immunopathogenesis of atopy in cats has strong similarities with that of AD in humans and dogs.

Urticaria – Angioedema – Anaphylaxis

Immunologically-mediated urticaria, angioedema, and anaphylaxis all are Type I hypersensitivity disorders and can be thought of as the same disease with a variation in severity and target organ. Nonimmunologic mechanisms can also cause these disorders and the resulting disorders are clinically indistinguishable from the allergic reactions.

Urticaria are focal superficial anaphylactic reactions where wheals (hives) develop in the skin. Lesions may be single or multiple and may affect the whole body. Angioedema reactions can be thought of as deep wheals. Deep blood vessels are affected and the edema causes diffuse swelling, typically of one area such as the head. Anaphylaxis is a severe systemic allergic reaction. In pets, the gastrointestinal tract is the shock organ and anaphylactic reactions cause contraction of the bowel smooth muscle and local vasodilation with splanchnic pooling of blood. As vasoactive substances are released into the circulation, generalized vasodilation can occur with hypotension and shock. Depending on the severity of the reaction, untreated anaphylaxis can be fatal.

These anaphylactic-type reactions are uncommon in the dog and are rare in the cat. Ingestants (foods, ornamental plants, insects), drugs, vaccines, and venoms from stinging or biting insects are the most common causes. In Europe (Italy, France, Belgium, and the Netherlands) the processionary caterpillar (*Thaumatopoea processionea*) is an increasing cause of urticaria, angioedema, or even anaphylactic reactions. The caterpillars develop into small butterflies, which produce eggs in oak trees in August and hatch to new caterpillars the following April. Their litter is bound on the branches of oak trees, may be more than 1 m in length, and is composed of tight spinnings of fecal material, sloughed skin, and caterpillars' hairs. Each caterpillar has approximately 700 000 to one million of these hairs, which contain substances responsible for the acute contact reaction after touching sensitive skin. Ingestion may be fatal. In man, contact with these caterpillars may result in a painful rash, blisters, or urticaria.

Factors important in man are shown in Table 2.1. Reactions to inhalant allergens, allergy vaccines, infections, physical stimuli (including excessive heat, cold, sunlight, and maybe even stress) have been recognized in pets. Type I hypersensitivity reactions may occur within minutes after the antibody combines with the antigen. Injected allergens (drugs, vaccines, venoms) will cause reactions in the sensitized patient almost immediately. Ingested allergens (e.g. foods, drugs) may not induce reactions for several hours and may persist for long periods until the allergen is completely absorbed or eliminated from the bowel. Pruritus may be mild to intense and depending upon the severity of the reaction the animal may become lethargic.

Urticarial reactions (Fig. 2.1) are characterized typically by widespread, asymptomatic wheals, which occur suddenly (in general within 30 minutes) and spontaneously regress, usually within 24–48 hours as long as exposure to the

Table 2.1 *Major etiologic categories of urticaria and angioedema*

Cause	Condition
Drugs	
Foods	
Inhalant allergens	
Infections	
Insect and arthropod bites and stings	
Penetrants and contactants	
Internal diseases	
Complement activation processes	Urticarial vasculitis
Genetic factors	Hereditary angioedema
	Familial cold urticaria
	Vibratory angioedema
	Familial localized heat urticaria
	Syndrome of urticaria, deafness, and amyloidosis
	Erythropoietic protoporphyria
	C3b deficiency
Physical factors	Dermatographism
	Delayed pressure urticaria
	Cold urticaria
	Localized heat urticaria
	Cholinergic urticaria
	Cold-induced cholinergic urticaria
	Solar urticaria
	Aquagenic urticaria
	Exercise-induced anaphylaxis
Psychogenic factors	

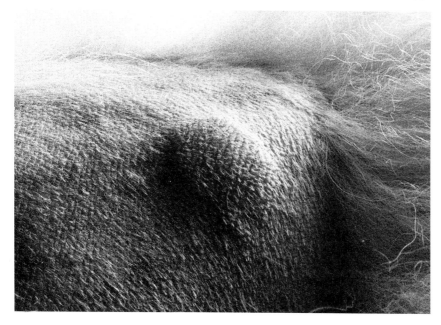

Figure 2.1   *A wheal caused by the intradermal injection of flea antigen in a hypersensitive patient.*

allergen is eliminated. In long-haired animals, the reaction may not be observed. In short-haired pets, the lesions are obvious (Figure 2.2). The papular lesions of folliculitis can sometimes be confused for urticaria. Urticarial lesions are typically not exudative and hairs cannot be easily epilated from them, but folliculitis has both of these features.

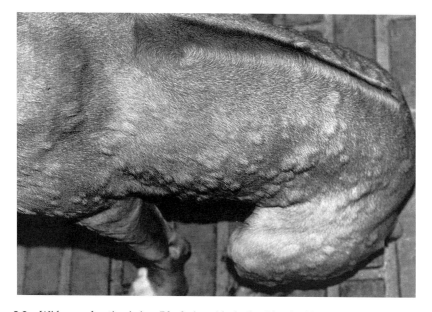

Figure 2.2   *Widespread urticaria in a Rhodesian ridgeback with a food hypersensitivity.*

Angioedema involves the edematous swelling of a larger part of the body and will spontaneously regress. Animals whose head or neck are involved (Figure 2.3) should be watched carefully as the respiratory tract may become obstructed as a result of laryngeal tissue swelling. Anaphylactic reactions produce shock and are true medical emergencies.

For each of these disorders, the offending agent should be identified as subsequent exposures can produce more severe reactions. Mild reactions (asymptomatic urticaria, angioedema of a nonvital part of the body) require no treatment. Antihistamines will have no effect on preexisting lesions, but may prevent the development of new lesions. Glucocorticoids are beneficial; in acute cases the intravenous route of administration may be preferable. Serious reactions (anaphylaxis, angioedema of the larynx) may require the concomitant use of epinephrine (1:1000) at a dose of 0.1–0.5 ml subcutaneously or intramuscularly plus shock therapy if necessary. After the reaction has resolved, the offending agent should be avoided. If the animal is drug sensitive, say to penicillin, that drug should be avoided and all similar drugs (semisynthetic penicillins and cephalosporins) should be avoided or used with caution since cross-reactivity can occur.

Atopic Disease

Atopy is a genetically determined predisposition to spontaneously develop Type I hypersensitivities to aeroallergens, which are normally innocuous substances. Siblings inherit the allergic predisposition from their parents, but are not necessarily allergic to the same allergens. Genetics confers the ability to hyperreact while environmental exposure determines which allergens are significant. In man, the

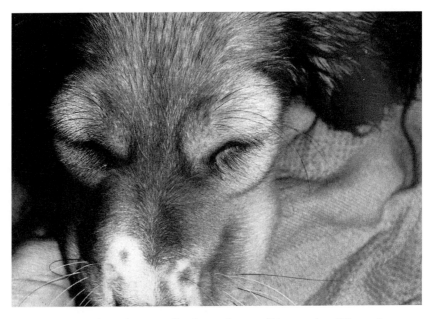

Figure 2.3 *Facial angioedema due to an allergic reaction to a distemper–hepatitis vaccine.*

term atopy is used to describe a triad of asthma, hay fever, and AD. In pets, atopy historically described a pruritic dermatitis associated with the inhalation of pollen, fungal, or environmental allergens. However, the respiratory route of exposure is the subject of investigation. In people with AD, there is substantial evidence for transcutaneous antigen exposure (Bruijnzeel-Koomen *et al.*, 1988; Frank and McEntee, 1995; Mudde *et al.*, 1995). In dogs with atopy, such a route is plausible since the most commonly affected sites (muzzle, feet, flexor and extensor sites) are likely to come into contact with environmental allergens and are subject to continuous minor trauma.

Clinical and immunologic data support the concept that canine atopy is an inherited immunologically influenced disease, but several publications (Peters *et al.*, 1982; Schwartzman *et al.*, 1983; Willemse *et al.*, 1985b) suggest that the IgE–mast cell theory may be too simplistic. As viral diseases or vaccinations (Frick and Brooks, 1983) can influence the cell-mediated immune system and, therefore, IgE production indirectly, environmental factors may also be important. Breeding experiments have clearly indicated that the IgE response is genetically controlled and that the offspring can be segregated into high and low responders (DeWeck *et al.*, 1997).

Canine atopy

Atopy is the second most common allergic skin disease of the dog. The true incidence of the disease in the dog population is unknown, but estimates vary from 3–15%. A higher incidence (30%) has been reported for referral practices, which indicates the refractory nature of the condition. The disorder has been recognized worldwide.

Sociologic data

Atopic disease can be recognized in any dog of any breeding, but because of the genetic predisposition, the disorder is recognized more frequently in certain breeds or families. Many reports fail to compare the incidence of the disease in a breed to the frequency of that particular breed in the general population so the true breed incidence is difficult to assess. In the USA in the 1980s, a breed predilection was reported for the Boston terrier, Cairn terrier, dalmatian, English bulldog, English setter, Irish setter, Lhasa apso, miniature schnauzer, pug, Sealyham terrier, Scottish terrier, West Highland white terrier, the wire haired fox terrier, and the golden retriever (Scott, 1981; Schick and Fadok, 1986; Scott *et al.*, 1995). In Europe at that time, a predisposition was observed for the German shepherd dog, poodle, and boxer (Willemse and Van den Brom, 1983). Recent data show a predisposition for Labrador retrievers, West Highland white terriers and boxers in the UK (Sture *et al.*, 1995), for bull terriers, chow-chows, West Highland white terriers, and boxers in Germany (Koch and Peters, 1994), for Labrador retrievers, Tervueren shepherd dogs, Pyrenean shepherd dogs, all types of setters, and fox terriers in the southwestern part of France (Carlotti and Costargent, 1994), for Labrador retrievers, golden retrievers, German shepherd dogs, and West Highland white terriers in the Netherlands (Willemse, 1996), for West Highland white terriers, boxers, fox terriers, German shepherd dogs, Labrador and golden retrievers, and Cairn terriers in Sweden (Ohlén, 1992), and for Labrador retrievers and cocker spaniels in Wisconsin and northern Illinois (DeBoer, 1993). Mongrels can also be affected.

Limited breeding studies show that the progeny of atopic dogs are more likely to develop atopic signs, but the mode of inheritance is unknown. If the conscientious breeders of a certain breed of dog are aware of the inherited predisposition to atopic disease, careful breeding programs can decrease the incidence of the disease in a practice area. Alternatively, poor breeding scruples can increase the incidence. Increased popularity of a specific breed is likely to increase the incidence of atopy because the population base increases and monetary considerations encourage the unrestricted breeding of unfit dogs. The increasing frequency of atopy in the Shar Pei bespeaks to the detrimental effect of breed popularity or uniqueness.

Atopy can be recognized in any dog of any breed, even mongrel dogs. Spontaneously atopic signs may develop in multiple unrelated dogs of different breeds within the same household. These findings suggest that factors other than genetics may be important. An increased incidence of atopy has been reported for females (Scott *et al.*, 1995) while other studies refute these findings (Carlotti and Costargent, 1994; Sture *et al.*, 1995). Since estrogens can elevate intracellular cGMP levels and consequently destabilize cells, an increased incidence in females would be plausible.

Threshold theory

The pathogenesis of IgE-mediated allergic disorders has been explained by Katz (1978) by means of the 'allergic breakthrough' and imbalance in normal 'damping' of IgE. It is postulated that the normal damping is regulated by T cell subsets, IL levels, and nonspecific suppressor factors of allergy. If the threshold of the damping mechanism is lowered to a level insufficient to control IgE antibody synthesis, exposure to an allergen would result in an 'allergic breakthrough'. Once the response entered the allergic zone, it would remain there until the damping mechanism renormalized, leading to a return of the IgE antibody response at the nonallergic level. At that point, normal balance between the threshold activity of the damping mechanism and IgE antibody synthesis would be restored. Experiments have provided evidence for a comparable phenomenon in dogs (Frick and Brooks, 1983), suggesting that attenuated live virus vaccines may selectively deplete suppressor T lymphocytes, thereby leading to a naturally occurring 'allergic breakthrough'.

Each animal will tolerate some level of a pruritic stimulus without itching. If the stimulus exceeds the animal's threshold, itching will occur. The threshold for pruritus is very individualized and can be raised or lowered by psychological changes as well as by physiological alterations associated with nutrition, systemic disease, environmental changes, or concomitant allergies (e.g. atopy, food hypersensitivity, or flea bite allergy). Nervous or highly strung animals tend to itch sooner or more intensely than mellow dogs. A subclinical atopic pruritus may become clinical if the animal develops a secondary disorder such as seborrhea, bacterial folliculitis, bacterial hypersensitivity, or *Malassezia* dermatitis. Stress may be a reason for clinical exacerbations, even in dogs successfully maintained on hyposensitization.

History

A detailed history is the single most important factor in the diagnosis and management of an atopic case. It provides the key information to determine if the animal's symptoms have an allergic basis and, if so, what the most likely allergens are. There is no ideal way to take an allergy history, but the owner's observations, the pet's medical record, and the veterinarian's own questioning all provide valuable information. Many clinicians ask the owner to fill out a history sheet before the animal is taken to an examination room. An example of such a form is shown in Table 2.2. The duration of the problem, the age at onset, the course of the disease, the seasonality of the problem, information about litter mates, nature and distribution of the signs, and the animal's response to medical therapy are important points to review with the owner. Questioning should also focus on the presence of other pets, dietary regimen, walking and indoor living environment, bedding, flea control programs, and previous treatments and their effect. Sometimes it is necessary to remove the pet from the owner so that the owner can concentrate on the history. If the client is referred or has been treated by other veterinarians, the owner should bring a copy of the pet's medical record. Once the client has provided the necessary information, the clinician should review it before the pet is examined so that confusing points can be clarified and additional information can be obtained during the examination. It is useful to list the owner's complaints and observations in chronologic order so patterns can be identified.

It is generally agreed that in dogs with atopy, the age at onset is early. In 75% of dogs, the first symptoms are seen before three years of age (Scott, 1981; Willemse and Van den Brom, 1983). The signs during the first year may have been so mild that the dog required no treatment and the owner may forget this episode. The owner should be questioned about earlier mild signs. Seasonal or perennial atopics will usually show an intensification of their signs during certain periods and these should be noted. Willemse and Van den Brom (1983) reported that approximately 27% of his patients developed their signs by one year of age while Scott (1981) found that 64% of his cases developed their signs in this period. Although rare, some highly inbred atopic dogs will show significant symptomatology within the first six months of life (LMR/WHM). After three years of age, the incidence of onset of atopy decreases and the condition infrequently starts in dogs older than six years of age. Dogs who are moved frequently as young animals may not show significant clinical signs until they are older dogs. True sudden onset of atopic disease in an older dog who has been in the same environment all of his life probably reflects some change in or insult to his immune system.

As in humans, atopy in dogs tends to be a chronic or chronically-relapsing dermatitis (Willemse and Van den Brom, 1983; Scott *et al.*, 1995). The latter study showed the disease to be present for more than one year in approximately 80% of the animals, whereas 33% of the dogs were affected for more than three years. Seasonal exacerbations are reported for 30–40% of the dogs with atopy. The progression from seasonal to nonseasonal disease occurs in 15% of dogs (Scott *et al.*, 1995). Van Stee (1983) made an interesting observation that a higher proportion of atopic dogs were born during the months of May, August, and December. This statistically significant increased incidence of atopy in dogs born during the onset of the major pollen seasons suggests that dogs may be particularly susceptible to primary sensitization during the first four months of life. Birth during nonpollen seasons would tend to disfavor the development of sensitization while birth during pollen periods may increase the incidence of sensitization. This point would have impact on breeding programs. Aeroallergens exist in the external and internal environment, but there are many more 'pollens' than internal allergens. Accordingly, most atopic dogs would be expected to first show signs of disease

Table 2.2 *Allergy history questionnaire.*

Owner's Name:_____Date: _____

Pet's Name:_____Breed:_____Age:_____Sex: _____

Primary Complaint: _____

If itching (scratching, rubbing, chewing, biting, licking) Where? _____

_____Face_____Feet_____Armpits_____Rear_____Generalized

Respiratory (wheezing, sneezing, coughing)? _____

Date or age first noticed: _____

Are symptoms worse:_____Spring_____Summer_____Fall_____Winter _____Year Round

Are symptoms getting worse?_____Yes_____No _____

What aggravates symptoms? _____

What helps symptoms? _____

Do any of the following occur?_____Sores_____Scabs_____Scaling_____Hair Loss

_____Odor_____Redness_____Watery Eyes_____Ear Problems_____Sweating

_____Hives_____Convulsions_____Drinks Excessive Water_____Ravenous Appetite

_____Vomiting_____Diarrhea_____Weight Loss_____Weight Gain

When did you last see a flea on your pet? _____

What do you normally feed your pet (type and brand)? _____

Is your pet allergic to any food?_____Yes_____No   Specify _____

Allergic to drug or medication?_____Yes_____No   Specify _____

Do you have other pets?_____Yes_____No_____Cats_____Dogs_____Birds _____Other

Do you know of any relatives of this pet that have skin problems? _____

_____

Does any human member of household have skin problems? Yes_____No_____

Where does this pet sleep? _____

Other illnesses and dates: _____

Does bathing help or aggravate? _____

Previous medications (brand):_____Shampoos_____Dips_____Sprays

_____Powders_____Ointments_____Tablets or Capsules

Last dose given_____Response_____

Injection_____Date_____Response _____

Previous veterinarian(s)_____

Previous tests/skin scrapings_____Cultures _____

Blood_____Other _____

Previous diagnosis:_____

What do you think is cause of this problem?

during the pollination season. Scott (1981) reported that 78% of his atopic patients first showed signs of disease in the spring to fall while 22% developed signs during the winter.

A personal or family history of atopy may also contribute to the diagnosis (Schwartzman, 1984). In the progeny of brother-to-sister matings of atopic dogs, 30 of 56 animals developed immediate skin test reactivity to inhalant allergens, and 13 dogs showed clinical evidence of atopic disease. Interestingly, in all dogs skin test reactivity developed before the onset of clinical signs. The latter did not occur before 13 months of age. Although the familial nature of the disease is well known, the mode of inheritance is unclear in both man and dogs (Vriesendorp *et al.*, 1975; Hanifin, 1982). Vriesendorp *et al.* (1975) found no relationship between serologically recognized DL-A groups (the major histocompatibility genetic region in dogs) and atopy. Although it was hypothesized that the DL-A haplotype 9,4 might offer protection against the disease and haplotype 3,R15 might be associated with a greater susceptibility, the statement has never been confirmed.

Glucocorticoids are usually so effective in the early stages of canine atopy that failure to improve with adequate steroid therapy makes the diagnosis of atopy less tenable. Secondary pyodermas and *Malassezia* infections (White *et al.*, 1997) are common in atopic dogs and these infected animals do not respond well to steroid therapy. Owners of steroid nonresponsive atopic suspects should be questioned carefully about the drug regimen used and the state of the dog's skin when the steroids were used.

The owner should be questioned carefully about sudden flairs in the animal's condition. Allergen levels can vary from day to day and, accordingly the dog's level of pruritus can change. Changes in the intensity of the pruritus associated with varying aeroallergen levels occur gradually over a 3–7 day period and not suddenly. Dogs who suddenly worsen have probably developed a secondary pyoderma, or *Malassezia* dermatitis, or have picked up fleas or another parasite.

Some suspected atopic dogs itch less when they are hospitalized or boarded at a kennel. This decrease in pruritus could reflect the avoidance of a local allergen, poor observation, or an increase in the pet's allergic threshold via stress. Improvement in the patient's condition while it is away from home does not prove or disprove atopy.

Diagnostic criteria of AD

In an attempt to provide consistency in the diagnosis of AD in humans, the concept of major and minor diagnostic features was introduced (Hanifin and Lobitz, 1977; Hanifin and Rajka, 1980). According to the established criteria at least three of the following major features must be present:

- pruritus;
- a typical morphology and distribution including flexural lichenification in adults and facial and extensor involvement in infants and children;
- a tendency towards chronic or chronically relapsing dermatitis;
- a personal or family history of atopy (asthma, allergic rhinitis, AD).

In addition, three or more of the following minor features must be present:

- early age of onset;
- immediate skin test reactivity;

- elevated serum IgE concentrations;
- xerosis;
- a tendency towards cutaneous infections;
- impaired cell-mediated immunity;
- recurrent conjunctivitis;
- cheilitis;
- a tendency towards nonspecific hand or foot dermatitis;
- facial pallor, facial erythema, and orbital darkening;
- food intolerance or intolerance to wool and lipid solvents;
- itch when sweating;
- course influenced by environmental or emotional factors;
- white dermographism and delayed blanch.

In dogs, pruritus has been considered a hallmark of AD and is typically manifested by foot licking and nose or head rubbing (Scott *et al.*, 1995). Since the occurrence of primary cutaneous lesions has never been firmly established in dogs or in man (Hanifin and Rajka, 1980), it may be that all the cutaneous changes are secondary to itch-induced scratching. This hypothesis is supported by Willemse and Van den Brom (1983) who found that although all of the dogs had signs of face rubbing and foot licking, only 67% had cutaneous lesions in the facial and pedal areas. In mild cases, one may only see broken hairs or salivary (rust colored) discoloration of the fur. Chronically affected skin will be hairless or hypotrichic, lichenified, and hyper-pigmented. The most frequently observed skin morphology includes erythema, papular reactions, crusts and lichenification. Although lichenified skin is seen in over 80% of the animals with AD, it does not appear to be related to the presence of immediate skin test reactivity. In addition, there is no apparant age-related difference in the distribution or morphology.

Some owners will deny a history of pruritus until they are told that licking or rubbing is a sign of itching. Some clients, especially first time dog owners, do not recognize that some level of itching can be normal (physiologic pruritus). Physiologic pruritus is described as a sharp well-defined pruritic sensation that is frequent but intermittent throughout the day. A normal dog can scratch occasionally, but it should be for brief periods of time and should not interrupt normal activity. A dog that itches frequently, focuses attention on one spot, keeps the owner awake, or will stop eating or playing to scratch has pathologic pruritus.

An occasional allergic dog will be presented with a history of pruritus of variable intensity, but with absolutely no skin changes to support the complaint. Once one is sure that the owner understands the concept of physiologic pruritus, all cases of nonlesional pruritus should be evaluated for allergy before the complaint is dismissed as a psychological problem of the owner or the dog.

The classical atopic dog is described as one that itches at his face, ears, feet, and axillary regions, but a wide variety of signs can be recognized (Figures 2.4 and Plate 1). Most reports do not give a detailed description of the distribution of the lesions, so comparison is difficult. In a study of 100 atopic dogs (Scott, 1981), it was reported that the initial most commonly involved pruritic sites were:

- ventrum only (35%);
- face, feet, and ventrum (22%);

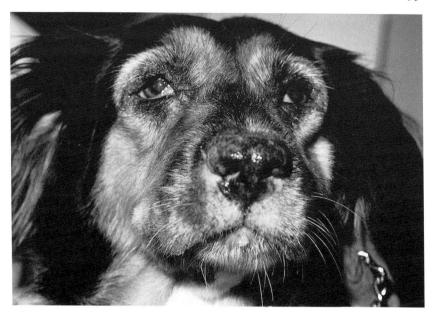

Figure 2.4 *An atopic dog with periocular self-trauma, conjunctivitis, and rhinorrhea.*

- face and ventrum (12%);
- face and feet (10%);
- feet (10%)
- face only (5%).

As the disease became more chronic, 42% of the dogs had generalized pruritus while the percentage of dogs who itched at their face, feet, and ventrum increased to 31%. A detailed frequency distribution of the symptomatology based on the evaluation of 208 dogs with AD (Willemse and Van den Brom, 1983) is shown in Table 2.3. Similar trends can be seen. As far as the distribution is concerned, the most commonly affected areas were the muzzle and the periocular area (60%), the feet (70%) and to a lesser extent the axillae (35%), the extensor side of the carpal joint (40%), and the flexural side of the tarsal joint (30%). Involvement of extensor and flexural surfaces was only observed in dogs where the atopic symptoms were associated with immediate skin test reactivity.

Although noncutaneous signs are uncommon in atopic dogs, conjunctivitis, reverse sneezing, rhinitis and asthma-like symptoms may occur. In one author's (LMR) practice, many dogs with keratoconjunctivitis sicca have been skin tested, show positive reactions, and respond to hyposensitization. Other minor diagnostic features of AD in man do occur in dogs with atopy. It is the authors' clinical impression that stress and sweating contribute considerably to the total amount of itch in atopic dogs. Increased sweating (hyperhidrosis) has been observed in about 10% of atopic dogs (Scott, 1981; Willemse and Van den Brom, 1983). Whether this sweating is the result of emotional stress or is an isolated phenomenon has not been investigated.

Xerosis or generalized dryness of the skin is commonly found in animals with AD

Table 2.3   *Frequency of signs and symptoms as observed in 208 dogs having atopic dermatitis by clinical definition (Willemse and Van den Brom, 1983)*

Symptoms	Number of dogs with immediate skin test reactivity ($n = 170$)	%	Number of dogs without immediate skin test reactivity ($n = 38$)	%
Pruritus, face rubbing, paw-and-feet licking	170	100.0	38	100.0
Bilateral conjunctivitis	51	30.0	11	28.9
Sweating	41	24.1	9	23.7
Sneezing	38	22.4	9	23.7
Discoloration of coat	13	7.6	3	7.9
Cutaneous involvement	161	94.7	37	97.4
Lichenification	143	84.1	33	86.8
Superficial pyoderma	45	26.5	4	10.5
Seborrhea	39	22.9	9	23.7
Affected skin regions				
Digits	124	72.9	28	73.7
Head	101	59.4	24	63.2
Extensor aspect carpal joint	70	41.2	0	0
Axillaries	60	35.3	7	18.4
Flexor aspect tarsal joint	52	30.6	0	0
Groins	31	18.2	7	18.4
Ear flaps	29	17.1	6	15.8
Abdomen	27	15.9	6	15.8
Flexor aspect elbow joint	12	7.1	2	5.3

and has been seen in association with the presence of staphylococcal skin infections (Scott, 1981; Willemse and Van den Brom, 1983). In addition, the incidence of superficial pyoderma was significantly higher in dogs with atopic symptoms with immediate skin test reactivity than in dogs with clinical manifestations but without a positive skin test. Although the presence of pyoderma in conjunction with AD in man is sometimes thought to be related to a decreased cell-mediated immunity with impaired chemotaxis (Hanifin, 1982), this has not been found in dogs. Recurrent conjunctivitis has often been seen in atopic dogs (Scott, 1981; Willemse and Van den Brom, 1983). Whether this reflects the presence of a hay fever-like phenomenon is uncertain. However, the improvement of many animals with the topical application of cromoglycate supports the idea. Cheilitis, facial erythema, and orbital darkening are noticed occasionally, but may be present in other diseases.

Special mention must be made of otitis externa, pododermatitis, acute moist dermatitis (hot spots), and acral pruritic nodules (lick granulomas). Otitis externa is a common finding in atopic dogs, occurring in up to 80%, and will be the initial complaint in 45% (Griffin, 1993; Scott *et al.*, 1995; Muse *et al.*, 1996). The ears are erythematous, waxy, edematous, and pruritic. Unless a secondary infection is superimposed on the allergic otitis, the condition is minimally exudative. Secondary bacterial or *Malassezia* overgrowth or infection is common and worsens the otic symptomatology. Resolution of any secondary infection will decrease the exudation, but not the pruritus unless the otic preparation contains glucocorticoids. Pedal pruritus with resultant pododermatitis is observed in 30–40% of dogs with AD (Scott, 1981; Willemse and Van den Brom, 1983). Most atopic dogs traumatize regions of their body and do not focus their attention on just one spot. However, a few atopic dogs are presented for recurrent episodes of acute moist dermatitis or an acral pruritic nodule. Careful examination of the history and patient will show that the dog itches elsewhere, but at a level where it is not noticed by or of concern to the owner. Dogs with true recurrent episodes of acute moist dermatitis are unlikely to be atopic. The condition is more likely to be associated with flea infestation, flea bite hypersensitivity, or pruritic folliculitis. The acral pruritic nodule is a focal area of disease on one or more limbs with a wide variety of causes. Atopic dogs do not usually itch at just one leg, but many dogs itch more intensely at one side of their body than the other. If the dog fixates on one spot, say the extensor aspect of the carpal joint, an acral pruritic nodule may be created. However, if the dog is an atopic, other symptoms should be seen.

It is apparent that most of the diagnostic criteria suggested by Hanifin and Rajka (1980) for humans may be used in dogs. Accordingly, a modification of these criteria was proposed for the definite diagnosis of canine atopic dermatitis (Willemse, 1986). Major features are:

- pruritus;
- facial or digital involvement;
- lichenification of the flexor surface of the tarsal joint or the extensor surface of the carpal joint;
- a chronic or chronically-relapsing dermatitis;
- an individual or family history of atopy;
- a breed predisposition.

Minor features are:
- onset of symptoms before the age of three years;
- immediate skin test reactivity to inhalant allergens;
- elevated serum concentrations of allergen-specific IgGd;
- elevated serum concentrations of allergen-specific IgE;
- xerosis;
- recurrent superficial staphylococcal pyoderma;
- recurrent *Malassezia* infection (White *et al.*, 1997);
- recurrent bilateral otitis externa (Muse *et al.*, 1996);
- bilateral recurrent conjunctivitis;
- facial erythema and cheilitis;
- sweating.

Although these criteria are not used by all dermatologists, there is an increasing tendency to do so. Dogs are considered to be atopic if they meet at least three of the major and three of the minor features. The major features can be used as a tool to standardize the selection of animals for *in vivo* and *in vitro* allergy testing.

Differential diagnosis

The list of differential diagnoses can be small or extensive depending on the history and physical findings. A list of commonly pruritic disorders of the dog is given in Table 2.4. Dogs with nonlesional pruritus are candidates for atopic disease, food hypersensitivity, early flea bite hypersensitivity, intestinal parasite hypersensitivity, contact dermatitis, hookworm dermatitis, or *Pelodera* dermatitis. The reader is referred to the appropriate chapters for a complete description of the allergic disorders.

When lesions are present, the list of differential diagnoses expands to include sarcoptic mange, flea bite hypersensitivity, bacterial folliculitis with or without a hypersensitivity component, seborrhea, *Malassezia* infection, and the various immune-mediated disorders. The concomitant occurrence of food hypersensitivity or contact allergy in dogs with AD is uncommon. It may be that food allergy or food intolerance are part of the atopic complex in some dogs or is a triggering factor for atopy. An argument in favor of this hypothesis is that food allergies are often seen before one year of age, and AD after that period of life. In addition, it is of interest, that in dogs with atopy, immediate skin reactivity to food store mite extracts has been found (Vollset, 1986).

Diagnostic tests

The diagnosis of atopy is based on the history, physical findings, elimination of the appropriate differential diagnoses, and allergy testing, which correlates with the history. If allergy testing cannot be done, the other diagnostic steps should be taken to make the tentative diagnosis as firm as possible. Patients referred for allergy testing should be thoroughly evaluated for other allergic and nonallergic causes of pruritus before the referral.

Skin scrapings should be done on all cases. Blood work is usually unrewarding as eosinophilia is uncommon in dogs. Total serum IgE measurement is of little value as the concentrations in normal and atopic dogs often overlap. Skin biopsies show a superficial perivascular dermatitis, which is not specific for atopic disease but will support that diagnosis.

Dogs with pyoderma or *Malassezia* infection should be treated appropriately to determine the significance of the infection. Atopic dogs are frequently secondarily infected and the infection intensifies or masks the signs of the atopic disease. Treatment of the secondary infection should lessen, but not eliminate the pruritus in an atopic dog. If the pruritus is completely eliminated with the treatment, the diagnosis of atopy is less likely. The authors (LMR, WHM) have seen dogs whose only sign of atopic disease was a recurrent generalized pruritic pyoderma. Antibiotic therapy resolved both the pyoderma and the pruritus, but the problem would recur. Skin testing showed significant reactions and immunotherapy resolved the problem. In these instances, the dogs were below their threshold level until the pyoderma appeared.

Since multiple forms of allergy can coexist in the same patient, all appropriate forms of allergy should be investigated. All nonseasonal atopic suspects should be checked for food hypersensitivity before skin testing. As previously mentioned, the definitive diagnosis of atopy is made by allergy testing, which correlates with the history. Approximately 80% of dogs with AD exhibit immediate skin test reactivity (after 20 minutes) to aeroallergens (Scott, 1981; Willemse and Van den Brom, 1983; Carlotti and

Table 2.4 *Pruritic disorders of the dog*

Disease	Primary lesions present	Level of pruritus	Response of pruritus to glucocorticoids	Sites of predilection
Atopy	No	Mild to intense	Excellent	Face, ears, feet, axillae, anywhere
Flea bite hypersensitivity	Yes	Moderate to intense	Good to excellent	Lower back, thighs, ventrum
Food hypersensitivity	No	Moderate to intense	Variable	As in flea bite hypersensitivity or atopy, anywhere
Hormonal hypersensitivity	No	Intense	Poor	Lower back, perineum, ventrum
Contact dermatitis	No	Moderate	Poor to good	Feet, ventrum, perineum
Internal parasite hypersensitivity	No?	Moderate to intense	Poor to good	Flanks, lower back, perineum
Drug hypersensitivity	Yes	Variable	Poor	Anywhere
Psychogenic pruritus	No	Mild to intense	Poor	Feet, flank folds, perineum, tail
Sarcoptic mange	Yes	Intense	Poor	Ears, elbows, hocks, ventrum
Cheyletiella dermatitis	Variable	None to intense	Good	Dorsum
Otodectic mange	No	Mild to moderate	Good to excellent	Ears, trunk
Demodicosis	Yes	Variable	Poor to good	Face, feet, anywhere
Pelodera dermatitis	No	Moderate to intense	Good	Feet, ventrum, perineum
Hookworm dermatitis	Yes	Moderate to intense	Poor to good	Feet, ventrum, perineum
Bacterial folliculitis	Yes	None to moderate	Poor to good	Anywhere
Bacterial hypersensitivity	Yes	Moderate to intense	Poor	Anywhere
Seborrhea complex	Variable	Mild to intense	Good	Face, ears, intertriginous areas, anywhere
Immune-mediated disorders	Yes	None to intense	Poor to good	Head, feet, ventrum, anywhere
Subcorneal pustular dermatosis	Yes	Mild to intense	Poor	Face, trunk
Cutaneous lymphomas	Variable	Moderate to intense	Poor to good	Face, anywhere

Costargent, 1994; Koch and Peters, 1994; Sture *et al.*, 1995). Late-phase IgE/IgGd-like reactions 2–8 hours after the injection are occasionally seen (Kristensen, 1994; Mason and Lloyd, 1996). Sensitivity to one allergen is uncommon. Multiple sensitivities are the rule. Multisensitivity occurs in approximately 60% of the animals. Allergens commonly reported to be important include pollens of grasses, trees, and weeds (5–30%), dandruff extracts of dogs, cats, and poultry, human dandruff, molds, house dust, house dust mites (20–80%), and storage mites such as *Acarus siro* (20–75%) and *Tyrophagus putrescentiae* (24–75%) (Vollset, 1986; DeBoer, 1993; Carlotti and Costargent, 1994; Koch and Peters, 1994; Sture *et al.*, 1995; Willemse, 1996). Willemse and Van den Brom (1983) showed a lower number of positive skin test reactions to multiple allergens in dogs over six years of age (P<0.001).

Although allergy testing will usually confirm the diagnosis, the real purpose for the testing is to start an immunotherapy protocol. If immunotherapy is inappropriate, there is limited value in doing the allergy tests. However, the testing might convince the pet owner that the dog is suffering from atopy and with confirmation of the diagnosis, the owner might be more likely to follow therapeutic recommendations.

Feline atopy

Although there are increasing reports about AD-like problems in cats (Reedy, 1982; Willemse, 1992; Anderson, 1993; Scott, 1995; Codner, 1986), it remains unclear exactly what feline atopy is. Cats with various cutaneous disorders have shown skin test reactivity to aeroallergens, among which house dust mites are most common. For the state of the art on the immunopathogenesis of feline atopy the reader is referred to the introductory parts of this chapter (Powell *et al.*, 1980; DeBoer *et al.*, 1993; Foster *et al.*, 1994; Roosje and Willemse, 1995; Roosje *et al.*, 1995a; Roosje *et al.*, 1995b; Roosje *et al.*, 1996).

The clinical presentation of atopy in the cat is not as clearcut as it is in the dog. Atopic cats can show lesional or nonlesional pruritus. Apart from miliary dermatitis, AD may include head and neck pruritus with or without rhinitis or conjunctivitis, traumatic alopecia mimicking psychogenic alopecia, generalized pruritus, lesions of the eosinophilic granuloma complex, facial excoriations, and generalized exfoliative dermatitis (Reedy, 1982; Anderson, 1993; Roosje and Willemse, 1995; Scott *et al.*, 1995). If lesions of the eosinophilic granuloma complex are seen, they usually occur in conjunction with other skin lesions, especially those of miliary dermatitis. Much of the data presented on so-called atopic cats deal with miliary dermatitis or alopecia due to excessive grooming.

The age at onset is very variable ranging from six months to 8.5 years, with most below the age of two years. No sex predilection has been mentioned. As in dogs, pruritus seems to be a hallmark for atopy-like problems in cats. Atopic cats can exhibit their symptoms seasonally or perennially. Since severely pruritic cats will mutilate their bodies, they are often presented to veterinary dermatologists early in the course of the disease so the true seasonality can be difficult to determine.

Diagnosis
The diagnosis of feline AD is usually based on a compatible history and physical examination, results of skin tests, response to glucocorticoids, histopathology, and the

exclusion of other cutaneous diseases such as food hypersensitivity, dermatophytosis, parasitic diseases, and flea bite allergy (Reedy, 1982; Willemse, 1992; Scott *et al.*, 1995). Similar to the findings in man (Soter, 1989), dermatohistopathologic examination of 'atopic' cat skin shows perivascular and interstitial dermal infiltrates consisting of mast cells, eosinophils, lymphocytes, and macrophages (Gross *et al.*, 1992). Histopathology does not reliably distinguish between the lesions of flea allergy, atopy, or food allergy (Gross *et al.*, 1992). It has been hypothesized that the various cutaneous manifestations (including also indolent ulcers and eosinophilic plaques) reflect different stages of the disease (Willemse, 1992). The diagnostic approach depends on the clinical presentation. Skin scrapings, fecal flotations, and fungal cultures should be run in all cases. The next step depends on the clinical presentation and history. Where appropriate, flea bite hypersensitivity should be excluded by an extensive flea control program and dietary allergy should be investigated by a dietary restriction.

Although skin testing is commonly performed in cats (Moriello and McMurdy, 1989; Bevier, 1990; Anderson, 1993; Codner, 1996) there are various problems in testing this species. Skin reactions are difficult to interpret and inconsistent, and stress influences skin test reactivity considerably (Willemse *et al.*, 1993). Serologic testing has not been properly evaluated in this species. Hence, its diagnostic value is questionable.

References

Anderson RK. *In vitro* testing for feline atopic disease. *Proc. 10th Ann. Congress Eur. Soc. Vet. Derm.* Congress Organisation, Aalborg (Denmark), p. 72, 1993.

Baldwin CI, De Medeiros F, Denham DA. IgE responses in cats infected with *Brugia pahangi. Parasite Immunol.* **15:** 291–296, 1993.

Bevier DE. The reaction of feline skin to the intradermal injection of allergenic extracts and passive cutaneous anaphylaxis using serum from skin test positive cats. In Von Tscharner C, Halliwell REW (eds) *Advances in Veterinary Dermatology.* Baillière Tindall, London, pp. 126–136, 1990.

Bruijnzeel-Koomen CAFM, Van Wichen DF, Spry CJF, *et al.* Active participation of eosinophils in patch test reactions to inhalant allergens in patients with atopic dermatitis. *Br. J. Dermatol.* **118:** 229–238, 1988.

Bruijnzeel-Koomen C, Mudde G, Bruijnzeel P, *et al.* IgE receptors on Langerhans' cells: their significance in the pathophysiology of atopic eczema. In Ruzicka T, Ring J, Przybilla B (eds) *Handbook of Atopic Eczema.* Springer Verlag, Berlin, pp. 154–165, 1991.

Butler JM, Peters JE, Hirshman CA, *et al.* Pruritic dermatitis in asthmatic basenji-greyhound dogs: a model for human atopic dermatitis. *J. Am. Acad. Dermatol.* **8:** 33–38, 1983.

Carlotti DN, Costargent F. Analysis of positive skin tests in 449 dogs with allergic dermatitis. *Eur. J. Comp. Anim. Pract.* **4:** 42–59, 1994.

Codner EC. Reactivity to intradermal injections of extracts of house dust mite and flea antigen in normal cats and cats suspected of being allergic. *12th Proc. Ann. .Meeting AAVD/ACVD.* Congress Organisation, Las Vegas, Nevada, pp. 26–27, 1996.

DeBoer DJ. Intradermal skin testing and response to hyposensitization in atopic dogs from the north central United States. *Proc. 10th Ann. Congress Eur. Soc. Vet. Derm.* Congress Organisation, Aalborg (Denmark), p. 267, 1993.

DeBoer DJ, Saban R, Schultz KT, *et al*. Feline IgE: Preliminary evidence of its existence and crossreactivity with canine IgE. In Ihrke PJ, Mason SI, White SD (eds) *Advances in Veterinary Dermatology*, Volume 2. Pergamon Press, Oxford, pp. 51–62, 1993.

DeWeck AL, Mayer P, Schiessl B, *et al*. Genetics and regulation of the IgE response leading to experimentally induced atopic-like dermatitis in beagle dogs. *Proc. Ann. Meeting AAVD/ACVD*. Nashville (USA), pp. 76–77, 1997.

Frank LA, McEntee MF. Demonstration of aeroallergen contact sensitivity in dogs. *J. Vet. Allergy Clin. Immunol.* **3:** 75–80, 1995.

Frick OL, Brooks DL. Immunoglobulin E antibodies to pollens augmented in dogs by virus vaccines. *Am. J. Vet. Res.* **44:** 440–445, 1983.

Foster AP, Duffus WPH, Shaw SE, *et al*. Studies on the isolation and characterization of a cat reaginic antibody. *10th Proc. Ann. Meeting AAVD/ACVD*. Congress Organisation, Charleston (USA), p. 62, 1994.

Griffin CE. Otitis externa and otitis media. In *Current Veterinary Therapy*. Mosby–Yearbook, St Louis, pp. 245–262, 1993.

Gross TL, Ihrke PJ, Walder EJ. *Veterinary Dermatopathology*. Mosby Yearbook, St. Louis, pp. 122–123, 1992.

Halliwell REW. The sites of production and localization of IgE in canine tissues. *Ann. NY Acad. Sci.*, **254:** 476–488, 1975.

Hanifin JM. Atopic dermatitis. *J. Am. Acad. Dermatol.* **6:** 1–13, 1982.

Hanifin JM, Lobitz WC. Newer concepts of atopic dermatitis. *Arch. Dermatol.* **113:** 663–670, 1977.

Hanifin JM, Rajka G. Diagnostic features of atopic dermatitis. *Acta. Derm. Venereol. (Stockholm)* **92:** 44–47, 1980.

Helton Rhodes K, Kerdel F, Soter NA. Investigation into the immunopathogenesis of canine atopy. *Sem. Vet. Med. Surg. (Small Anim.)* **2:** 199–201, 1987.

Katz DH. The allergic phenotype: manifestation of 'allergic breakthrough' and imbalance in normal 'damping' of IgE antibody production. *Immunol. Rev.* **41:** 77–108, 1978.

Kleinbeck ML, Hites MJ, Loker JL, *et al*. Enzyme linked immunosorbent assay for measurement of allergen-specific IgE antibodies in canine serum. *Am. J. Vet. Res.* **50:** 1831–1839, 1989.

Koch HJ, Peters S. 207 Intrakutantests bei Hunden mit Verdacht auf atopische Dermatitis. *Kleintierpraxis* **39:** 25–36, 1994.

Kristensen F. Der allergische Hund Inhalations und Kontaktallergene. *Proc 40. Jahrestagung Fachgruppe Kleintierkrankheiten der Deutschen Veterinärmedizinischen Gesellschaft*. Congress Organisation, Dresden (Germany), pp. 27–36, 1994

Leung DYM, Rhodes AR, Geha RS. Enumeration of T-cell subsets in atopic dermatitis using monoclonal antibodies. *J. Allergy Clin. Immunol.* **67(6):**450–455, 1981.

Lever R, Turbitt M, Sanderson A, *et al*. Immunophenotyping of the cutaneous infiltrate and of the mononuclear cells in the peripheral blood in patients with atopic dermatitis. *J. Invest. Derm.* **89:** 4, 1987.

Mason IS, Lloyd DH. Evaluation of compound 48/80 as a model of immediate hypersensitivity in the skin of dogs. *Vet. Derm.* **7:** 81–83, 1996.

Moore PF, Rossito PV, Danilenko DM, *et al*. Monoclonal antibodies specific for canine CD4 and CD8 define functional T-lymphocyte subsets and high-density expression of CD4 by canine neutrophils. *Tissue Antigens* **40:** 75–85, 1992.

Moriello KA, McMurdy MA. The prevalence of positive intradermal skin test reactions to flea extract in clinically normal cats. *Comp. Anim. Pract.* **19:** 298–302, 1989.

Mudde GC, Bheekha R, Bruijnzeel–Koomen CAFM. IgE-mediated antigen presentation. *Allergy.* **50:** 193–199, 1995.

Muse R, Griffin C, Rosenkrantz WS. The prevalence of otic manifestations and otitis externa in allergic dogs. *12th Proc. Ann. Meeting AAVD/ACVD.* Congress Organisation, Las Vegas, Nevada pp. 33–36, 1996.

Nimmo Wilkie JS, Yager JA, Wilkie BN, *et al.* Abnormal cutaneous responses to mitogens and a contact antigen in dogs with atopic dermatitis. *Vet. Immunol. Immunopathol.* **28:** 97–106, 1991.

Nimmo Wilkie JS, Yager JA, Wilkie BN, *et al.* Changes in cell-mediated immune response after experimentally-induced anaphylaxis in dogs. *Vet. Immunol. Immunolopathol.* **32:** 325–338, 1992.

Ohlén BM. Projekt allergitester i Sverige. *Svensk. Veter. Tidning.* 1992; **44:** 365–371.

Olivry T, Moore PF, Affolter VK, *et al.* Langerhans' cell hyperplasia and surface IgE expression in canine atopic dermatitis. *11th Proc Ann Meeting AAVD/ACVD.* Congress Organisation, Santa Fe (New Mexico), pp. 36–37, 1995.

Olivry T, Moore PF, Naydan DK. Characterization of the inflammatory infiltrate in canine atopic dermatitis. *11th Proc Ann Meeting AAVD/ACVD.* Congress Organisation, Santa Fe (New Mexico), p. 3, 1995b.

Parish WE. The clinical relevance of heat-stable, short-term sensitizing anaphylactic IgG antibodies (IgG S-TS) and of related activities of IgG4 and IgG2. *Br. J. Dermatol.* **105:** 223, 1981.

Pène J, Rousset F, Brière F, *et al.* IgE production by normal human B-cells induced by alloreactive T cell clones is mediated by IL-4 and suppressed by IFN-γ *J. Immunol.* 1988; **141:** 1218–1224.

Peters JE, Hirshman CA, Malley A. The basenji-greyhound dog model of asthma: leukocyte histamine release, serum IgE, and airway response to inhaled antigen. *J. Immunol.* **129:** 1245–1249, 1982.

Powell MB, Weisbroth SH, Roth L, *et al.* Reaginic hypersensitivity in *Otodectes cynotis* infestation of cats and mode of mite feeding. *Am. J. Vet. Res.* **41:** 877–882,1980.

Reedy L. Results of allergy testing and hyposensitization in selected feline skin diseases. *J. Am. Anim. Hosp. Assoc.* **18:** 618, 1982.

Rhodes KH, Kerdel F, Soter NA. Comparative aspects of canine and human atopic dermatitis. *Sem. Vet. Med. Surg. (Small Anim.)* **2:** 166–172, 1987.

Rockey JH, Schwartzman RM. Skin sensitizing antibodies: a comparative study of canine and human PK and PCA antibodies and a canine myeloma protein. *J. Immunol.* **98:** 1143–1151, 1967.

Roosje PJ, Willemse T. Cytophilic antibodies in cats with miliary dermatitis and eosinophilic plaques: passive transfer of immediate-type hypersensitivity. *Vet. Quart.* **17:** 66–68, 1995.

Roosje PJ, Thepen T, Van Kooten PJS, *et al.* Investigations on the CD4/CD8 ratio and cytokine production in lesional skin and peripheral blood of cats with allergic dermatitis. *Abstract 4th International Vet. Immunol. Symp.* Davis (USA), p. 166, 1995a.

Roosje PJ, Van Kooten PJS, Thepen T, *et al.* A role of Th2 cells in the pathogenesis of allergic dermatitis in cats? Abstracts of Joint Congress of the British and Netherlands Society for Immunology, Brighton (UK), December 6–8 1995. *Immunology* **86(Suppl. 1):** 98–W3.3, 1995b.

Roosje PJ, Whitaker-Menezes D, Goldschmidt MH, *et al.* MHC Class II⁺ and CD1A⁺ cells in lesional skin of cats with allergic dermatitis. *Book of Abstracts, 3rd World Congress on Veterinary Dermatology.* Congress Organisation, Edinburgh (UK), p. 59, 1996.

Schick RO, Fadok VA. Response of atopic dogs to regional allergens: 268 cases (1981–1984). *J. Am. Vet. Med. Assoc.* **189:** 1493–1496, 1986.

Schwartzman RM. Immunologic studies of progeny of atopic dogs. *Am. J. Vet. Res.* **45:** 375–378, 1984.

Schwartzman RM, Rockey JH, Halliwell REW. Canine reaginic antibody. Characterization of the spontaneous anti-ragweed and induced anti-dinitrophenyl reaginic antibodies of the atopic dog. *Clin. exp. Immunol.* **9:** 549–569, 1971.

Schwartzman RM, Massicot JG, Sogn DD, *et al.* The atopic dog model: report of an attempt to establish a colony. *Int. Archs. Allergy Appl. Immunol.* **72:** 97–101, 1983.

Scott DW. Observations on canine atopy. *J. Am. Anim. Hosp. Assoc.* 1981; **17:** 91–100.

Scott DW, Miller WH, Griffin CG. *Small Animal Dermatology.* W.B. Saunders, Philadelphia, pp. 518–523, 1995.

Sinke JD, Thepen T, Bihari IC, *et al.* Immunophenotyping of skin-infiltrating T-cell subsets in dogs with atopic dermatitis. *Book of Abstracts 3rd World Congress on Veterinary Dermatology.* Congress Organisation, Edinburgh (UK), p. 46, 1996.

Soter NA. Morphology of atopic eczema. *Allergy* **44:** 16–19, 1989.

Sture GH, Halliwell REW, Thoday KL, *et al.* Canine atopic disease: the prevalence of positive intradermal skin tests at two sites in the north and south of Great Britain. *Vet. Immunol. Immunopathol.* **44:** 293–308, 1995.

Szentivanyi A. Beta-adrenergic theory of the atopic abnormality in bronchial asthma. *J. Allergy Clin. Immunol.* **42:** 203–232, 1968.

Thomsen MK, Kristensen F, Elling F. Species specificity in the generation of eicosanoids: emphasis on leukocyte-activating factors in the skin of allergic dogs and humans. In Ihrke PJ, Mason IS, White SD (eds) *Advances in Veterinary Dermatology*, Volume 2. Pergamon Press, Oxford, pp. 63–78, , 1993.

Uehara M. Heterogeneity of serum IgE levels in atopic dermatitis. *Acta. Derm. Venereol. (Stockholm)* **66:** 404–408, 1986.

Van der Heyden FL, Wierenga EL, Bos JD, *et al.* High frequency of IL4-producing CD4⁺ allergen-specific T lymphocytes in atopic dermatitis lesional skin. *J. Invest. Dermatol.* **389:** 394, 1991.

Van Stee EW. Risk factors in canine atopy. *Calif. Vet.* **4:** 8–10, 1983.

Vollset I. Immediate type hypersensitivity in dogs induced by storage mites. *Res. Vet. Sci.* **40:** 123–127, 1986.

Vriesendorp HM, Smid-Mercx BMJ, Visser TP, *et al.* Serological DL-A typing of normal and atopic dogs. *Transpl. Proc.* **7:** 375–377, 1975.

White SD, Bourdeau P, Blumstein P, *et al.* Comparison via cytology and culture of carriage of *Malassezia pachydermatis* in atopic and healthy dogs. In Kwochka K, von Tscharner C, Willemse T (eds) *Advances in Veterinary Dermatology*, Volume 3. Butterworth Heinemann, 1997 (in press).

Wierenga EA, Snoek M, Jansen HM, *et al.* Human atopen-specific Types 1 and 2 helper T cell clones. *J. Immunol.* **144:** 4651–4656, 1990.

Willemse A. Atopic skin disease: a review and a re-consideration of diagnostic criteria. *J. Small Anim. Pract.* **27:** 771–778, 1986.

Willemse T. Feline Atopie. Sinn oder Unsinn? *Kleintierpraxis.* **37:** 129–132, 1992.

Willemse T. Canine atopic dermatitis. *Proc 3rd World Congress Vet. Derm.* Congress Organisation, Edinburgh (UK), 44–48, 1996.

Willemse A, Van den Brom WE. Investigations of the symptomatology and the significance of immediate skin test reactivity in canine atopic dermatitis. *Res. Vet. Sci.* **34:** 261–265, 1983.

Willemse A, Noordzij A, Rutten VPMG, *et al.* Induction of non-IgE anaphylactic antibodies in dogs. *Clin. Exp. Immunol.* **59:** 351–358, 1985.

Willemse A, Noordzij A, Van den Brom WE, *et al.* Allergen specific IgGd antibodies in dogs with atopic dermatitis as determined by the enzyme linked immunosorbent assay (ELISA). *Clin. Exp. Immunol.* **59:** 359–363, 1985.

Willemse T, Vroom MW, Mol JA, *et al.* Changes in plasma cortisol, corticotropin, and melanocyte-stimulating hormone concentrations in cats before and after physical restraint and intradermal testing. *Am. J. Vet. Res.* **54:** 69–72, 1993.

Yager JA. The skin as an immune organ. In: Ihrke PJ, Mason IS, White SD (eds) *Advances in Veterinary Dermatology*, Volume 2. Pergamon Press, Oxford, pp. 3–32, 1993.

Zachary CB, Allen MH, MacDonald DM. *In situ* qualification of T-lymphocyte subsets and Langerhans' cells in the inflammatory infiltrate of atopic eczema. *Br. J. Dermatol.* **112:** 149–156, 1995.

3

Aeroallergens and Aerobiology

Introduction

Aeroallergens are airborne particles such as pollens, house dust, mold spores, and animal danders that are capable of eliciting an allergic reaction in a susceptible individual. They are complex particles containing many molecular components, only some of which are allergenic. Most allergens have two or more antigenic determinants. Allergens are typically water soluble proteins or glycoproteins with a molecular weight ranging from 10–70 kD and vary in size from 2–60 μm. Larger particles have trouble reaching the terminal bronchioles and penetrating the mucous membranes. For a particle to be a significant aeroallergen, it must be antigenic, present in sufficient amounts, and dispersible.

Aerobiology

Aerobiology is the science of the origins, release, transport, and surface impact of windborne biologic particles. Pollens and mold spores are typically studied, but other aeroallergens such as animal danders can also be considered. Pollen or mold spore release is affected by climate (wind, humidity, and temperature), geography, and vegetation. Once a particle is airborne, it is subject to the effects of wind velocity, turbulence, rain, gravity, and atmospheric pressure. Dry warm conditions with brisk winds favor pollen transfer and pollens can travel several hundred miles. The pollen count in the vicinity of the plant is much higher and much more significant. Rainfall is thought to clean the air, but the cleansing effect depends on the duration of the rain and the droplet size. During thunderstorms, the raindrops are typically large and will not remove much pollen. The droplet size of prolonged rains is typically smaller and such rains effectively clear the air. Storms, whether they are brief or prolonged, can prevent pollens from reaching high altitudes and can concentrate the allergens lower to the ground.

Pollens and mold spores can be identified by their electron microscopic appearance (Figure 3.1) and can be collected and counted by a variety of methods. Most windborne pollen grains are yellowish, roughly spherical bodies with an average diameter of 14–60 μm and often have globules of surface lipid. The outermost envelope, or excrine, of the pollen is often prominently sculptured and may bear apertures as circular spores (porate), elongated furrows (colpate), or both (colporate).

So-called 'pollen counts' are available from local weather bureaus, health departments, or private human allergists in some areas. These data are most valuable for identifying which pollens and mold spores occur in a geographic area. If quantitative

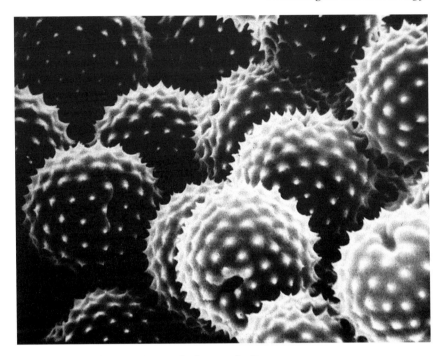

Figure 3.1 *Scanning electron micrograph of ragweed pollen.*

methods are used, the concentration of the various aeroallergens can also be determined. Gravitational methods are the simplest, but have many drawbacks. A slide coated with a soft glycerine jelly is exposed to the air for 24 hours and then the pollens are identified by their morphology and their numbers are counted. Slide placement is very important since wind velocity and direction greatly affect which pollens will be in the area. As small particles are less affected by gravity, this method favors the collection of large particles. Since airflow is unknown, gravitational pollen counts are, however, not reliable. Volumetric methods involve the use of machinery, which samples the air in known volumes. Smaller pollens will be collected with these methods and the pollen counts tend to be more reliable. Pollen counts are most helpful in determining which pollens are in a geographic area. When pollen counts are low, many allergic patients will experience less intense symptoms, but symptomatology is not directly related to the pollen count. Individual sensitivity combined with the local concentration of pollens is very important. Most pollens never reach the air, but fall to the ground near the plant. Since dogs and cats are low to the ground and constantly sniff, they are exposed to many more pollens than man. Preliminary data suggest that transcutaneous sensitization to pollens may be a route of exposure (Frank and McEntee, 1995).

Pollen Aeroallergens

Pollen grains are essential for the reproduction of seed plants. Pollen transfer is accomplished by insects (entomophilous pollination), the wind (anemophilous pollination), or a combination of both. Entomophilous pollination typically occurs for plants producing single, showy, colorful and fragrant flowers. These plants have local allergenic potential for people or animals in their immediate vicinity, but are insignificant away from the plant since their pollens are large, heavy, have an adhesive coating, and are produced in small amounts. Anemophilous plants are typically drab with multiple, small, inconspicuous, and odorless flowers. Because of the relative inefficiency of wind pollination, these plants can liberate millions of pollen grains.

Air pollen levels depend on the number of plants in an area and the efficiency of pollen release. Although some plants forcibly eject their pollens, most just drop the pollen. Pollens can fall to leaves or to the ground. Pollens caught in vegetation are subject to wind dispersal while pollen on the ground is lost. Dogs or cats who wander through fields are exposed to massive pollen loads from the ground.

For a pollen to be a major allergen, it should be allergenic, windborne, buoyant, and produced in large quantities by abundant, widely distributed plants. Ragweed is the best known example of a pollen that meets all five criteria. In man, dandelion is not important because although it is allergenic and abundant, it is rarely airborne.

Pollen shedding is not uniform throughout the day because it is affected by air temperature, humidity, and wind velocity. Rapidly moving air of low humidity promotes pollination. Typically, the best conditions for pollination occur at midday and in the afternoon when the air is warm and dry. Many plants have mechanisms to prevent pollen release when the humidity is high. Short ragweed pollen release is affected by diminishing day length, overnight rainfall, and temperature. As the overnight temperature rises and the humidity decreases, pollen release is triggered 1–3 hours after sunrise. Airborne levels increase 2–4 hours later as pollens on the plant leaves dry out and become windborne. Because of their buoyancy, airborne pollens can travel for hundreds of miles. Ragweed pollens have been detected at altitudes of 17 000 feet and as far as 400 miles from land. Again, local concentrations are much more important.

Plant growth obviously affects plant pollination. Dry cool growing conditions limit plant numbers while warm wet conditions encourage heavy plant growth. Within any one of the botanical zones of the USA, there are certain growing seasons for the various plants. As a general rule, trees pollinate first in the spring, followed by grasses and then weeds. Molds, depending on their method of spore release, tend to peak during wet conditions in the spring and fall. During the early growing season, pollen production is scant. Air pollen levels peak during the middle of the growing season and then gradually decrease. Although pollen grains are reproductively viable for only a few hours, their allergenicity lasts much longer. Frost will terminate pollination by killing the plant, but already released pollens will linger on dead plants and on the ground. In warmer climates, some plants will continue to pollinate year round, although pollen levels will vary with the season and local weather conditions. The geographic distribution and occurrence of the source plant have a major influence on the allergenic importance. Many grasses, for example *Phleum pratense* (timothy grass), and *Lolium perenne* (perennial ryegrass) and some weeds, for example *Artemisia* spp. (mugwort) occur worldwide, partly explaining their allergenic importance. Other plants frequently occur in specific but extensive habitats where they give rise to allergies, for example *Betula verucosa* (birch) in temperate northern hemisphere areas, *Parietaria* spp. in the more dry southern Europe, and *Ambrosia* spp. (ragweeds) in the central part of North America. Massive pollinations from locally found plants can also cause an allergic response for those in the immediate area, for example the fields of *Secale cereale* (cultivated rye). Some plants do not pollinate yearly, for example *Fagus* spp. (beech) (D'Ammato *et al.*, 1991).

The botanical classification of plants can be helpful in determining the allergenic potential of a plant. Plants are described by their order, family, genus, and species. For some plants, subspecies or varieties also exist. In large families, related genera may be grouped as tribes. Closely related plants may share some common antigens and may be cross-reactive.

Grasses

Grasses constitute approximately 20% of the earth's vegetation cover. There are approximately 400 genera of grasses with at least 4500 species. Several hundred of the 4500 are cultivated by man and these are of greatest allergenic significance. During the growing season, grass pollens are common in all habitats throughout the world, and grass pollens are responsible for between 10 to 30% of all human IgE-mediated allergies.

In the temperate regions of the USA, the peak pollen period for grasses is from mid-May to mid-July. Throughout the northeastern two-thirds of the USA and southern Canada, the bulk of windborne grass pollen is derived from bluegrass (Canada and June or Kentucky), orchard grass, timothy grass, and red top grass. The rye grasses, Italian or perennial, are also important. Bermuda grass is a major pollen source throughout the southern half of the USA and along the Pacific Coast and pollinates year round.

In Europe most widely distributed grasses associated with grass pollen allergies are *Poa pratensis* (Kentucky), *Festuca eliator* (meadow fescue), *Dactylis glomerata* (orchard), *Lolium perenne* (perennial rye), and *Phleum pratense* (timothy). In addition *Agropyron repens* (quack grass) is common in mid and south France and the Mediterranean area, whereas in central Europe, Germany, the UK, northern France, the Benelux, and Scandinavia *Anthoxantum odoratum* (sweet vernal), *Holcus lanatus* (velvet), and *Agrostis alba* (redtop) may also be the cause of pollinosis. In those parts of Europe with a mild Mediterranean climate pollination occurs mainly between April and September. In areas with a moderate climate, the pollination season is usually between May–June and August. People allergic to multiple grasses share skin test and radioallergosorbent test (RAST) positivity to *Lolium perenne* (perennial rye) and *Dactylus glomerata* (orchard) (Ree *et al.*, 1992, 1994; Roberts *et al.*, 1994).

Most temperate zone grasses, except Bermuda grass, have some allergenic cross-reactivity. Grass pollen typically contains at least two, but usually more antigens. Some are specific for the individual pollen while others are common to the entire family. Rye grass has four group antigens, but one is nonallergenic or weakly allergenic. Rye Group I antigen, or one very similar to it, is found in most, if not all grasses, except Bermuda grass. Group II antigen is prominent in rye, fescue, orchard and velvet grasses, while timothy and sweet vernal are relatively deficient.

Rapid advances have been made in the past few years in allergen characterization and sequence determination by chemical and molecular biologic approaches. An allergen from a single species may consist of several closely similar molecules. These similar molecules are designated as isoallergens when they share the following common biochemical properties: similar molecular size; identical biological function, if known (e.g. enzymatic action); and at least 67% identity of amino acid sequences. The recommendation that a minimum of 67% of the sequences be identical before two allergens are assigned to the same group is only a guideline. There are likely to be borderline cases. For example, the ragweed allergens *Amb a 1* and 2 share 65% amino acid sequence identity. These allergens were assigned to different groups because of their different immunochemical properties before their sequences were known. Allergens from different species of the same or a different genus which share the above-mentioned common biochemical properties are considered to belong to the same group and the sequence identity requirement can be less than 67% as is the case for allergens of the same species. For example, *Amb a 5* and *Amb t 5* from short and giant ragweed pollens have about 45% sequence identity, and also have similar tertiary structures. Other examples are the minor pollen allergens *Amb a 10, Poa p 10*, and *Lol p 10* from ragweed, Kentucky blue grass, and ryegrass, respectively. Although their sequences are not known, they are assigned to the same allergen group as they clearly have the same biologic function of cytochrome c (World Health Organization, 1995).

Weeds

Weeds are small annual plants that grow wild and have little or no agricultural or decorative value. The most important allergic group is the Compositae family, which includes 20 000 or more species and is divided into 14 tribes. The ragweed tribe (*Ambrosia*) is most important, and ragweed is the major cause of hay fever in man in the USA.

More than a dozen ragweed species are found in North America, but six are of major significance: short, giant, slender, western, southern, and false (bur) ragweeds are widely distributed in the USA and adjacent Canada. Short and giant ragweed are the most prolific sources of pollen. Ragweed pollen contains approximately 14 soluble proteins and polypeptide antigens, but they are not all significant allergens. For short ragweed, at least five separate allergens have been identified. These allergens vary in their molecular weight, physical and chemical characteristics, speed of extractability, and heat lability. Certain patients will react to some antigens while others will not. The bulk of the allergenic activity is believed to be associated with a simple globular protein called antigen E. Antigen E is 200 times more active than whole ragweed extract. The allergenic role of ragweed is increasing in Europe, in particular in the eastern central European region: Hungary, the former Yugoslavia, the Czech Republic, Slovakia, and the eastern most part of Austria. There are also occasional reports of ragweed pollen in Switzerland and France. Other portions of the Eurasian land mass, Australia, Africa, and Great Britain remain essentially free of ragweed. *Ambrosia artemisiifolia* (short ragweed) and *A. eliator* are the most common species in Europe, although *A. trifida* (giant ragweed), *A. maritima*, and *A. psilostachya* (western ragweed) have also been reported from this area (D'Ammato *et al.*, 1991).

The pollens of the *Iva* species are similar in appearance and allergenic activity to ragweed. Rough marsh elder, burweed marsh elder (prairie ragweed), and poverty weed may cross-react in ragweed sensitive patients. The same may be true for cockleburs.

The tansy tribe includes the sages, sagebrushes, wormwoods and mugworts. The most common species in Europe are *Artemisia vulgaris* (mugwort), which is abundant throughout the continent, and *A. verlotorum* and *A. annua* (annual sagebrush), predominantly in the southern half of Europe (D'Ammato *et al.*, 1991). Members of the dandelion tribe include dandelions, asters, goldenrods, sneezeweed, and dog fennel. Cultivated members include chrysanthemums, dahlias, and marigolds. These weeds and flowers are typically insect pollinated and are not of major windborne significance except in the vicinity of the plant. Ragweed sensitive patients may show a sensitivity to members of the dandelion tribe.

The goosefoot (Chenopodiaceae) family includes Russian thistle, burning bush (*Kochia*), salt bushes, smotherweeds, greasewood, lamb's quarter, and Mexican tea. This family is especially important in the Mediterranean area, although *Chenopodium album* (lamb's quarter) is also relevant in northern France, the Benelux countries, the UK and Scandinavia (D'Ammato *et al.*, 1991). The amaranth (Amaranthaceae) family includes pigweed and western waterhemp. These families produce similar pollens and some investigations suggest strong interfamilial as well as intrafamilial similarities in the allergens. Sorrels and docks belong to the Polygonaceae family and seem to cross-react.

Although plants of *Parietaria* have been identified in California, it is a well-known allergy-inducing plant typical of the Mediterranean area. In particular, it is the most important allergenic plant in some regions bordering the Mediterranean such as southern Italy and the coast of Spain. The genus *Parietaria* (pellitory-of-the-wall) belongs to the family of Urticaceae, together with the allergenically unimportant *Urtica dioica* (nettle). *Parietaria officinalis* and *P. judaica* are the most common species. *P. officinalis* grows mainly in the hilly and mountain areas (under 1000 m of altitude) of Spain, France, northern Italy, Austria, Bulgaria, Czech Republic, Slovakia, Rumania, and Russia. *P. judaica* grows in coastal Mediterranean areas, particularly on walls in the towns of Spain, southern France, Italy, former Yugoslavia, Albania, and Greece. It also grows in some other European regions, such as the UK, where it was introduced in the Middle Ages by monks (D'Ammato *et al.*, 1991).

Over 90 weed and garden plant pollen extracts are available, but the nature of the allergens of these flowers are not well defined. Ragweed antigen E activity has been found in the various ragweed species, marsh elders and cockleburs so these pollens may cross-react. Plants within the same tribe also may cross-react.

Trees

In general, the period of pollination of deciduous trees is short and occurs shortly before, during, and shortly after leaf development. In more temperate climates, tree pollination is concluded by late spring. In warmer areas, this season may be extended. In some areas, conifers, especially mountain cedar, pollinate in the winter. Tree pollens are less significant allergens, than weed and grass pollens.

Two classes of trees, the Gymnospermae and the Angiospermae, are of allergenic significance. The Gymnospermae include the conifers, which produce vast amounts of pollens. Essentially, two major types of pollens are released by this class. Pines, spruces, firs, true cedars, black hemlock and golden larch release large (i.e. 50–90 μm), coarsely surfaced grains, while representatives of the cypress–juniper family, yew family and the bald cypress–sequoia family share spherical pollen grains, 20–35 μm in diameter. In man, the conifers, which produce large pollens, are of uncertain but probably limited allergic significance. The families that produce the smaller pollens tend to be more important. Mountain cedar, red cedar and ornamental yews and junipers are examples of important conifers in the USA. The allergenic importance of Cupressaceae pollen in Europe is limited to France and Italy: *Cupressus sempervirens* (Italian cypress), *C. arizona* (Arizona cypress), and *C. glabra*. Other species belonging to the Cupressaceae and mainly important in the south of France are *Juniperus occidentalis* (western juniper) and *Thuja orientalis* (thuja). In humans in 80% of the cases, skin tests to *J. communis* correlated with skin tests to *C. sempervirens*. With *T. orientalis*, the correlation was 60%. Pollination of the Cupressaceae in Europe begins in January and ends in mid- to late March (D'Ammato *et al.*, 1991).

The Angiospermae are the conventionally flowering trees with many families and species. The Salicaceae family includes two genera: the willows (*Salix*) and the poplars and aspens (*Populus*). The pollens of the two genera are dissimilar morphologically and probably in allergic content as well. The *Populus* genus includes the poplars, aspens, and cottonwoods.

The Juglandaceae family includes the *Carya* and *Juglans* genera. The *Carya* genus includes the hickories and pecans while the *Juglans* genus includes the walnuts and butternuts. The Betulaceae family includes the hazelnut and filbert (*Corylus*), the birches (*Betula*) and the elders (*Alnus*). All over Europe *Corylus* spp., *Betula* spp., *Alnus* spp. together with *Quercus* spp. are considered allergenically important. Clinical and laboratory observations have provided evidence of allergenic cross-reactivities between *Betula* spp. and many tree pollens. For human patients with tree pollen allergy, more than 90% with a positive clinical history will give positive skin prick tests or RAST when tested against birch pollen (D'Ammato *et al.*, 1991).

The Fagaceae family includes the oaks (*Quercus*), the beeches (*Fagus*) and chestnuts (*Castanea*). Oak pollens are morphologically very similar. The Ulmaceae family includes the elms (*Ulmus*) and hackberries (*Celtis*). The Oleaceae family includes the ashes (*Fraxinus*) and the olive tree (*Olea*). In Europe olive pollen (*Olea europaea*) has been recognized as one of the most important allergenic pollens in Mediterranean Europe. There the pollen season is very short, lasting not more than 40 days in May to June, but is very intensive. The Aceraceae family includes maples and box elders. Insect pollination occurs to varying degrees in this family. The mulberry family (Moraceae) includes the mulberries (*Morus* and *Broussonetia*), hemp (*Cannabis*), hops (*Humulus*) and Osage orange (*Maclura*). In Japan, sugi pollen (*Cryptomecia japonica*), a relative of bold cypress, is very important.

At present, tree pollens are thought to be antigenically different. If tree mixtures are to be used for testing or immunotherapy, species from one family should be grouped together.

Fungal (Mold) Allergies

Fungi are universal in distribution and fungal spores can comprise the bulk of the suspended allergenic particles in an area depending on the weather conditions and land usage. Most fungi of allergic significance are nonpathogenic saprophytes. Fungi reproduce by sexual and/or asexual methods. Many of the common allergenic fungi reproduce asexually. All fungi require oxygen for growth and grow best under warm and humid conditions. The majority of fungi become dormant at subfreezing temperatures, but can survive prolonged freezing. Atmospheric moisture not only affects fungal growth and sporulation, but also spore dispersal. Although the general atmospheric humidity can be very low, fungi can find free water for growth and sporulation in damp areas and can therefore be found almost anywhere.

Some fungi shoot their spores into the environment and this process requires free water. High air concentrations of these spores occur with rainfall or fog or during the hours of darkness when the humidity tends to increase. Levels of *Fusarium*, *Phoma* and *Cephalosporium* peak with precipitation. Most fungi of allergic significance disperse their spores in dry conditions. Spore dispersal increases as air speed increases and humidity decreases. Maximum levels occur during sunny afternoon periods. Species of *Cladosporium* (formerly *Hormodendrum*), *Alternaria*, *Aspergillus*, *Epicoccum*, *Helminthosporium*, *Penicillium* and *Rhizopus* use dry spore dispersal. Once a spore is airborne, it is subject to the same atmospheric processes as pollens.

Fungi are common indoors and outdoors. Certain species are typically field molds while others will grow both inside and outside. Accordingly, symptomatology may be seasonal or perennial. Seasonal symptoms tend to peak in mid-summer and persist until well after a killing frost. Perennial symptoms can occur because most houses, especially those that are damp, have fungi growing in them. *Penicillium*, *Aspergillus*, *Rhizopus*, and *Mucor* are common indoor 'mildew' isolates. The following discussion highlights some important features of some fungi.

Alternaria grows on organic debris in the soil and parasitizes the leaves, stems, flowers, and fruits of many vegetables, cereal grains, and ornamental plants. The spores are common in the air from late spring to fall, especially from noon until 3 p.m. In man, *Alternaria* is considered the most clinically reactive airborne fungus especially in dry warm climates. *Aspergillus* is a common soil fungus and also grows in stored foods and on wet surfaces inside bathrooms, basements, and drip pans of refrigerators. *Aureobasidium (Pullaria)* is a soil saprophyte that grows on decaying vegetation. Spore concentration peaks in the afternoon. The fungus also grows on caulking compounds so it can be found in bathrooms. It is also found on paper, lumber and paints. *Cladosporium* grows on organic debris in the soil and on dead leaves, but can also be found on leather, rubber, cloth, paper, and wood products. This type of spore is very common in the air, especially in areas with a temperate climate, with peak air concentration levels seen from mid-summer through to December. The major allergens of *Alternaria (Alt a I)*, *Cladosporium* and *Aspergillus* have been identified (Bessot *et al.*, 1994). Peak daily levels occur between 11 a.m. and 3 p.m. *Curvularia* is a common parasite of grasses, and spores are dispersed by lawn-mowing activities. *Epicoccum* is widespread in temperate regions, especially in grasslands and agricultural areas. It colonizes decaying vegetable matter, plant leaves, uncooked fruit, and textiles. Peak concentrations occur in late summer and the fall. *Fusarium* species are parasitic on vegetable and field crops and the fungus can be found on stored fruits and vegetables like cucumbers, tomatoes, and potatoes. Spore dispersal requires rain so spores are common in the air after rain. *Helminthosporium* is a prevalent outdoor fungus of grasses and cereal grains. Grain threshing releases large quantities of these spores. Natural spore release peaks around 2 p.m. *Mucor* is a soil saprophyte, especially of leaf litter and organic debris, and can be found on animal wastes. Spore levels in the air tend to be low. *Penicillium* is a fungus of the soil, fruits, breads, cheeses, and other foods. Airborne levels outside are low, but are plentiful inside during the winter. Exposure can also occur by the ingestion of the various blue-veined cheeses. Patients allergic to this mold do not necessarily have an increased sensitivity to penicillin drugs. *Phoma* is found on certain green plants and on paper products like books and magazines. *Rhizopus* is a common saprophyte of organic soil debris outside and can be found on cured meats, root vegetables, and bakery goods inside. *Stemphyllium* parasitizes leaves and stems of vegetable crops and can also be found in decaying plant material, damp paper, canvas, and cotton fabric. Skin test cross-reactivity with *Alternaria* has been noted. Spores are fewer in number than *Alternaria* spores and are found during the daytime in the summer months.

Many more fungi exist than are listed above and may be of allergenic significance. Fungi contain weak antigens, which do not appear to cross-react with rare exception. Mold allergens are prepared by different methods and those prepared from the powdered spore material are more active antigenically than those prepared from the mycelium. One batch of a mold allergen can vary significantly from the next batch. These factors have made it difficult to determine the true incidence and significance of mold sensitivity in pets.

In one author's experience (TW), molds are of no importance in dogs with atopic dermatitis. Skin threshold concentrations were determined at 1% (w/v) concentration with 95% confidence intervals between 0.1–12% (Willemse and Van den Brom, 1983). Molds tested were *Alternaria tenuis, Cladosporium fulvum, C. herbarum, Mucor mucedo, Rhizopus nigricans, Pullaria pullulans, Penicillium notatum*, and *Aspergillus fumigatus*. Although occasional reactions were seen in the early 1980s, in the subsequent ten year period Willemse has never found any positive skin test reaction in atopic dogs. Hence, these allergens are no longer part of the skin test panel.

The other two authors are not in agreement about the insignificance of molds. The reasons for this disagreement are not known, but may relate to differences in the American and European dog populations, the allergens used, or environmental differences. Both Reedy and Miller frequently find significant intradermal and serologic reactions to various fungal allergens in their atopic patients. Since most commercial serologic allergy tests in the USA show a high frequency of fungal reactions, the true meaning of the serologic results is unclear. The intradermal results are more convincing. Reactions in seemingly appropriate frequencies are seen and historical correlation is high. However, since molds are ubiquitous and release their allergenic spores during periods when other aeroallergens are prevalent, the question remains as to whether the mold reactions are clinically significant or not. Immunotherapy studies could answer the question. Two groups of dogs would be needed. The first would be 'mold only' allergic dogs and the second would include dogs allergic to molds and other aeroallergens. For the 'mold only' group, the immunotherapy vaccine would contain all the appropriate molds. For the second group, the molds would not be included in the vaccine. In a double-blinded placebo-controlled study with large numbers of dogs in both groups, the importance of fungal antigens in canine atopy could be determined. Unfortunately, neither author has a sufficient number of 'mold only' dogs to perform the study.

Environmental Allergens

This group of allergens includes dusts, danders, feathers, furniture stuffings, and a variety of other allergens. These allergens are typically associated with indoor symptoms. Depending on the animal's sensitivity, the signs may be seasonal or perennial. Although indoor allergens are present year round, their relative concentrations are lower during the spring and summer months because houses are more open. As winter approaches, the windows and doors are closed and the concentrations start to increase.

House dust

House dust is an important common universal and controversial aeroallergen that is actually a heterogenous ill-defined substance. House dust contains dust mites, storage mites, animal danders, molds, insect debris, bacteria, fibrous material of plant and animal origin, food remnants, and many other substances. With its vastly different consituents, it can scarcely be regarded as a distinct allergen. With its crudeness, its use in allergy testing and immunotherapy has been questioned. Dusts from different parts of the world have a similar antigenicity. House dust extracts tend to be irritating and must be used carefully to avoid false-positive reactions. In man, there appears to be some uniqueness to house dust antigen that cannot be explained by its various ill-defined constituents.

House dust mites are free-living arachnids that appear to be an important allergenic component of house dust. These mites live on epidermal debris from people and animals, yeasts, molds, and remnants of household foods. There are more than 36 species of mites in dust, but *Dermatophagoides farinae* and *D. pteronyssinus* (Figure 3.2) appear to be most important. In general, *D. farinae* is more common in the USA and *D. pteronyssinus* predominates in Europe, Asia, and Africa. The two species do not seem to interbreed and have both shared and unique antigenic determinants. Dust mites thrive in houses with wall-to-wall carpeting, high humidity, and temperatures of 17–24°C. More mites are found in damp (humid) houses than in dry homes as the relative humidity must be above 60% for suitable reproduction. The number of live mites generally increases in a home from August through to November. More mites are found on the surfaces of mattresses than on the floor since epidermal cells are concentrated on the mattresses. Mite allergenicity does not depend on the viability of the mite as mite excreta and dead mites are also allergenic. The vigor of household cleaning or extermination does not appear to affect mite recovery rates. Two major groups of mite allergens have been identified. Group I allergens are 25 kD and are primarily found in mite feces. The allergenicity of the feces appears to be independent of the mite's food source. Group II allergens are essentially of somatic origin and have molecular weights of 15 kD. The ratio of group I to group II allergens in feces ranges from 20–33. Both groups of allergens are proteolytic enzymes. Biochemical studies have demonstrated *Der p I* to be a cysteine protease, and *Der p II* a lysozyme. For both *D. pteronyssinus* and *D. farinae* groups of allergens have been identified. In the air, group I and group II allergens are mainly carried by particles larger than 10 µm, which only become airborne when disturbed (e.g. by vacuum cleaning) (Bessot *et al.*, 1994).

Noli *et al.* (1996) evaluated the significance of reactions to crude extracts and purified fractions of the house dust mites *D. pteronyssinus (Der p I* and *Der p II)* and *D.*

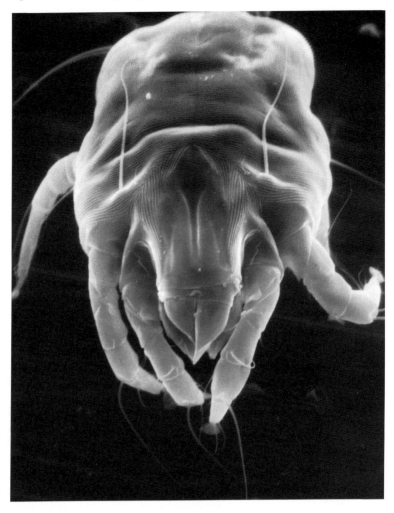

Figure 3.2   *Scanning electron micrograph of* Dermatophagoides pteronyssinus. *(Courtesy T.A.E. Platts-Mills, University of Virginia, Charlottesville.)*

farinae (Der f I and *Der f II)* in dogs with clinical manifestations of atopic dermatitis. In 13 healthy control dogs and eight dogs with atopic dermatitis immediate skin test reactivity was determined to serial dilutions of *Der p I, Der p II, Der f I* and *Der f II*. In addition, allergen-specific IgGd antibodies were determined by means of an enzyme-linked immunosorbent assay (ELISA) and Western blot. The results suggest that in contrast to findings in humans and despite immediate skin test reactivity in some dogs, *Der p I, Der p II, Der f I* and *Der f II* are unlikely major allergens in dogs with atopic dermatitis. Only serum of atopic dogs consistently binds a 90 kD polypeptide of *D. farinae*, as shown by Western blot analysis.

The allergenicity of house dust increases when it is stored for several months before it is extracted. Inoculation of sterile dust samples with live house dust mites increases the skin test reactivity of the extract and the increase in reactivity parallels the numbers of mites in the preparation. Most human patients who react to dust antigen also react to mite antigen, but at much lower concentrations. Reactivity to dust mites has been reported in veterinary medicine, but the rate is lower than in man. In animals and man, dust mites are a major source of house dust allergen, but not the only source.

Other dusts such as barn dust and wood dust may be important depending upon the animal's exposure. In addition to the house dust mites, there are a variety of anatomically different mites of the tyroglyphid family (storage mites), which are found in large numbers in stored hay, cereal products, and house dust. Predominant species include *Acarus siro*, *Glycyphagus destructor*, and *Tyrophagus putrescentiae* (Platts-Mills and Chapman, 1987; Platts-Mills and de Weck, 1989). Storage mites have been recognized to cause asthma, allergic rhinitis, and atopic disease in farmworkers, bakers, (Tee, 1994) and the urban population (Wraith *et al.*, 1979; Luczynska *et al.*, 1990; Tee, 1994). The mites have been isolated from the dust of houses with high humidity and allergic persons inhabiting these dwellings showed larger wheals to storage mites than to *D. pteronyssinus* (Wraith *et al.*, 1979). One of these storage mites, *Tyrophagus putrescentiae*, seems to be an important antigen, both to man (Green and Woolcock, 1978; Luczynska *et al.*, 1990; Tee, 1994) and the dog (Vollset, 1986; Koch and Peters, 1994). Positive skin reactions to this mite have been obtained in up to 80% of asthmatic human patients (Green and Woolcock, 1978) and in 23.7% of atopic dogs (Koch and Peters, 1994). Also *T. putrescentiae* crude extract-specific IgGd antibodies are frequently observed in dogs with clinical symptoms compatible with atopy (Willemse, 1994).

Unlike *Dermatophagoides* spp. where antigenic fractions and DNA sequences have been determined, only limited information is available about *T. putrescentiae* (Arlian *et al.*, 1984; Johansson *et al.*, 1994). Arlian *et al.* (1984) found that *T. putrescentiae* mite bodies extracts shared several antigens with *T. putrescentiae* feces. Further identification of allergenic components in *T. putrescentiae* extracts was carried out using sodium dodecyl sulfate–polyacrylamide gel electrophoresis (SDS–PAGE) and immunoblotting (Johansson *et al.*, 1994). The highest frequency of IgE binding was to a 16 kD component of *T. putrescentiae*.

Epidermal allergens

Animals and man constantly shed hair and dead epidermal cells into the environment. Hair is considered to be a minor allergen because it is less soluble and less airborne. Accordingly, the popularly held belief that short-haired or non-shedding animals are 'hypoallergenic' is incorrect. Epidermal cells or danders are proteins with multiple antigenic determinants and are often contaminated with saliva, serum, or urine, which can increase the antigenicity of the dander. It has been shown that dander extracts vary depending on the method of extraction and that there are probably allergens specific for one breed of animal. A person sensitive to dog dander can be more sensitive to one breed of dog than another independent of the dog's hair length or shedding pattern. This phenomenon is suspected, but not proved for other species of animals.

Cat allergen

For humans, cats are more allergenic than dogs. In the USA, it is estimated that 2% of the population is allergic to cats. Immunochemical studies have shown that the major allergen from cat pelts is *Fel d I*. This allergen is more potent than pure epidermal extracts and differs from serum proteins. It is found mainly in the sebaceous glands of the skin, but also in high concentration in the salivary glands. *Fel d I* is stored on the skin and fur and its concentration is ten times greater at the root of the hair than at the tip. It is found in all breeds, but amounts vary between individuals in and between different breeds. Male cats have higher concentrations than females. Allergens are also present in the voided urine and serum. *Fel d I* is a polypeptide with a molecular weight of 35–39 kD on size extraction high performance liquid chromatography (HPLC) and 17–18 kD on SDS–PAGE. It is especially abundant in dust from carpets and upholstered furniture. Cat allergens are so widespread that they are part of our daily environment. There is hardly a dwelling without *Fel d I* in its dust. In contrast to mite allergens, cat allergens remain suspended in the air for extended periods of time, even without disturbance (Luczynska *et al.*, 1990; Charpin *et al.*, 1991; Duffort *et al.*, 1991; Bessot *et al.*, 1994). The grooming habits of the cat cause it to spread these allergens over its body and therefore increase its allergenicity. Drugs such as atropine, which decrease salivary secretions, inhibit spreading of the antigen.

Dog allergen

Dog allergens are found mainly in skin, but are also present in serum and saliva (Schou, 1993). A major allergen, *Can f I*, has been purified (Schou *et al.*, 1991). It is a polypeptide with a molecular weight of 22–25 kD. Albumin is another allergen of importance and the reason for cross-reactions between cat and dog extracts (Boutin *et al.*, 1988). The concentration of *Can f I* may vary within and between breeds. Dog allergens can be present in high concentrations in an environment to which dogs have no access (Dybendal *et al.*, 1989). The significance of a strong reaction to dog dander in a dog is uncertain.

Human allergen

One person typically produces 5 g of dander/week, so animals are exposed to high concentrations of this allergen. Surveys from veterinarians indicate that reactions to human dander are seen in up to 50% of dogs. This antigen is no longer available in the USA and its absence may explain why some classically atopic dogs are skin test negative.

Other epidermal allergens

Extracts from the camel, cow, deer, fox, gerbil, goat, guinea pig, hamster, horse, mink, monkey, mouse, pig, rabbit, rat, and seal are available commercially. These allergens probably include not only epidermal antigens, but also serum, salivary, or urinary antigens. A major allergen is found in mouse urine (*Mus m I*) and rat urine (*Rat n I*), and some human patients allergic to horses react not only to epidermal antigens, but also to serum proteins.

Since the use of horse and cattle hair as furniture stuffing or carpet matting is decreasing, the incidence of reactivity should be decreasing. Pets in rural environments can be exposed to farm animals and could develop sensitivities to them. Direct contact with the animal is not necessary to develop sensitivity. One of the authors (TW) has seen dogs hypersensitive to horse dander extracts when the dogs were never directly exposed to horses. In these cases, the horse dander was brought home with the owner or the owner's children from horse stables or riding schools.

Sheep's wool

The true allergenicity of sheep's wool is debatable since wool is an irritating substance and extracts contain not only wool, but also dusts and danders from humans and other animals. Although skin test reactivity to wool is common in the dog, the significance of wool as an aeroallergen is uncertain. The authors no longer test with wool.

Feather allergens

Exposure to feathers in pillows, comforters, jackets, and quilts or by handling birds is known to cause respiratory and cutaneous allergic disease. Aged feathers are more allergenic than freshly plucked feathers. Since antigenicity increases with age and many human patients show a strong correlation between skin test reactivity to feathers and house dust, it is theorized that house dust mites are responsible for the allergenicity of feather extracts. Work in patients with feather-induced hypersensitivity pneumonitis and chemical extraction studies show that feather extracts differ from house dust extracts.

Most commercial feather extracts are mixtures of chicken, goose, and duck feathers since these are common types of feathers used for stuffings. The degree of antigenic cross-reactivity between these feathers and those from pets and wild birds is unknown. The authors have recognized dogs allergic to the household parrot as proven by isolation (LMR/WHM) or skin test reactivity to parrot feathers' extract (TW). These dogs reacted to mixed feather extract. In the rare 'feather-only' allergic dogs, immunotherapy with mixed feather antigen has been successful (LMR/WHM).

Kapok

Kapok is the moisture-resistant seed hair from the kapok tree used as a stuffing for furniture, mattresses, and aquatic life jackets or cushions. The use of synthetic fibers has markedly decreased the use of kapok. As for house dust and feathers, the allergenicity of kapok increases with age because of house dust mite contamination and biologic deterioration.

Cottonseed and flaxseed

The water-soluble proteinaceous material from cottonseeds can contaminate inexpensive cotton stuffing and cause allergic signs, but the increasing use of synthetic fibers has decreased the incidence of reactivity to cottonseed.

Pyrethrum

Pyrethrums are widely used botanical insecticides produced from the flower heads of the *Chrysanthemum cinerarie-folium* plant. These plants are members of the Compositae family and are related botanically to ragweed. Patients allergic to ragweed may also be reactive to pyrethrum insecticides. Clinical allergy to these insecticides appears to be very low.

Tobacco

Tobacco smoke can be irritating and it will cause many pets to sneeze. Inhalant allergies to tobacco smoke are rare, but do occur. Since Scott (1981) reported a high incidence of false-positive reactions to tobacco, skin test results must be evaluated critically. One author (WHM) has seen two dogs who were apparently allergic to marijuana smoke.

Insect allergens

Insect hypersensitivity is typically due to the bite or sting of the insect rather than the inhalation of insect-associated allergens (Chapter 9). In humans, cockroach antigen appears to be a significant allergen and quite distinct from house dust. This allergen seems to have a less important role in Europe than in the USA. The prevalence of cutaneous sensitization to cockroach in atopic patients is about 10% in Europe, 53% in the USA and 46% in Asia (Bidat *et al.*, 1993). Two major allergens have been identified: *Bla g I* and *Bla g II*. Cockroach allergens are mainly found in the exoskeleton and feces. Inhalation of insect debris from the caddis fly and mayfly also causes allergic symptoms. Nesbitt (1978) reported a 60% skin test reactivity of urban dogs to cockroach antigen. Its significance is not clear. Griffin *et al.* (1993) tested ten dogs with histories of insect exposure to multiple types of insects with allergenic extracts of cockroach, black fly, house fly, black ant, and red ant. They found no skin test reactions to cockroach allergen, but antigen-specific IgE was detected in six of the ten dogs. Similar discrepancies were found for the other extracts. In a study of 40 flea-positive dogs (Willis, 1994), 17 dogs reacted to multiple insect and arachnid extracts. The most common reactants were black ant, horse fly, and black fly extracts. The incidence of mosquito bite hypersensitivity in dogs is unknown, but a report from Germany (Koch and Peters, 1994) showed 14% of a group of 207 dogs to be positive.

Other allergens

Various gums, glues, and fibers are available for allergy testing. Their allergenicity is questionable. Very likely these substances are irritants and should be used for patch testing animals with clinical manifestations of contact allergy. If the animal's exposure history indicates that one of these allergens may be important, the animal should be patch tested (see Chapter 8).

In general, indoor plants are minimally allergenic since they do not produce pollens. However, their moist pots are sites for mold growth and some plant parts can be allergenic. Leaf parts from *Ficus benjamina*, the weeping fig, and nectar secretions from *Abutilon striatum*, the flowering maple, are probably significant allergens (LMR/WHM).

Allergen Preparation

Simply stated, allergy extracts are prepared by collecting the material, extracting the 'allergens' and mixing them with preservatives. The collecting and manufacturing techniques can vary from laboratory to laboratory. Additionally, the allergenicity of one batch of an allergen can be significantly different from the next batch even if it is produced by the same company. This variability reflects our ignorance of what the major antigenic determinants are in the various allergens and the biologic variability of pollens. Until all allergens are defined, all extracts should be purchased from the same laboratory to maintain as much consistency as possible.

Pollen extracts are prepared by collecting the pollen, cleaning it if possible, and drying to prevent bacterial or fungal contamination. Before extraction, pollens are often defatted with various ethers and techniques. Careless defatting can remove some of the potential allergens. Fungal antigens are typically made from dried ground powders of the mycelial mat, but sometimes only the growth medium or the mat plus the growth medium are used. Allergens are extracted from the crude materials by using saline types of solutions to which other agents can be added. Once the extraction is completed, the allergen can be freeze-dried or diluted to the necessary strength. Sterility checks are run on each batch and after each vial is produced.

To inhibit microbial contamination, preservatives are added to the extracts. Commercially, either 0.2–0.4% phenol or 50% glycerin is used. Some laboratories offer extracts preserved with 0.03% human serum albumin, but these have not been studied in animals. Preservatives not only inhibit microbial growth, but also affect the stability of the extracts.

Stability of Allergenic Extracts

Allergenic extracts are dated biologic materials and will start to lose potency within weeks to months of the manufacturing date. The loss of potency is related to time, temperature, the concentration of the allergen, the preservative used, and the presence of interfering substance such as the plastic syringe used for intradermal injection. Outdated extracts should not be used, but the use of allergens close to their expiration date is also questionable since they are not at their original potency.

Extract potency is greatly affected by the preservative used. Allergenic extracts preserved with 50% glycerin are most stable, while phenol-preserved extracts are least stable. Preservation with 10% glycerin or 0.03% human serum albumin gives intermediate results. Since glycerinated extracts can cause false-positive skin test reactions, they are not recommended for use in veterinary medicine.

The decay of phenol-preserved extracts is affected by time, temperature, and the concentration of the allergen. Old extracts lose biologic potency and the degradation products formed can be irritating. Refrigeration is the primary retardant of decay. Periodic exposure of antigens, especially those diluted to skin test strength, to room temperature increases the potency loss. Diluted extracts preserved with phenol can lose 50% of their original activity by one year.

Proteolytic enzymes that are naturally present in an extract or introduced by bacterial contamination will lower the potency. This is especially true in mold extracts. Contaminated vaccine may be dangerous so any vaccine with changing physical characteristics should be discarded. Very concentrated allergens (1:10 weight to volume (W/V) or 40 000 protein nitrogen units (PNU)/ml) tend to precipitate when stored over 3–6 months. Precipitated extracts are not as potent, and may be antigenically different, and should be discarded.

Standardization of Allergenic Extracts

The composition of allergy extracts is very variable due to variations in for example collection techniques and extraction techniques and unfortunately no uniform method of standardization exists. Only when an accurate measurement of biologic potency is available will uniform standardization be practical.

In the USA, extracts are sold either on a W/V basis or with the concentration indicated as PNU/ml. In Europe, concentrations of extracts are also expressed as Noon units (NU)/ml. This unit is commonly used for pollen extracts. The W/V concentration is determined by dividing the weight of the defatted allergen by the volume of the diluent. For example, 1 g of allergen diluted with 1000 ml of diluent yields a 1:1000 solution. The PNU concentration is determined by extracting the protein from the allergen with phosphotungstic acid. By definition, 1 mg of protein is equal to 100 000 PNU. 1 NU is defined as 1 ml of an extract made from 1 mg of pollen in 1 l of extracting fluid.

No method gives a true indication of biologic potency. With the PNU and NU method, one would have to assume that all proteins present were antigenically active and that there were no non-protein antigens. Neither of these assumptions is true. In the WV method, the amount of material present that is not protein is unknown. If significant amounts of non-protein material are present, the extract would probably be less potent than the concentration indicated. No method addresses the problems of the variability of antigenic determinants in various batches of crude allergens or the effect of extraction on the antigens.

A formula exists to estimate the PNU concentration of a W/V extract. 1 ml of a 1:50 W/V solution should contain approximately 10 000 PNU. According to this formula, 1 ml of a 1:1000 W/V solution should contain 500 PNU. 1 NU is considered to be similar to 1 PNU. Many investigators have indicated that house dust is too irritating for skin testing dogs at 1000 PNU/ml. Concentrations at or below 250 PNU/ml are necessary to limit the number of false-positive reactions. Histamine release assays, RAST, or RAST inhibition tests, crossed immunoelectrophoresis, isoelectric focussing, and ultraviolet absorption spectra are all used to measure antigenic potency and purity of extracts. Although the RAST test is not used commonly, the results seem to give a reliable indication of the potency of the extract. The authors suggest that allergens are purchased from the same manufacturer to avoid any inconsistencies.

Ultimately, the true test of biologic potency is the skin test reactivity of an allergen. Manufacturers of skin test strength allergens must be able to provide standardization data. Skin threshold concentrations should have been determined in healthy control dogs (Sture *et al.*, 1995) for all individual and mixed allergens. The concentration of batches that give fewer or more reactions than expected probably differs from that indicated.

Individual Versus Grouped Allergens

Allergens can be purchased as individual extracts or in stock mixtures. The use of mixtures for skin testing is controversial. The use of mixtures decreases the number of skin tests per animal and also decreases the cost of the allergens, but the reliability of the test results can be questionable. Scott (1981) reported poor correlation between mixed and individual allergens when he compared molds, epidermals, and weeds. The tendency was for his (and also the authors') patients to react to the individual allergen, but not to the group antigen. He did find that mixed grass, mixed ragweed, and mixed dust antigens were satisfactory, but one author (LMR) is unable to confirm this. Willemse and others (Nesbitt, 1978; Nesbitt *et al.*, 1984) have found that the correlation rate between individual and mixed antigens varies from 60–75%. Group allergens are prepared by mixing small amounts of each ingredient in the same vial. 1 ml of a five-allergen mixture at a strength of 1000 PNU/ml contains 200 PNU of each antigen. At skin testing, the animal would be injected with 10 PNU of each allergen instead of the 50 PNU that would be used if individual allergens were used. If more than five antigens are mixed together, the concentration of each allergen would be even lower.

Stock mixtures are not available with all allergens in them. If only mixtures are used, some important allergens may be overlooked.

Assuming that the mixtures used contain all the pertinent allergens, skin test reactions must be evaluated carefully. A negative reaction to a mixture could indicate that the animal is not sensitive to any of the allergens or that the concentration of the individual antigens is too low to cause a reaction. True positive reactions indicate that the animal is sensitive to one or more of the antigens in the mixture. If the animal is truly sensitive to all of the antigens, the use of that mixture for immunotherapy is valid. If the animal is only sensitive to one or several of the allergens, the concentration of the important allergens in the vaccine is lowered by the non-reactive substances.

If all allergens were antigenically unique, the use of large mixtures would be very questionable. Since some allergens share common antigens, some mixtures may be valid. Stock mixtures containing very dissimilar allergens such as house dust, epidermals, and mixed insects should not be used. Mixtures should only include similar antigens.

Mixed grass antigen is probably the most valid mixture since most grasses except Bermuda share at least one common antigen. Since ryegrass, meadow fescue, orchard grass, and velvet grass share two common antigens, these grasses should show significant cross-reactivity. Ideally, grasses should be tested for individually. If the circumstances necessitate the use of mixtures, one or two mixed suburban grass antigens should be used. In those areas where timothy or Bermuda grasses are prevalent, these allergens should be used separately.

The cross-reactivity of trees, weeds, and molds is questionable. Trees or weeds within the same family may cross-react while species within the same genus should be even more similar. People reactive to various trees from the Betulaceae (alder, birch, hazel), but also to other trees, share prick test reactions and positive RAST scores to *Betula* allergen (*Bet v 1*) (D'Ammato *et al.*, 1991). Ragweed pollens share antigens so mixed ragweed antigen should give valid results. Similarly, mixtures of rough pigweed, spiny pigweed, careless weed, and Palmer's amaranth; lamb's quarter, jerusalem oak, and mexican tea; yellow dock and sheep sorrel; rough marsh elder and burweed marsh elder; allscale, lenscale, and wingscale; and mugwort, wormwood, costal sage, and big sagebrush should be valid since these weeds are grouped by family and genus. Since plants of the *Ambrosia, Iva* and *Xanthium* genera all produce similar pollens and share some ragweed antigen E activity, mixtures of ragweed, cocklebur, and marsh elder could be valid. Members of the Chenopodiaceae and Amaranthaceae families are thought to be similar, so mixtures of lamb's quarter, mexican tea, russian thistle, burning bush (*Kochia*), and pigweed may be valid.

Nesbitt *et al.* (1984) correlated the number of positive and negative skin test reactions for four weed pairs and found a correlation of 59% for lamb's quarter and pigweed, 65% for mixed ragweed and rough marsh elder, 66% for mixed ragweed and cocklebur, and 62% for mixed ragweed and mugwort. These data show that weeds of different genera do not completely cross-react and that weeds from different families (lamb's quarter and pigweed) cross-react less than weeds from the same family (ragweed, marsh elder, cocklebur, and mugwort). The authors feel that the use of mixtures of weeds from different genera is not the best choice. Weeds should preferably be tested individually or as mixtures from the same genus.

The use of tree or mold mixtures should follow the same line. Mixtures of different species from the same genus should be most cross-reactive, while mixtures from different families should be least reactive. Nesbitt *et al.* (1984) tested a mold mixture of four fungi, two of which were from the Dematiaceae family while the other two were from the Moniliaceae family. When he compared the results of the mixed and individual allergens, his correlation ranged from 63–65%. If the two members of each family were completely cross-reactive, one would expect a higher correlation rate.

From the above discussion, it is clear that testing with individual allergens should give more accurate results. When mixtures are to be used, members from the same genus should be grouped together. Mixtures of allergens from the same family, but different genuses, may not be reliable. The botanic classification of important pollens is shown in Tables 3.1–3.4. These tables represent a compilation of the information supplied to the authors by different allergy companies in the USA and representative literature on pollens in Europe (D'Ammato *et al.*, 1991). Ideally, an animal that reacts to a mixed antigen should be tested for the individual components of the mixture to determine which allergens are significant. This obviously negates the advantages of using mixed allergens.

Nesbitt *et al.* (1984) noted that dogs that underwent immunotherapy with vaccines containing individual mold, grass, and tree allergens did better than dogs treated with vaccines containing mixtures. Nonreactive allergens in mixtures will decrease the concentration of the important allergens in the vaccine and may make the vaccine less effective. However, it is uncertain whether the presence of nonrelevant allergens or the effects of mold proteases were responsible for the decreased efficacy. Proteases can decrease the biologic activity of certain grasses and weed pollen extracts when coincubated in the same vial for 30 days (Rosenbaum, 1996).

Table 3.1 *Botanical classification of grasses of the Gramineae family*

Genus (common name)	Species	Common name	Synonyms	Pollinating period
Agrostis (Bentgrasses)	*tenuis*	Colonial bentgrass	Creeping bent	Late spring
	alba	Redtop	Herd's grass	Summer
Cynodon	*dactylon*	Bermuda	Devil, scutch, wire grass	Spring, summer, fall
Poa (bluegrasses)	*compressa*	Canada	English bluegrass, Wire grass	Summer
	pratensis	Kentucky	June grass, Meadow grass	Summer
	sandbergii	Sandberg		Late spring, summer
Bromus (bromegrasses)	*rigidus*	Broncho	Ripgut	Late spring
	carinatus	California bromegrass		Late spring, early summer
	secalinus	Cheat	Chess, rye-brome Cock-grass	Summer
	inermis	Bromegrass	Hungarian bromegrass	Summer
	unioloides	Southern chess	Soft chess	Summer
Phalaris (canary grasses)	*canariensis*	Canary grass		Late spring
	arundinacea	Reed canary		Summer
	minor	Small canary	Mediterranian	Spring
Festuca (fescues)	*eliator*	Meadow fescue	Tall fescue, Dover grass	Summer
	rubra	Red fescue		Summer
Sorghum	*halepense*	Johnson grass	Evergreen millet	Summer
Koeleria	*cristata*	Koeler's grass	June grass, Western June grass	Summer
Avena (oats)	*sativa*	Cultivated oat		Late spring
	barbata	Slender wild oat		Spring
	fatua	Wild oat		Spring and early summer
Dactylis	*glomerata*	Orchard grass	Dew grass, Hard grass, Cocksfoot	Late spring, early summer
Elymus (Wild ryes)	*triticoides*	Alkali rye	Beardless wildrye	Late spring
	cinereus	Giant wild-rye		Late spring, early summer
	glaucus	Western blue, Wild-rye		Early summer

(continued overleaf)

Table 3.1   *(continued)*

Genus (common name)	Species	Common name	Synonyms	Pollinating period
Lolium (ryegrass)	*multiflorum*	Italian ryegrass	Ryegrass	Summer
	perenne	Perennial ryegrass	English rye	Summer
Distichlis	*stricata*	Salt grass	Alkali grass	Summer
Sorghum	*vulgare* var *sudanense*	Sudan grass		Summer
Anthoxantum	*odoratum*	Sweet vernal grass		Spring
Phleum	*pratense*	Timothy grass	Herd's grass	Late spring, summer
Holcus	*lanatus*	Velvet grass	Soft grass, feather grass	Summer
Triticum	*aestivum*	Wheat		Early summer
Agropyron (wheatgrasses)	*repens*	Quackgrass	Quitchgrass	Early summer
	Smithii	Western wheatgrass	Bluejoint, bluestem	Summer

Table 3.2   *Botanical classifications of trees of allergic significance.*

Family (common name)	Genus	Species	Common name	Synonyms	Pollinating period
Aceraceae	*Acer*	*negundo*	Box elder	Ash-leaved maple Cut-leaed maple	Spring
	Acer	*macrophyllum*	Coast maple	Broad-leaved maple	Spring
	Acer	*saccharum*	Hard maple	Sugar, black, rock	Spring
	Acer	*rubrum*	Red maple	Scarlet, swamp, white maple	Early spring
	Acer	*saccharinum*	Silver maple	River, soft, swamp	Late winter
Betulaceae	*Alnus*	*sinuata*	Sitka alder	Wavy-leaved	Spring and early summer
	Alnus	*tenuifolia*	Slender alder	Mountain	Spring
	Alnus	*rugosa*	Tag alder	Hoary, speckled	Early spring
	Alnus	*rhombifolia*	White alder	Alder	Early spring
	Betula	*papyrifera*	Paper birch	Canoe	Spring
	Betula	*nigra*	Red birch	River, water	Spring
	Betula	*occidentalis*	Spring birch	California, black, mountain	Spring
	Betula	*pendula*	White birch	European white	Spring
	Corylus	*americana*	American hazelnut	Filbert, hazel	Early spring
	Corylus	*californica*	California hazelnut	California hazel	Early spring

Table 3.2 *(continued)*

Family (common name)	Genus	Species	Common name	Synonyms	Pollinating period
Fagaceae	*Fagus*	*grandifolia*	Beech		Spring
	Quercus	*macrocarpa*	Burr oak	Mossy cup	Spring
	Quercus	*kelloggii*	California black	Kellogg's oak	Spring
	Quercus	*agrifolia*	Coast live oak	Live oak	Spring
	Quercus	*gambelii*	Gambel oak, White oak	Rocky Mountain	Spring
	Quercus	*garryana*	Garry's oak, white	Oregon, western	Spring
	Quercus	*stellata*	Post oak	Iron	Spring
	Quercus	*rubra*	Red oak		Spring
	Quercus	*dumosa*	Scrub oak		Spring
	Quercus	*lobata*	Valley oak	White oak	Spring
	Quercus	*virginiana*	Virginia live oak	Eastern live, Texas live	Spring
	Quercus	*alba*	White oak		Spring
Hamamelideae	*Liquid-ambar*	*styraciflua*	Sweetgum	Liquidambar	Late spring
Juglandaceae	*Carya*	*pecan*	Pecan		Spring
	Carya	*ovata*	Shagbark hickory	Shag	Late spring
	Carya	*tomentosa*	White hickory	Mockernut	Late spring
	Juglans	*nigra*	Black walnut		spring
	Juglans	*regia*	English walnut	Persian	Spring
	Juglans	*hindsii*	California black walnut		Spring
	Juglans	*californica*	Southern California black walnut		Early spring
Leguminosae	*Acacia*	spp.	Acacia	Cassie, wattle	Late winter, spring
	Prosopis	*juliflora*	Mesquite, Honey locust	Honey Mesquite	Spring and summer
Moraceae	*Morus*	spp.	Mulberry		Spring
Myrtaceae	*Eucalyptus*	*globulus*	Eucalyptus	Gum tree	All seasons
Oleaceae	*Fraxinus*	*velutina*	Arizona ash		Spring
	Fraxinus	*pennsylvanica*	Green ash		Spring
	Fraxinus	*americana*	White ash		Spring
	Olea	*europaea*	Olive		Late spring
	Liqustrum	*vulgare*	Privet		Late spring

(continued overleaf)

Table 3.2 (*continued*)

Family (common name)	Genus	Species	Common name	Synonyms	Pollinating period
Pinaceae	*Juniperus*	*asheii*	Mountain cedar	Juniper, Mexican, rock	Winter
	Juniperus	*virginiana*	Red cedar	Red savin, Carolina cedar, pencil wood	Early spring
	Juniperus	*occidentalis*	Western juniper	Juniper	Spring
	Cupressus	*arizona*	Arizona cypress		Early spring
	Cupressus	*sempervirens*	Italian cypress		Late winter
	Cupressus	*macrocarpa*	Monterey cypress		Spring
	Pseudotsuga	*menziesii*	Douglas fir	Douglas spruce, Oregan pine	Spring
	Pinus	*contorta*	Lodgepole pine	Scrub pine	Late spring
	Pinus	*ponderosa*	Yellow pine	Bull, ponderosa	Late spring
	Pinus	*strobus*	Eastern white		Late spring
	Pinus	*monticola*	Western white		Late spring
Platanaceae	*Platanus*	*racemosa*	California sycamore	Planetree, western sycamore	Early spring
	Platanus	*orientalis*	Eastern sycamore	Planetree, button-ball, buttonwood	Spring
	Platanus	*acerifolia*	Maple leaf, Sycamore	London planetree, 'oriental' sycamore	Spring
Salicaceae	*Populus*	*tremuloides*	Aspen	Poplar, aspen, quaking aspen	Spring
	Populus	*balsamifera*	Balsam		Early spring
	Populus	*trichocarpa*	Black cottonwood		Early spring
	Populus	*deltoides*	Common cottonwood	Necklace poplar	Early spring
	Populus	*fremontii*	Fremont cottonwood	California	Early spring
	Populus	*alba*	White poplar	Abele, silver	Early spring
	Salix	spp.	Willow		Late winter, spring
Taxodiaceae	*Sequoia*	*sempervirens*	Redwood		Spring
Tiliaceae	*Tilia*	*americana*	Linden	Basswood, whitewood	Spring
Ulmaceae	*Ulmus*	*americana*	American elm	White elm	Early spring
	Ulmus	*pumila*	Evergreen elm	Chinese	Early spring
	Ulmus	*parvifolia*	Chinese elm	Evergreen elm, silver elm	Early spring
	Celtis	*occidentalis*	Hackberry	False elm, sugarberry hoop ash	Spring

Table 3.3 *Botanical classification of weeds of allergic significance.*

Family (common name)	Genus	Species	Common name	Synonyms	Pollinating period
Amaranthaceae	*Amaranthus*	*palmeri*	Careless weed		Summer
	Amaranthus	*retroflexus*	Rough redroot	Rough pigweed,	Summer
			Pigweed	Green amaranth	
	Amaranthus	*spinosus*	Spiny pigweed		Summer
	Amaranthus	*tamariscinus*	Waterhemp	Western waterhemp	Late summer
Chenopodiaceae	*Bassia*	*hyssopifolia*	Bassia	Five-hook bassia	Summer
	Beta	*vulgaris*	Sugar beet		Late spring, summer
	Sarcobatus	*vermiculatus*	Greasewood	Chico	Late spring, early summer
	Allenrolfea	*occidentalis*	Iodine bush	Burroweed	Summer
	Kochia	*scoparia*	Kochia	Burning bush, summer cypress, fireweed, belvedere	Summer
	Chenopodium	*album*	Lamb's quarter	White pigweed, pigweed	Spring and summer
	Chenopodium	*ambrosioides*	Mexican tea	Wormseed	Late summer, early fall
	Salicornia	*ambigua*	Pickleweed	Grasswort, samphire	Late spring, summer
	Salsola	*kali*	Russian thistle	Tumbleweed, saltwort	Summer
	Atriplex	*polycarpa*	Allscale	Desert sage	Late summer
	Atriplex	*wrightii*	Annual saltbush		Summer
	Atriplex	*serenana*	Bractscale		Summer
	Atriplex	*lentiformis*	Lenscale	Quailbrush	Late summer
	Atriplex	*confertifolia*	Sheepfat	Shadscale, spiny saltbush	Late spring, early summer
	Atriplex	*argentea expansa*	Silverscale	Silver orach	Summer
	Atriplex	*patula hastata*	Spearscale		Summer
	Atriplex	*canescens*	Wingscale	Shadscale	Summer
	Eurotia	*lanata*	Winter fat	Sweet sage	Late spring
Compositae	*Balsamorhiza*	*sagittata*	Balsam root		Spring
	Iva	*xanthifolia*	Burweed marsh elder	Prairie ragweed	Spring
	Iva	*ciliata*	Marsh elder	Rough marsh elder	Summer
	Iva	*angustifolia*	Narrowleaf Marsh elder	Small-flowered marsh elder	Late spring, summer
	Xanthium	*commune*	Cocklebur	Clotbur	Late summer

(continued overleaf)

Table 3.3   *(continued)*

Family (common name)	Genus	Species	Common name	Synonyms	Pollinating period
	Taraxacum	*officinale*	Dandelion		Spring, summer
	Solidago	spp.	Goldenrod		Late summer, early fall
	Ambrosia	*artemisiifolia*	Short ragweed	Low, common ragweed	Late summer, fall
	Ambrosia	*trifida*	Giant ragweed	Tall ragweed	Late summer, fall
	Ambrosia	*bidentata*	Southern ragweed		Late summer
	Ambrosia	*psilostachya*	Western ragweed		Late summer, early fall
	Franseria	*acanthicarpa*	False ragweed	Beachbur, beach sandbur	Spring, summer
	Franseria	*dumosa*	Desert ragweed	Burrobush, burroweed, desert bursage	Spring
	Ambrosia	*deltoidea*	Rabbit bush	Canyon ragweed, Arizona bursage	Spring
	Dicoria	*canescens*	Silver ragweed	Dicoria	Fall
	Artemisia	*annua*	Annual sagebrush	Sagewort, annual wormwort	Summer
	Artemisia	*tridentata*	Common sagebrush	Mountain sagebrush	Late summer, fall
	Artemisia	*dracunculus*	Green sagebrush	Dragon sagewort, Indian hair tonic	Summer
	Artemisia	*vulgaris*	Mugwort	California mugwort	Summer
	Artemisia	*frigida*	Pasture sagebrush	Carpet sage, prairie sage, estafiata	Summer, early fall
	Artemisia	*ludoviciana*	White sagebrush	Prairie sagebrush, wormwood	Late summer, early fall
	Artemisia	*absinthium*	Wormwood	Sagewort, absinth sage	Late summer
	Salicornia	*ambigua*	Pickleweed	Grasswort, samphire	Late spring, summer
Cruciferae	*Brassica*	*campestris*	Mustard	Field mustard	Spring and summer

Table 3.3   *(continued)*

Family (common name)	Genus	Species	Common name	Synonyms	Pollinating period
Plantaginaceae	*Plantago*	*major*	Common plantain	Greater plantain	Late spring, summer
	Plantago	*lanceolata*	English plantain	Buckhorn, ribgrass	Spring, summer
Polygonaceae	*Rumex*	*obtusifolius*	Bitter dock	Broadleaf	Summer
	Rumex	*acetosella*	Sheep sorrel	Sorrel dock, field sorrel, red sorrel	Late spring
	Rumex	*crispus*	Yellow dock	Curly dock	Summer
Urticaceae	*Urtica*	*dioica*	Nettle	Hoary nettle	Summer

Table 3.4   *Pollens of major importance in Europe and their pollination period.*

Pollen type	Region 1–1	Region 1–2	Region 2–1	Region 2–2	Region 3–1	Region 3–2[1]
Trees – shrubs						
Corylus ssp	Feb–May		March–April		March–April	April
Alnus spp	Feb–March				Feb–April	April–May
Quercus spp		April–May	April–May	May	May	
Betula spp			April–May		April–May	May–June
Salix spp			April–May			
Ulmus spp			March–April			
Castanea spp			June–July		June–July	
Cupressus spp	Jan–May	March–May				
Juniperus spp		March–May				
Thuja spp		March–May				
Platanus spp		March–May				
Olea europaea	May–June					
Weeds						
Chenopodium spp	May–Sept	May–August		Aug	Aug	Aug
Kochia scoparia	May–Sept					
Atriplex wrightii	May–Sept					
Salsola pestifer	May–Sept					
Parietaria spp	March–Sept	March–Sept	June–Sept	June–Sept		
Artemisia vulgaris	Aug–Sept	Aug–Sept	July–Aug	July–Aug	July–Aug	
A. annua	Sept–Oct					
A. verlotorum	Sept–Oct					
Rumex spp			June–Aug	June–Aug		
Plantago spp		June–Aug	June–July	June–July		
Urtica spp			June–Sept	June–Sept		
Ambrosia spp		Aug–Sept	Aug–Sept			

(continued overleaf)

Table 3.4   *(continued)*

Pollen type	Region 1–1	Region 1–2	Region 2–1	Region 2–2	Region 3–1	Region 3–2[1]
Grasses						
Poaceae[2]	April–Sept	April–Sept	May–Aug	May–Aug	May–Aug	June–Aug
Agropyron repens	April–Sept	April–Sept				

[1]Region 1–1: Mediterranean; 1–2: Mid/south France; 2–1: Central Europe and mid/north Germany; 2–2: UK; 3–1: Northern France and Benelux, 3–2: Scandinavia.
[2]See Tables 4.11–4–13 (Chapter 4).

Allergens of Significance in Veterinary Medicine

It is virtually impossible to compare the data from one veterinary dermatologist with the next since many different allergens, allergen concentrations, and techniques are used. Tables 3.5–3.10 show the incidence of skin test reactivity of dogs as found in the USA (Nesbitt, 1978; Nesbitt *et al.*, 1984; Schick and Fadok, 1986; Schou *et al.*, 1991) and in Europe (Willemse and Van den Brom, 1983; Vollset, 1986; Ohlén, 1992; Carlotti and Costargent, 1994; Koch and Peters, 1994; Willemse, 1994; Sture *et al.*, 1995). Since these studies only cover a limited geographic area, the reader is referred to Chapter 4 for a more precise description of important pollen allergens.

Table 3.5   *Skin test reactivity (%) of dogs to grass antigens.*

Allergen	New York[1]	New York[2]	Pacific Northwest[3]	Northern Florida[4]	Southern Florida[4]	Illinois[4]	North Carolina[4]
Mixed	30	53	85	21	39	29	18
June		48					
Orchard		50	82				
Timothy		47	76	34	46	22	29
Sweet vernal		40	84				
Red top		44					
Meadow fescue		45					
Bermuda				38	52	21	25
Bahia				45	61	19	29
Johnson				36	37	15	21
Salt				28	19	2	7
Rye		67	83				
Blue			89				
Velvet			76				

[1]Scott, 1981. [2]Nesbitt *et al.*, 1984. [3] Nesbitt *et al.*, 1978. [4]Schick and Fadok, 1986.

Table 3.6 *Skin test reactivity (%) of dogs to tree antigens*

Allergen	New York[1]	New York[2]	Pacific Northwest[3]	Northern Florida[4]	Southern Florida[4]	Illinois[4]	North Carolina[4]
Mixed	27	47	78				
Ash		35	71				
Birch		35	70				
Beech		29		21	19	11	14
Elm		36		21	24	5	11
Hickory		39		26	30	5	21
Maple		29	82				
Poplar		32		25	28	4	11
Oak		38	78				
Red cedar		39		38	40	13	25
Pine		32		26	9	9	14
Cottonwood			73				
Willow			79	34	24	12	11
Alder			79				
Walnut			56	30	27	7	21
Hackberry				30	28	15	21
Pecan				38	39	8	32
Palm				38	42	4	21
Live oak				42	39	4	14
Sycamore				23	28	2	14
Sweet gum				21	24	0	18
Acacia				32	36	1	14
Mango				17	28	2	7
Red mulberry				30	36	2	18
Orange				28	48	3	4
Pepper tree				34	36	2	14
Australian Pine				28	24	2	4

[1]Scott, 1981. [2]Nesbitt *et al.*, 1984. [3]Nesbitt, 1978. [4]Schick and Fadok,1986.

Table 3.7   *Skin test reactivity (%) of dogs to weed antigens.*

Allergen	New York[1]	New York[2]	Pacific Northwest[3]	Northern Florida[4]	Southern Florida[4]	Illinois[4]	North Carolina[4]
Mixed		63	80				
Lamb's-quarter	10	60	77	47	37	25	29
Cocklebur	13	59		34	42	32	32
English plantain	17	46	75	25	33	22	25
Rough marsh elder	10	62		42	48	33	32
Sheep sorrel	17	46	72	38	33	33	32
Pigweed	15	56	80	40	37	22	36
Mugwort		52					
Mixed ragweed	35	59		38	39	45	39
Yellow dock	17		78	47	55	33	29
Goldenrod	35			26	42	20	25
Dog fennel				32	40	24	36
Baccharis sp.				30	39	14	21
Kochia	17			43	45	25	36
Dandelion	22		76				

[1]Scott, 1981. [2]Nesbitt *et al.*, 1984. [3]Nesbitt, 1978. [4]Schick and Fadok,1986.

Table 3.8   *Skin test reactivity (%) of dogs to fungal antigens.*

Allergen	New York[1]	New York[2]	Pacific Northwest[3]	Northern Florida[4]	Southern Florida[4]	Illinois[4]	North Carolina[4]
Mixed		43	88				
Cladosporium (Hormodendum)	15	35	80				
Alternaria	25	37	79	15	15	21	18
Aspergillus	15	42		15	19	27	11
Penicillum	15	47	84	17	24	24	18
Botrytis	20	33					
Phoma	35	35					
Epicoccum	8	32					
Mucor	35	39					
Pullaria	40	42					
Helmintho-sporium	42	30					
Curvularia		38					
Rhodotorulus		40					
Fusarium	42	37					
Rhizopus	20	42					
Stemphyllium	8						

[1]Scott, 1981. [2]Nesbitt *et al.*, 1984. [3]Nesbitt, 1978. [4]Schick and Fadok,1986.

Table 3.9   *Skin test reactivity (%) of dogs to environmental antigens.*

Allergen	New York[1]	New York[2]	Pacific Northwest[3]	Northern Florida[4]	Southern Florida[4]	Illinois[4]	North Carolina[4]
House dust	35	64	71	68	49	34	39
House dust mite				62	46	34	46
Mixed epidermals	30	76					
Cat epithelium	30	71	67	36	18	1	18
Dog epithelium		74	56				
Horse epitheliulm		65	75				
Human epithelium	50		17				
Mixed feathers	35	76	51	11	15	25	32
Wool	35	59	63	21	24	27	32
Kapok	48	50	84	23	22	24	21
Cottonseed	25	53					
Tobacco	38		28				
Newsprint	30						

[1]Scott, 1981. [2]Nesbitt *et al.*, 1984. [3]Nesbitt, 1978. [4]Schick and Fadok, 1986.

Table 3.10 *Skin test reactivity (%) of atopic dogs to environmental allergens in Europe.*

Allergen	France[1] 1992	Sweden 1992	Norway 1985	Holland 1983	Holland 1994	UK[2] 1995	Germany[3] 1994
Dermatophagoides House dust	41.4	75.5	54.9	39.4	77.4	62.1 – 58.1	59.4
Dermatophagoides pteronyssinus	21.5	11.8	1.6	3.4	25.8	19.4	13.5
Dermatophagoides farinae	80.5	47.3	37.7		71.0	49.4 – 41.9	18.8
Moulds	9.4	5.4 – 13.8	3.3	4.3		8.0 – 12.9	
Dog dander	9.0	26.9	0.8	25.0	19.4		35.7
Cat dander	5.5	59.9	2.5	29.8	6.5		45.4
Human dander			41.8	39.8	32.3	67.8 – 54.8	66.2
Horse dander				13.0	1.6	26.4 – 38.7	43.0
Mixed feathers	3.9			13.0	4.8		6.3 – 7.2
Sheep's wool	1.9	18.2	0.8				3.9
Storage mites:							
Tyrophagus putrescentiae					77.4	35.6 – 35.5	23.7
Glycyphagus domesticus					22.6		26.6
Acarus siro					77.4	18.4 – 25.8	19.3
Grasses	1.9	6.3	4.1	21.2	12.9	29.9 – 25.8	6.8
Lolium perenne (perennial rye)	1.9						5.8
Phleum pratense (timothy)		5.9	8.2	10.6		14.9 – 16.1	
Poa pratensis (Kentucky)					12.6		4.3
Festuca eliator (fescue)	1.9					12.6	
Weeds	2.7–3.5	3.5–6.3	3.3	13.0	19.4	26.4 – 25.8	2.9 – 4.3
Artemisia vulgaris (mugwort)	3.5	3.5		10.1			4.8
Chenopodium album (lamb's quarter)							3.9
Plantago lanceolata (English plantain)	3.1						6.8
Rumex acetosella (sheep sorrel)							6.8
Trees	1.6–5.1	4.5	6.6	12.0	6.5	24.1 – 22.6	1.9 – 3.4
Quercus spp. (oak)	4.7					16.1	4.8
Betula spp. (birch)	3.5	5.4	5.7	6.8			

[1]Concerns Aquitane (southwest of France).
[2]Concerns Edinburgh and London area, respectively.
[3]References: Carlotti and Costargent (1994), Ohlén (1992), Vollset (1986), Willemse and Van den Brom (1983), Willemse (1994 and unpublished data), Sture *et al.* (1995), and Koch and Peters (1994), to columns 2–8, respectively.

References

Arlian LG, Geis DP, Vyszenski-Moher DL, Bernstein IL, Gallagher JS. Antigenic and allergenic properties of the storage mite *Tyrophagus putrescentiae*. *J. Allergy Clin. Immunol.* **74(2)**: 166–171, 1984.

Bessot JC, de Blay F, Pauli G. From allergen sources to reduction of allergen exposure. *Eur. Resp. J.* **7**: 392–397, 1994.

Bidat E, Chevalier MC, Croisier C, *et al.* L'apparition de la blatte dans la poussière de maison. *Rev. Fr. Allergol.* **33**: 22–29, 1993.

Boutin Y, Hebert H, Vrancken E, *et al.* Allergenicity and cross-reactivity of cat and dog allergenic extracts. *Clin. Allergy* **18**: 287–293, 1988.

Carlotti DN, Costargent F. Analysis of positive skin tests in 449 dogs with allergic dermatitis. *Eur. J. Comp. Anim. Pract.* **4**: 42–59, 1994.

Charpin C, Mata P, Charpin D, *et al.* Fel d I allergen distribution in cat fur and skin. *J. Allergy Clin. Immunol.* **88**: 77–82, 1991.

D'Ammato G, Spieksma FTM, Bonini S. *Allergenic Pollen and Pollinosis in Europe.* Science Publications, Oxford, 1991.

Duffort O, Carreirra J, Nito G, *et al.* Studies on the biochemical structure of the major cat allergen *Felis domesticus* I. *Mol. Immunol.* **28**: 301–309, 1991.

Dybendal T, Vik H, Elsayed S. Dust from carpeted and smooth floors. II. Antigenic and allergenic content of dust vacuumed from carpeted and smooth floors in schools under routine cleaning schedules. *Allergy* **44**: 401–411, 1989.

Frank LA, McEntee MF. Demonstration of aeroallergen contact sensitivity in dogs. *Vet. Allergy Clin. Immunol.* **3**: 75–80, 1995.

Green WF, Woolcock AJ. *Tyrophagus putrescentiae:* an allergenically important mite. *Clin. Allergy* **8**: 135–144, 1978.

Griffin CE, Rosenkrantz WS, Alaba S. Detection of insect/arachnid specific IgE in dogs: comparison of two techniques utilizing Western blots as the standard. In Ihrke PJ, Mason IS, White SD (eds), *Advances in Veterinary, Dermatology*, volume 2. Saunders Co., Philadelphia, pp. 263–269, 1993.

Johansson E, Johansson SGO, Van Hage-Hamsten M. Allergenic characterization of *Acarus siro* and *Tyrophagus putrescentia* and their crossreactivity with *Lepidoglyphus destructor* and *Dermatophagoides pteronyssinus*. *Clin. Exper. Allergy* **24**: 743–751, 1994.

Koch HJ, Peters S. 207 Intrakutantests bei Hunden mit Verdacht auf atopische Dermatitis. *Kleintierpraxis* **39**: 25–36, 1994.

Luczynska CM, Griffin P, Davies RJ, Topping MD. Prevalence of specific IgE to storage mites (*A. siro*, *L. destructor* and *T. longior*) in an urban population and crossreactivity with the house dust mite (*D. pteronyssinus*). *Clin. Exp. Allergy* **20**: 403–406, 1990.

Nesbitt GH. Canine allergic inhalant dermatitis: a review of 230 cases. *J. Am. Vet. Med. Assoc.* **172**: 55–60, 1978.

Nesbitt GH, Kedan, GS, Caciolo, P. Canine atopy. Part I: Etiology and diagnosis. *Comp. Cont. Ed.* **6**: 75–84, 1984.

Noli C, Bernadina WE, Willemse T. The significance of reactions to purified fractions of *Dermatophagoides pteronyssinus* and *Dermatophagoides farinae* in canine atopic dermatitis. *Vet. Immunol. Immunopathol.* **52**: 147–157, 1996.

Ohlén BM. Projekt allergitester i Sverige. *Svenks Veter Tidning* **44**: 365–371, 1992.

Platts-Mills ThAE, Chapman MD. Dust mites: Immunology, allergic disease and environmental control. *J. Allergy Clin. Immunol.* **80(6)**: 755–775, 1987.

Platts-Mills ThAE, de Weck AL. Dust mite allergens and asthma – A worldwide problem. *J. Allergy. Clin. Immunol.* **83(2)**: 416–427, 1989.

Ree R van, Driessen MNBM, Van Leeuwen WA, *et al.* Variability of IgE antibodies to group I and V allergens in eight grass pollen species. *Clin. Exp. Allergy* **22**: 611–17, 1992.

Ree R van, van Leeuwen, WA, Van den Berg, M, *et al.* IgE and IgG cross-reactivity among *Lol p I* and *Lol p II/III* – Identification of the C-termini of *Lol p I, II,* and *III* as cross-reactive structures. *Allergy* **49**: 254–261, 1994.

Roberts AM, van Ree R, Cardy SM, *et al.* A recombinant allergen from *Dactylus glomerata* with high sequence homology to *Lol p II* is cross-reactive with *Lol p I.* *Immunol.* **76**: 389–396, 1992.

Rosenbaum MR. The effects of mold proteases on the biological activity of pollen allergenic extracts in atopic dogs. *Proc. 12th Ann Members' Meeting Am. Acad. Vet. Derm. & Am. Coll. Vet. Derm.* Congress Organisation, Las Vegas, Nevada; pp. 20–21, 1996.

Schick RO, Fadok VA. Response of atopic dogs to regional allergens: 268 cases (1981–1984). *J. Am. Vet. Med. Assoc.* **189**: 1493–1496, 1986.

Schou C. Defining allergens of mammalian origin. *Clin. Exp. Immunol.* 1993; **23**: 7–14.

Schou C, Svendson U, Loewenstein H. Purification and characterization of the major dog allergen, *Can f I. Clin. Exp. Immunol.* **21**: 321–328, 1991.

Scott DW. Observations on canine atopy. *J. Am. Anim. Hosp. Assoc.* **17**: 91–1001, 1981.

Sture GR, Halliwell REW, Thoday KL, *et al.* Canine atopic dermatitis: the prevalence of positive intradermal skin tests at two sites in the north and south of Great Britain. *Vet. Immun. Immunopathol.* **44**: 293–308, 1995.

Tee RD. Allergy to storage mites. *Clin. Exper. Allergy*, **24**: 636–640, 1994.

Vollset I. Immediate type hypersensitivity in dogs induced by storage mites. *Res. Vet. Sci.* **40**: 123–127, 1986.

Willemse T, Van den Brom WE. Evaluation of the intradermal allergy test in normal dogs. *Res. Vet. Sci.* **32**: 57–61, 1982.

Willemse T, Van den Brom WE. Investigations of the symptomatology and the significance of immediate skin test reactivity in canine atopic dermatitis. *Res. Vet. Sci.* **34**: 261–265, 1983.

Willemse T. Hyposensitization of dogs with atopic dermatitis based on the results of *in vivo* and *in vitro* (IgGd ELISA) diagnostic tests. *10th Proc. Am. Coll. Vet. Derm.,* Congress Organisation, Charleston (USA), p. 61, 1994.

Willis EL. IgE mediated insect and arachnid hypersensitivity in the dog. *10th Proc. Ann. Memb. Meeting AAVD & ACVD,* Congress Organisation, Charleston, South Carolina, pp. 33–34, 1994.

World Health Organization. Allergen nomenclature: WHO/IUS Allergen Nomenclature Subcommittee World Health Organization, Geneva, Switzerland. *Clin. Exp. Allergy* **25**: 27–37, 1995.

Wraith DG, Cunnington AM, Seymour WM. The role and allergenic importance of storage mites in house dust and other environments. *Clin. Allergy* **9**: 545–561, 1979.

4

Allergy Testing

Introduction

Allergy testing is used to identify the causative allergens in animals suspected to have atopy on the basis of their clinical manifestations. Once the allergens are identified, specific therapy of avoidance and/or immunotherapy can be initiated. Allergy testing is a valuable tool in all cases as it is convinces owners that their pet suffers from atopy. In addition, many pet owners want to know exactly which allergens are important for their pet. Allergy testing is mandatory when immunotherapy is appropriate, but is also important in mono-allergy patients (e.g. hypersensitivity to house dust mites) where avoidance may become a therapeutic option. If symptomatic treatment is the only therapeutic modality that will be used, allergy testing may be declined by a pet owner because it has no therapeutic benefit.

Both *in vivo* and *in vitro* methods of allergy testing are available. *In vitro* testing involves serum measurement of immunoreactants involved in the allergic reaction. *In vivo* allergy testing revolves around the induction of a small scale allergic reaction by the intentional exposure of the patient to a minute amount of allergen. *In vitro* testing is discussed later in this chapter.

In the clinical situation *in vivo* allergy testing in dogs and cats is carried out via the skin, although theoretically such tests can also be carried out via the conjunctivae, or nasal or bronchial mucosa. The skin is the only practical site as it is readily accessible, easily observed, easily tested, and a large number of tests can be performed safely at one time. Skin test reactivity only indicates skin sensitivity. The clinical significance of test reactions must be determined by correlating the reactions with the history.

Allergen Purchase

Allergens can be purchased from various laboratories in different strengths and volumes. The allergens used for skin testing should also be used for immunotherapy. Uniform standardization of allergens does not exist and extracts of the same allergen can differ from company to company. Companies offering skin test-strength antigens should be able to show that their allergens have been biostandardized. In other words, the allergens should have been tested in healthy animals in order to determine the skin test concentration to which no reactivity can be observed. This threshold concentration is suitable for testing atopic animals.

When the decision to carry out skin testing is made, one must decide whether concentrated or skin test-strength antigens are to be ordered. If skin test-strength antigens are used, separate vaccines for immunotherapy must also be bought from the antigen supplier. Because of government sterility requirements, custom-made vaccines will take at least one month before they are received.

The purchase of concentrated antigens gives one the flexibility of making one's own skin test antigens as well as vaccines for immunotherapy. Concentrated allergens come in different strengths and volumes. The higher the concentration and the larger the volume, the lower the cost on a protein nitrogen unit (PNU)/ml basis. Very concentrated allergens tend to precipitate out and should not be purchased unless the vial is to be used within six months. A concentration of 20 000 PNU/ml is most appropriate.

The decision to buy diluted or concentrated allergens is not only an economic decision. Allergens purchased must be used before their expiration date. If only a few patients are to receive a hyposensitization vaccine, the allergens will expire before they are used. In this case the veterinarian will have to absorb the cost or the cost of each vaccine will be very high. It is impossible to calculate the exact number of cases needed to reach the break-even point, but if fewer than 15 vaccines are to be made each year, it would not be economic to purchase concentrated allergens. If 15–30 vaccines are made each year, the cost of the allergens will be recovered with a small profit for the veterinarian. As the number of yearly vaccines increases the cost per vaccine decreases to the point where the vaccine can cost 50% of that charged by the antigen supplier. On the other hand, the purchase of diluted allergens in skin threshold concentrations has the advantage that the allergens are always at the correct concentration. Purchasing concentrated allergens obliges the veterinarian to carry out the serial dilutions him or herself and mistakes can easily be made. Since healthy animals are not usually available to test each new batch, errors in testing can result. In Europe, veterinarians buy diluted allergens while in the USA, most practitioners buy concentrated allergens instead.

Selection of Test Antigens

Approximately 425 non-food allergy extracts are available commercially. Obviously it is impossible to test for all of these allergens. Certain allergens are not found in some floristic zones and can be eliminated from consideration, but the number remaining will still be excessive.

Figure 4.1 shows a map of the botanic or floristic zones of the USA and Tables 4.1–4.10 list important pollen allergens found in each region. The data were tabulated from materials supplied by major allergen companies in the USA. These lists should not be considered all inclusive or exclusive. As each region is quite large, some pollens are not found in all states or countries. For example, Bermuda grass is listed in USA region 1, but it is restricted to the southern portions of Pennsylvania and New Jersey. Even in one area of a particular zone, the pollens of prevalence can vary greatly as the degree and nature of urban development affects the types and numbers of plants present. In agricultural areas, cultivated crops of corn, rye, barley, oats, wheat, alfalfa, castor bean, and sugar beets may be significant allergens for pets. Tables 4.11–4.13 present similar information for different areas of Europe (Driessen *et al.*, 1988; D'Ammato *et al.*, 1991; Carlotti and Costargent, 1994; Koch and Peters, 1994; Sture *et al.*, 1995). Only the most important pollens are given. The lists

TEN POLLINATION ZONES

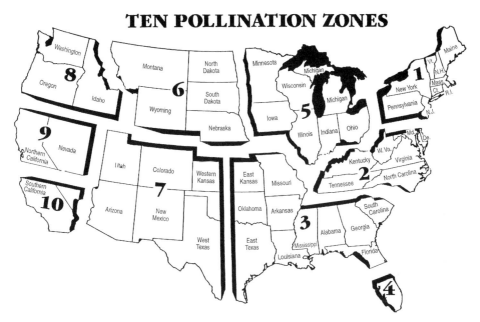

Figure 4.1   *Botanical zones of the USA.*

do not pretend to be complete. All over Europe, airborne pollen of grasses is very common, followed by Urticaceae pollen. In western Europe, aproximately 50% of all airborne pollen comes from these two taxa. More centrally in Europe, trees such as birch and alder predominate over weeds. This tendency becomes even more prominent in the nordic countries. In the family of Compositae, the allergenic role of ragweed is increasing in Europe (D'Ammato *et al.*, 1991). The area covered by this plant is extending in some European areas, particularly France, Austria, Hungary, northern Italy, and the former Yugoslavia.

The allergy laboratories and the personnel at the local weather bureau, health department, medical school, or veterinary college can aid in antigen selection. Perhaps the best source of accurate local information is the human allergist as area pollens that are important in man are probably important in pets. Another option is the purchase of test panels developed by the allergen supplier that are appropriate for various regions. It is common in Europe to purchase a complete test panel. Important local fungal antigens such as barn molds, can be identified by exposing malt agar culture plates to the air for one hour. Standard mycologic techniques are used to identify all growths. The importance of fungal or mold allergens in atopy in pet animals is questionable. Hard evidence on their significance, for example evaluation on the effect of hyposensitization in animals with exclusive mold allergy, are not available. Nevertheless, many dermatologists including the North American authors, use mold allergens in their standard test panel. In contrast, one of the authors (TW) did not find any reaction to mold allergens over a 10-year period and excluded these allergens from the standard allergy test panel.

Since there are vast numbers of regional allergens, any skin test set is incomplete, but will hopefully include all or most of the important allergens. Because the botanic and climatic conditions in an area change, the importance of a particular allergen

Table 4.1   *Pollens of importance – USA region 1 (Maine, New Hampshire, Vermont, Massachusetts, Rhode Island, Connecticut, New York, New Jersey, Pennsylvania).*

Grasses	Trees and shrubs	Weeds
Bermuda	Alder, tag	Cocklebur
Blue, Kentucky	Ash, white	Dock, yellow
Brome, smooth	Ash, green	Goldenrod
Fescue, meadow	Aspen	Kochia
Johnson	Beech	Lamb's quarter
Orchard	Birch, white	Marsh elder
Quack	Birch, cherry	Mugwort
Red top	Birch, red	Pigweed, rough
Rye, perennial	Birch, yellow	Pigweed, spiny
Rye, Italian	Birch, paper	Plantain, English
Sweet vernal	Box elder	Ragweed, giant
Timothy	Cedar, red	Ragweed, short
Velvet	Cottonwood, common	Sorrel, sheep
	Elm, American	Wormwood
	Hackberry	
	Hazelnut, American	
	Hickory, white	
	Hickory, shagbark	
	Hickory, shellbark	
	Maple, red	
	Maple, sugar	
	Maple, silver	
	Mulberry, red	
	Oak, black	
	Oak, bur	
	Oak, red	
	Oak, white	
	Pine, eastern white	
	Sweet gum	
	Sycamore, American	
	Walnut, black	
	Willow	

Table 4.2   *Pollens of importance – USA region 2 (Maryland, Delaware, District of Columbia, Virginia, West Virginia, Kentucky, North Carolina, Tennessee).*

Grasses	Trees and shrubs	Weeds
Bermuda	Alder, tag	Cocklebur
Blue, Kentucky	Ash, white	Dock, yellow
Brome, smooth	Ash, green	Dog fennel
Fescue, meadow	Aspen	Goldenrod
Johnson	Bayberry	Lamb's quarter
Orchard	Beech	Marsh elder
Quack	Birch, red	Mugwort
Red top	Box elder	Pigweed, rough
Rye, perennial	Cedar, red	Pigweed, spiny

Table 4.2   *(continued)*

Grasses	Trees and shrubs	Weeds
Rye, Italian	Cottonwood, common	Plantain, English
Sweet vernal	Cypress, bald	Ragweed, giant
Timothy	Elm, American	Ragweed, short
Velvet	Hackberry	Sorrel, sheep
	Hazelnut, American	Wormwood
	Hickory, white	
	Hickory, shagbark	
	Hickory, shellbark	
	Maple, red	
	Maple, sugar	
	Maple, silver	
	Mulberry, red	
	Mulberry, white	
	Mulberry, paper	
	Oak, black	
	Oak, red	
	Oak, water	
	Oak, Virginia live	
	Oak, white	
	Oak, post	
	Pecan	
	Pine, Virginia scrub	
	Pine, loblolly	
	Pine, shortleaf	
	Sweet gum	
	Sycamore, American	
	Walnut, black	
	Willow	

Table 4.3   *Pollens of importance – USA region 3 (South Carolina, Georgia, Northern Florida, Alabama, Mississippi, Louisiana, Arkansas, East Texas, Oklahoma, East Kansas, Missouri).*

Grasses	Trees and shrubs	Weeds
Bahia	Alder, tag	Careless weed
Bermuda	Ash, white	Cocklebur
Blue, Kentucky	Ash, green	Dock, yellow
Brome	Bayberry	Dog fennel
Fescue, meadow	Beech	Goldenrod
Johnson	Birch, red	Kochia
Orchard	Box elder	Lamb's quarter
Quack	Cedar, red	Marsh elder
Red top	Cottonwood, common	Pigweed, rough
Rye, perennial	Cypress, bald	Pigweed, spiny
Rye, Italian	Elm, cedar	Plantain, English
Sweet vernal	Elm, American	Ragweed, giant
Timothy	Hackberry	Ragweed, short

(continued overleaf)

Table 4.3   *(continued)*

Grasses	Trees and shrubs	Weeds
Velvet	Hazelnut, American	Ragweed, southern
	Hickory, white	Sorrel, sheep
	Hickory, shagbark	Water hemp, western
	Hickory, shellbark	
	Maple, red	
	Maple, sugar	
	Maple, silver	
	Mesquite	
	Mulberry, red	
	Mulberry, white	
	Mulberry, paper	
	Oak, white	
	Oak, post	
	Oak, red	
	Oak, black	
	Oak, water	
	Oak, Virginia live	
	Pecan	
	Pine, Virginia scrub	
	Pine, loblolly	
	Pine, shortleaf	
	Sweet gum	
	Sycamore, American	
	Walnut, black	
	Willow	

Table 4.4   *Pollens of importance – USA region 4 (South Florida)*

Grasses	Trees and shrubs	Weeds
Bahia	Bayberry	Baccharis
Bermuda	Box elder	Cocklebur
Johnson	Hackberry	Dock, yellow
Rye, Italian	Maple, red	Dog fennel
Salt	Melaleuca	Goldenrod
	Mulberry, red	Lamb's quarter
	Mulberry, white	Marsh elder
	Oak, live	Pigweed, rough
	Palm	Pigweed, spiny
	Pine, Australian	Plantain, English
	Pine, longleaf	Ragweed, short
	Pine, slash	Sorrel, sheep
	Sweet gum	
	Willow	

Table 4.5 *Pollens of importance – USA region 5 (Ohio, Michigan, Indiana, Illinois, Wisconsin, Minnesota, Iowa.)*

Grasses	Trees and shrubs	Weeds
Bermuda	Alder, tag	Cocklebur
Blue, Kentucky	Ash, white	Dandelion
Brome	Ash, green	Dock, yellow
Canary, reed	Aspen	Goldenrod
Johnson	Beech	Kochia
Fescue, meadow	Birch, red	Marsh elder, burweed
Orchard	Box elder	Mugwort
Quack	Cedar, red	Nettle
Rye, perennial	Cottonwood, common	Pigweed, rough
Rye, Italian	Elm, American	Pigweed, spiny
Sweet vernal	Hazelnut, American	Ragweed, giant
Timothy	Hickory, shagbark	Ragweed, short
Velvet	Hickory, shellbark	Ragweed, western
Western wheat	Hickory, white	Russian thistle
	Maple, red	Sorrel, sheep
	Maple, sugar	
	Maple, silver	
	Mulberry, red	
	Oak, white	
	Oak, bur	
	Oak, red	
	Oak, black	
	Pecan	
	Pine, eastern white	
	Pine, red	
	Sycamore, American	
	Walnut, black	
	Willow	

Table 4.6 *Pollens of importance – USA region 6 (North Dakota, South Dakota, Nebraska, Montana, Wyoming).*

Grasses	Trees and shrubs	Weeds
Blue, Kentucky	Ash, green	Cocklebur
Brome	Aspen	Dock, yellow
Canary, reed	Box elder	Kochia
Fescue, meadow	Cedar, red	Lamb's quarter
Grama	Cedar, Rocky Mountain	Marsh elder, burweed
Orchard	Cottonwood, common	Nettle
Quack	Elm, American	Plantain, English
Red top	Oak, bur	Poverty weed
Rye, perennial	Willow	Ragweed, false
Rye, Italian		Ragweed, giant
Timothy		Ragweed, short
Western wheat		Ragweed, western

(continued overleaf)

Table 4.6   *(continued)*

Grasses	Trees and shrubs	Weeds
Wild rye		Russian thistle
		Sagebrush, common
		Sagebrush, white
		Scale, wing
		Sorrel, sheep
		Water hemp, western

Table 4.7   *Pollens of importance – USA region 7 (West Kansas, West Oklahoma, West Texas, Colorado, New Mexico, Arizona, Utah).*

Grasses	Trees and shrubs	Weeds
Bermuda	Ash, green	Careless weed
Blue, Kentucky	Ash, Arizona	Cocklebur
Brome	Aspen	Dock, yellow
Canary, reed	Box elder	Iodine bush
Fescue, meadow	Cedar, salt	Kochia
Grama	Cedar, mountain	Lamb's quarter
Johnson	Cedar, Rocky Mountain	Marsh elder
Orchard	Cottonwood, common	Marsh elder, burweed
Quack	Cottonwood, Fremont	Pigweed, rough
Red top	Cypress, Arizona	Plantain, English
Rye, perennial	Elm, American	Poverty weed
Rye, Italian	Elm, Chinese	Ragweed, false
Timothy	Juniper, pinchot	Ragweed, giant
Western wheat	Juniper, oneseed	Ragweed, short
Wild rye	Juniper, Utah	Ragweed, western
	Mesquite	Russian thistle
	Mulberry, white	Sagebrush, common
	Mulberry, red	Sagebrush, pasture
	Mulberry, paper	Sagebrush, white
	Oak, Virginia live	Saltbrush, annual
	Oak, gambel	Scale, all
	Olive	Scale, lens
	Pecan	Scale, wing
	Sycamore, American	Sheepfat
	Walnut, Arizona	Sorrel, sheep
		Water hemp, western

Table 4.8   *Pollens of importance – USA region 8 (Washington, Oregon, Idaho).*

Grasses	Trees and shrubs	Weeds
Bermuda	Alder, red	Cocklebur
Blue, Kentucky	Alder, white	Marsh elder, burweed
Brome	Ash, Oregon	Dock, yellow
Canary, reed	Aspen	Kochia

Table 4.8 *(continued)*

Grasses	Trees and shrubs	Weeds
Fescue, meadow	Birch	Lamb's quarter
Oat	Box elder	Mugwort
Orchard	Cedar, Rocky Mountain	Nettle
Quack	Cottonwood, black	Pigweed, rough
Red top	Elm, American	Plantain, English
Rye, perennial	Elm, Chinese	Poverty weed
Rye, Italian	Hazelnut spp.	Ragweed, false
Salt	Juniper, Utah	Ragweed, giant
Sweet vernal	Juniper, western	Ragweed, western
Timothy	Maple, coast	Russian thistle
Velvet	Oak, Garry	Sagebrush, mugwort
Western wheat	Oak, California black	Sagebrush, common
Wild rye	Pine, western yellow	Sagebrush, white
	Pine, white	Scale, wing
	Walnut, black	Sheepfat
	Walnut, English	Sorrel, sheep
	Willow	

Table 4.9 *Pollens of importance – USA region 9 (Northern California, Nevada except extreme southern portion).*

Grasses	Trees and shrubs	Weeds
Bermuda	Alder, white	Cocklebur
Blue, Kentucky	Ash, Oregon	Dock, yellow
Brome	Birch	Greasewood
Canary, reed	Box elder	Iodine bush
Fescue, meadow	Cedar, Rocky Mountain	Kochia
Johnson	Cedar, salt	Lamb's quarter
Oat	Cottonwood, black	Mugwort
Orchard	Cottonwood, Fremont	Pigweed, rough
Quack	Elm, American	Plantain, English
Red top	Elm, Chinese	Poverty weed
Rye, perennial	Elm, Siberian	Ragweed, false
Rye, Italian	Hazelnut	Ragweed, western
Salt	Juniper, western	Russian thistle
Sweet vernal	Juniper, California	Sagebrush, white
Timothy	Maple, coast	Sagebrush, common
Velvet	Oak, coast live	Scale, lens
Western wheat	Oak, California black	Scale, wing
Wild rye	Oak, California scrub	Sheepfat
	Pine, western yellow	Sorrel, sheep
	Pine, white	
	Walnut, black	
	Walnut, southern California black	
	Walnut, English	
	Willow	

Table 4.10   *Pollens of importance – USA region 10 (Southern California, extreme southern Nevada).*

Grasses	Trees and shrubs	Weeds
Bermuda	Acacia	Careless weed
Blue, Kentucky	Ash, Arizona	Burrobush
Brome	Birch	Cocklebur
Fescue, meadow	Cottonwood, black	Dock, yellow
Johnson	Cottonwood, Fremont	Iodine bush
Oat	Cypress, Arizona	Kochia
Orchard	Elm, American	Lamb's quarter
Red Top	Elm, Chinese	Pigweed, rough
Rye, perennial	Elm, Siberian	Plantain, English
Rye, Italian	Eucalyptus	Poverty weed
Timothy	Maple, coast	Ragweed, desert
Velvet	Box elder	Ragweed, false
Wild rye	Mesquite	Ragweed, western
	Mulberry, white	Russian thistle
	Mulberry, paper	Sagebrush, coast
	Oak, California scrub	Sagebrush, common
	Oak, coast line	Scale, lens
	Oak, valley	Scale, all
	Olive	Scale, wing
	Pine, Australian	Sheep sorrel
	Pine, western yellow	
	Sycamore, western	
	Walnut, black	
	Walnut, southern California black	

Table 4.11   *Pollens of major importance – Europe region 1 (Mediterranean and the mid and south France).*

Mediterranean	Mid and south France
Trees and shrubs	
Corylus spp. (hazel)	*Quercus* spp. (oak)
Alnus spp. (alder)	*Cupressus* spp. (cypress)
Cupressus sempervirens (Italian cypress)	*Juniperus occidentalis* (western juniper)
Cupressus arizona (Arizona cypress)	*Thuja occidentalis* (thuja)
Cupressus glabra (cypress)	*Platanus orientalis* (eastern sycamore)
Olea europaea (olive)	*Broussonetia papyrifera*
Weeds	
Chenopodium album (lamb's quarter)	*Artemisia vulgaris* (mugwort)
Chenopodium berlandieri (goose foot)	*Parietaria officinalis* (pellitory-of-
Kochia scoparia (burning bush)	the-wall)
Atriplex wrightii (annual saltbush)	*Plantago lanceolata* (English plantain)
Salsola pestifer (Russian thistle)	*Ambrosia artemisiifolia* (short ragweed)
Parietaria officinalis (pellitory-of-the-wall)	
Parietaria judaica	
Artemisia vulgaris (mugwort)	
Artemisia verlotorum (sagebush)	
Artemisia annua (annual sagebush)	

Table 4.11   *(continued)*

Mediterranean	Mid and south France
Grasses	
Poa pratensis (Kentucky grass)	*Poa pratensis* (Kentucky grass)
Festuca eliator (meadow fescue)	*Festuca eliator* (meadow fescue)
Dactylis glomerata (orchard)	*Dactylis glomerata* (orchard)
Lolium perenne (perennial rye)	*Lolium perenne* (perennial rye)
Phleum pratense (timothy)	*Phleum pratense* (timothy)
Agropyron repens (quackgrass)	*Agropyron repens* (quackgrass)

Table 4.12   *Pollens of major importance – Europe region 2 (Central Europe, northern Germany, UK).*

Central Europe and northern Germany	UK
Trees and shrubs	
Corylus spp. (hazel)	*Quercus alba* (white oak)
Quercus spp. (oak)	
Castanea spp. (chestnut)	
Betula spp. (birch)	
Salix spp. (willow)	
Ulmus spp. (elm)	
Weeds	
Parietaria judaica (pellitory-of-the-wall)	*Parietaria judaica* (pellitory-of-the-wall)
Rumex acetosa (field sorrel)	*Rumex crispus* (yellow dock)
Rumex acetosella (sheep sorrel)	*Chenopodium album* (lamb's quarter)
Artemisia vulgaris (common mugwort)	*Artemisia vulgaris* (common mugwort)
Ambrosia artemisiifolia (short ragweed)	*Urtica dioica* (nettle)
Ambrosia elatior	*Plantago lanceolata* (English plantain)
Plantago lanceolata (English plantain)	
Taraxacum officinale (dandelion)	
Urtica dioica (nettle)	
Grasses	
Poa pratensis (Kentucky)	*Poa pratensis* (Kentucky)
Festuca eliator (meadow fescue)	*Festuca eliator* (meadow fescue)
Dactylis glomerata (orchard)	*Dactylis glomerata* (orchard)
Lolium perenne (perennial rye)	*Lolium perenne* (perennial rye)
Anthoxantum odoratum (sweet vernal)	*Anthoxantum odoratum* (sweet vernal)
Phleum pratense (timothy)	*Phleum pratense* (timothy)
Holcus lanatus (velvet)	*Holcus lanatus* (velvet)
Agrostis alba (redtop)	*Agrostis alba* (redtop)

Table 4.13   *Pollens of major importance – Europe region 3 (Northern France, Benelux, Scandinavia (including Denmark).*

Northern France and Benelux	Scandinavia
Trees and shrubs	
Alnus spp. (alder)	*Betula* spp. (birch)
Corylus spp. (hazel)	*Alnus* spp. (alder)

(continued overleaf)

Table 4.13   *(continued)*

Northern France and Benelux	Scandinavia
Betula spp. (birch)	*Corylus* spp. (hazel)
Fagus spp. (beech)	*Ulmus* spp. (elm)
Quercus spp. (oak)	
Castanea spp. (chestnut)	
Carpinus spp. (hornbeam)	
Weeds	
Artemisia vulgaris (common mugwort)	*Artemisia vulgaris* (common mugwort)
Chenopodium album (lamb's quarter)	*Chenopodium album* (lamb's quarter)
Grasses	
Poa pratensis (Kentucky)	*Poa pratensis* (Kentucky)
Festuca eliator (meadow fescue)	*Festuca eliator* (meadow fescue)
Dactylis glomerata (orchard)	*Dactylis glomerata* (orchard)
Lolium perenne (perennial rye)	*Lolium perenne* (perennial rye)
Anthoxantum odoratum (sweet vernal)	*Anthoxantum odoratum* (sweet vernal)
Phleum pratense (timothy)	*Phleum pratense* (timothy)
Holcus lanatus (velvet)	*Holcus lanatus* (velvet)
Agrostis alba (redtop)	*Agrostis alba* (redtop)

can also change. All skin test results should be kept in a tabular form and reviewed at least yearly. Allergens with a low incidence of reactivity of approximately 5% are not of major importance and can be replaced with a new allergen. The elimination of an allergen with a low reactivity means that an important allergen will be missed in a small number of animals.

Tables 4.14–4.16 list the allergens the authors presently use in their skin testing. Although most animals examined by the authors will be tested for all allergens, skin testing gives the veterinarian great flexibility. Animals with summer allergies may not have to be tested for indoor antigens. The authors use many different allergens for testing. These sets were developed over a number of years and reflect the nature of the practices, the importance of the various allergens in each area, and a number of other factors. As a general rule, satisfactory information can be obtained with 25–30 well selected allergens. If a complete test panel cannot be purchased, the beginner should select approximately 20 of the most important local pollens (grasses, weeds, and trees) and add four or five molds, if appropriate, for the region. House dust, important epidermals (e.g. human, cat, dog), storage mites, and mixed feathers should be included as well as a positive and negative control. In Europe where storage mite extracts are available, they should be a standard part of a test panel. The most important representatives of these mites are *Glycyphagus domesticus* (Glycyphagidae), *Acarus siro* and *Tyrophagus putrescentiae* (Acaridae) (Vollset, 1986; Lee, 1994). These allergens are not currently available in the USA. The incidence of immediate skin test reactivity in atopic dogs to one of these allergens is 22.6–26.6% for *Glycyphagus domesticus* (Koch and Peters, 1994; Willemse, 1994), 23.7–77.4% for *Tyrophagus putrescentiae* (Koch and Peters, 1994; Willemse, 1994; Sture *et al.*, 1995), and 19.3–77.4% for *Acarus siro* (Koch and Peters, 1994; Willemse, 1994). As one becomes familiar with the initial test set and allergy testing in general, shortcomings of the test antigens will become obvious and allergens can be added or dropped as

Table 4.14 Skin test antigens (as used in Dr Reedy's referral practice).

Grasses	Weeds	Trees and shrubs	Molds	Miscellaneous
Johnson	Ragweed	Mountain cedar	*Alternaria*	House dust
Bermuda	Cocklebur	Elm	*Hormodendrum*	Mixed feathers
Rye	Marsh elder	Mesquite	*Penicillium*	Cat epithelium
Kentucky blue	Careless weed	Oak	*Aspergillus*	Cockroach
Orchard	Sage	Box elder		Flea
Timothy	Kochia			House dust mite
Bahia	Russian thistle			
Quack	Yellow dock			
	Lamb's quarter			
	English plantain			

Table 4.15 Skin test antigens – College of Veterinary Medicine, Cornell University.

Grasses	Weeds	Trees and shrubs	Molds	Miscellaneous
Alfalfa	English plantain	Ash mix	*Alternaria*	House dust
Kentucky blue	Lamb's quarter	Birch mix	*Aspergillus* mix	Kapok
Orchard	Pigweed mix	Elm mix	*Epicoccum*	Flea
Perennial rye	Cocklebur	Maple–Box elder mix	*Fusarium* mix	Mixed feathers
Timothy	Marsh elder	Eastern oak mix	*Curvularia*	Cottonseed
Redtop	Goldenrod	White pine	*Helminthosporium*	Cat epithelium
Sweet vernal	Ragweed mix	White poplar	*Hormodendrum*	
Meadow fescue	Dock–sorrel mix	American beech	*Mucor* mix	
Brome	Dandelion	Black walnut	*Penicillium* mix	
Quack	Kochia	Eastern sycamore	*Pullaria*	
	Mugwort	Red cedar	*Phoma*	
	Wormwood	White alder	*Rhizopus* mix	
		Bayberry	*Stemphyllium*	
			Botrytis	
			Cephalosporium	

Table 4.16 *Skin test antigens – Utrecht University Faculty of Veterinary Medicine.*

Grasses	Weeds	Trees and shrubs	Miscellaneous
Cynodon dactylon (Bermuda)	Artemisia vulgaris (mugwort)	Betula spp. (birch)	Dog dander
Dactylis glomerata (orchard)	Urtica dioica (nettle)	Alnus spp. (alder)	Cat dander
Anthoxantum odoratum	Solidago virgaurea (goldenrod)	Corylus spp. (hazel)	Human dander
Phleum pratense (timothy)	Chenopodium album (lamb's quarter)	Quercus spp. (oak)	Mixed feathers[1]
Holcus lanatus (velvet)	Taraxacum officinale (dandelion)	Fagus spp. (beech)	Whole body flea
Poa pratensis (Kentucky)	Rumex acetosella (sheep sorrel)	Ulmus spp. (elm)	Storage mites[2]
Lolium perenne (perennial rye)	Plantago lanceolata (English plantain)	Populus spp. (poplar)	Dermatophagoides pteronyssinus
	Ambrosia eliator (small ragweed)	Salix spp. (willow)	Dermatophagoides farinae
	Brassica napus (rape)	Fraxinus spp. (ash)	Barn dust
	Chrysantemum spp. (ox-eye)	Acer glutinosa (maple)	

[1] Other epidermals pending the history.
[2] Tyrophagus putrescentiae, Acarus siro, Glycyphagus domesticus.

needed. With a new allergy test set, the test results should be reviewed every few months for the first year to make sure that the concentration of the antigens is correct and that the testing technique is not resulting in false-negative or false-positive reactions.

Since the number of allergy test sites is limited, the use of mixtures is tempting. Scott (1981) reported a good correlation between the results obtained with mixed and individual allergens for grasses, ragweed, and house dust, but a poor correlation for mixed molds, mixed epidermals, and mixed weeds. He found that dogs who had negative reactions to the mixed antigens could show positive reactions to one or more components of the mixture if the allergens were tested individually. Nesbitt *et al.* (1984) studied this point more extensively and found dissimilar results. He reported that in general he found more reactivity with the mixed antigens than with the individual allergens. He correlated the percentage of reactivity for the mixed and individual allergens and found a range of 56–77% for trees; 60–67% for weeds; 61–75% for grasses; 61–73% for molds; and 67–77% for epidermals. These data are very difficult to interpret, but taken at face value suggest that depending upon the allergen group, mixtures will give reliable results from 56–77% of the time. However, the most crucial test in deciding between the applicability of mixtures versus individual allergens is the experiment comparing the result of hyposensitization in two groups of dogs sensitive to either pollen mixtures or individual pollens. Until these data are developed, a rational conclusion on the value of mixtures for testing cannot be made. As mentioned in Chapter 3, mixtures of grasses and pollens from the same genus may be used.

Another aspect for discussion concerns the use of crude allergen extracts versus purified extracts. Most allergens consist of (glyco)proteins and polysaccharides and only a small part acts as an allergenic component. The remaining parts are probably responsible for nonspecific reaction in skin tests or *in vitro* allergy tests. For example, two major groups have been identified in mite allergens: Group I allergens are 25 kD, thermolabile proteins primarily found in mite feces; Group II allergens are essentially of somatic origin, have molecular weights of 15 kD, and are heat-resistant proteins. Group I and II mite allergens are proteolytic enzymes. Biochemical studies have demonstrated *Der p I* (the first purified fraction of *Dermatophagoides pteronyssinus*) to be a cysteine protease, and *Der p II* a lysozyme (Bessot *et al.*, 1994). In dogs *Der p I*, *Der p II*, *Der f I* (the first purified fraction of *D. farinae*), and *Der f II* do not seem to play a crucial role. However, a 90 kD polypeptide was found to be IgGd-specific in atopic dogs (Noli *et al.*, 1996). Rapid advances have been made in the past few years on allergen characterization and sequence determination by chemical and molecular biologic approaches. As a consequence, the amino acid sequence of numerous allergens including grass, weed, and tree pollens, mites, animal danders, and fungi are known (World Health Organization, 1995). Future research in veterinary dermatology will no doubt focus on the importance of these purified allergens.

Positive and negative controls are included in each skin test to determine the reactivity of the skin and to grade the skin test reactions. The negative control should be the diluent solution used to dilute the allergens. Most diluents are phosphate-buffered saline with 0.2 or 0.4% phenol added. Although it is rare, the diluent can irritate the skin of some dogs and cause false-positive reactions, which negates the remainder of the test. The positive control is used to determine the reactivity of the patient's skin. Most allergists in the USA use histamine phosphate at a strength of 1:100 000, whereas in Europe a 0.01% solution is most commonly used. Histamine tests the inflammatory response capability of the skin and not the lability of the mast cell. If the histamine reaction is poor, the skin test is invalid as far as negative reactions are concerned. Alternatively, a good histamine reaction does not guarantee that the negative skin test results are valid. The wheals caused by positive reactions to antigens are immunologically mediated and involve mast cell degranulation. Glucocorticoids stabilize cell membranes and this stability can apparently persist for some time.

A compound 48/80 is used by some allergists as a positive control. This compound stimulates mast cell degranulation and mimics immunologic degranulation. Not only is histamine released, but other inflammatory mediators are also included so the irritability of the skin is tested in a more natural fashion. A poor response to 48/80 can indicate that the skin has a poor inflammatory response potential or that the mast cells are decreased in number or reactive capability. A recent study (Mason and Lloyd, 1996) in dogs showed that compound 48/80 rapidly elicits dose responsive increases in skin thickness. The histologic changes in mast cell morphology, together with the induced tissue eosinophilia indicate that these changes might be mediated, at least in part, by mast cell degranulation. The accumulation of eosinophils, neutrophils, and mononuclear cells in histological specimens 6 hours and 30 hours after injection of compound 48/80 suggest that a late-phase reaction is also induced. For dogs, a concentration of 5 μg/ml has been suggested for skin testing.

The ideal positive control would be an antibody directed against reaginic antibody (IgE and/or IgGd). This antisera would cause immunologic mast cell degranulation. One author (WHM) used anti-IgE as a positive control and found it to be a better indicator of the reactivity of the dog than histamine. Unfortunately, this antisera is not available commercially.

Regardless of which positive control is used, if its reaction is poor, the remainder of the skin test is questionable. Positive reactions may be valid, but negative reactions are uninterpretable. With histamine, the maximum reaction occurs 8–10 minutes after the injection. With 48/80 or anti-IgE, the wheal reaches maximum size in 15–30 minutes (Mason and Lloyd, 1996). A good positive control reaction should be approximately 12–20 mm in diameter.

Test Antigen Concentration

If an allergen is too concentrated, it will cause a reaction in a nonallergic individual. The threshold concentration of an allergen is the maximum concentration at which a minimum, possibly zero, number of nonallergic animals will develop skin test reactions. Accordingly, the concentration of the test allergens should be such that no false-positive reactions occur. If the concentration is too low, allergic patients may not react, resulting in false-negatives. Therefore, the concentration should be adjusted so that the incidence of false-positive reactions is less than 10%.

Willemse and Van den Brom (1982) found that the skin threshold concentration for house dust, house dust mite, and human dandruff were the same in the dog as in man. For animal danders, pollen mixtures, and fungi, they found that the threshold concentration for the dog was ten times higher than it was in man. For pollens, a concentration of 1000 Noon units/ml was ideal for testing dogs. This is approximately equivalent to 500 PNU/ml. In another study on dogs (August, 1982), 90 normal dogs were tested with various concentrations of allergens and an acceptable threshold concentration of 1500 PNU/ml was found for ragweed, cocklebur, cotton linters, nylon, kapok, pyrethrum, and various mixtures. For house dust, a mold mixture, and a household insect mixture, a concentration of 250 PNU/ml was too irritating. These data show the variability in irritability of allergens.

In a study on cats (Bevier, 1990), test concentrations between 250 and 1250 PNU/ml were suggested depending upon the pollens involved. House dust extract was an irritant in a substantial percentage of cats at all tested concentrations ranging from 25–1500 PNU/ml. The threshold concentration for a 1:1 mixture of *D. farinae* and *D. pteronyssinus* appeared to be greater than 1:1000 W/V (Codner, 1996), which differed from the threshold concentration reported for house dust mites in the dog of 1:50 000 W/V (Codner and Tinker, 1995).

Most veterinary dermatologists use a concentration of 1000 PNU/ml for skin testing with most allergens. House dust and house dust mite extracts are known irritants and should be used at a strength of 250 PNU/ml or less. Other questionably irritating allergens are *Rhizopus nigricans*, sheep's wool, silk, animal danders, and mixed feathers. For these antigens, a strength of 250 or 500 PNU/ml has been suggested by some authors.

Initially, all allergens should be used on some normal dogs. If the reactivity for any one allergen is 10% or more, the concentration should be decreased. Ideally each new batch of allergens should be tested on normal dogs to make sure that the new antigens are not irritating. This is typically impossible and not necessary if the allergens are purchased from the same reputable allergy laboratory. Again, allergy test results should be kept in a tabular form and an indication should be made when a new batch of allergens is used. If there is a sudden increase or decrease in reactivity of a specific allergen, that allergen should be checked for e.g., concentration, dating and contamination.

Stability of Test Antigens

Allergens are biologic products that lose potency with time. Outdated extracts should be discarded. Loss of potency is affected by the nature of the preservative used, the concentration of the allergenic solution, the temperature, adhesion of allergenic components to plastic syringes, and the time. Also mixing of molds and pollen extracts may reduce the biologic activity of certain grass and weed pollen extracts when co-incubated in the same vial for 30 days. Such a decrease is due to mold extract proteases (Rosenbaum, 1996). Glycerinated extracts tend to lose potency less rapidly, but are not satisfactory for intradermal skin testing. In 1993, Campbell published some preliminary data, suggesting that skin-test strength allergens stored in plastic syringes lost potency more rapidly then allergens stored in glass syringes. Johnson (1995) corroborated the superiority of glass syringes, but showed that plastic syringes were satisfactory when syringes were changed frequently. Both of these studies were preliminary and further more detailed studies are awaited. Until such data are available, it would seem prudent to change the allergens stored in plastic syringes at least every 14 days.

Allergens kept at 35°C will lose approximately 50% of their antigenicity within seven days. To minimize the temperature-dependent loss of potency, allergens, especially those at skin strength, should be kept refrigerated. When the allergens are removed from the refrigerator for use, they should be kept cool with refrigerator packs available from the supplier.

One author (LMR) tested 20 dogs with two sets of antigens to determine what effect storage time had on skin test reactivity. One set was freshly made while the other was constantly refrigerated at 4°C for 30 days. A correlation of only 20% was seen. In those cases where fresh and dated allergens gave dissimilar results, the dated extracts gave false-negative results in 40% of the cases. Equally as interesting was the false-positive rate of 40% with the dated extracts. It would appear that stored antigens can not only lose potency, but can also undergo degradation, which can make them irritating. Another author (TW) has carried out a similar study with various allegenic extracts kept at 4°C or at room temperature for various store periods ranging from four weeks to 12 months. Stability in terms of reliable skin test results was present for nine months in those allergens stored at 4°C, whereas the allergens stored at room temperature lost their allergenicity after eight weeks. Obviously these data are very dissimilar and probably relate to differences in for example the antigens and preservatives used. This highlights the need to keep allergy test results in a tabular fashion. The point of allergen instability should become apparent when positive reactions start to decrease. Until a clinician develops the stability data for his or her own clinical situation, the recommendations from the allergen's manufacturer should be followed. When skin-test strength allergens are made 'in house', two authors (LMR, WHM) believe that the solutions should be replaced every 30–60 days.

Factors Affecting Skin Testing

Technique, allergen preparation, drugs, inherent host factors, and the season of the year can affect skin test results and cause false-positive or false-negative reactions. The most common reason for questionable test results is drug interference. Anti-inflammatory or immunosuppressive drugs decrease the reactivity of the skin and interfere with the interpretation of skin tests. Positive results obtained in the face of drug therapy are valid while negative results are open to question.

Diphenhydramine can suppress skin testing for 1.9 days, chlorpheniramine for 2.5 days, and hydroxyzine for 4.3 days. The authors suggest that all antihistamines are withdrawn for at least 7–10 days, but preferably 14 days, before skin testing. In man, glucocorticoids are not believed to interfere with allergy testing, but this is not so in the dog. The duration of the blocking effect of steroids is variable and depends on inherent host factors, the drug used, the dosage, route, and frequency of administration, and, most importantly, the duration of treatment. Since steroids are absorbed from topical preparations, even otic medications, all routes of administration must be considered. Patients who have been given oral glucocorticoids intermittently or for two weeks or less, can typically be skin tested after withdrawal of the drug for two weeks. When injectable drugs have been given, the withdrawal period is longer and is at least four weeks, but more typically, 6–8 weeks. The authors have seen cases where a valid skin test could not be obtained for at least four months after steroid withdrawal. When drug interference from steroids or other therapeutic agents may be a problem, the animal should be tested with the positive and negative controls before the complete skin test is started. If the skin reactivity is weak (i.e. with the formation of a poorly circumscribed flat histamine wheal) the complete skin test should be postponed for at least two weeks.

Inherent host factors also affect skin test results. Schwartzman (1984) showed that very young dogs were less reactive than young adult dogs and Willemse and Van den Brom (1983) found a significantly lower frequency of test reactions in dogs over six years of age. Young dogs could be less reactive because of their short periods of sensitization. Decreased reactivity of the skin with advancing age is recognized in man. Willemse's data from dogs support this observation and he offers the explanations of decreased antibody synthesis, alterations in the effector system, or changes in target organ sensitivity or responsiveness. August (1982) found a lower reactivity in adult dogs aged 1–4 years that could not be explained. He also noted an overall reduction in reactivity in animals with darker coats. Conflicting findings have been reported by Bevier (1990) who found that cats younger than 1½ years of age had a significantly higher response to allergens than older cats; a lower response was seen in cats with dark coats.

Pregnancy, stress, and serious internal diseases can reduce the reactivity of the skin. Healthy dogs that struggle violently during skin testing could release enough endogenous glucocorticoid and catecholamine to reduce or completely block skin reactivity. Two authors (LMR, WHM) have seen examples where satisfactory skin test results could not be obtained until the dog was tranquillized. In contrast, the other author (TW) has never experienced this stress-induced alteration of skin testing (taking a diminished histamine reaction as control) while testing highly stressed dogs.

It has been demonstrated that nonsedated dogs show a significant rise in their post-testing plasma cortisol concentrations (Frank *et al.*, 1992). However, since all the authors have tested many nonsedated excitable dogs with good results, the question on the need for sedation in skin testing remains unanswered. Since sedation makes the testing go more smoothly and quickly, two authors (LMR, WHM) routinely sedate all healthy dogs.

In man, maximum skin test reactivity occurs between 7 p.m. and 11 p.m. while the weakest reactivity occurs at 7 a.m. This probably is due to the circadian variation in plasma cortisol concentration. It is not known if this occurs in dogs, but seasonal variations in reactivity do occur.

Immunoglobulins, IgE, and/or IgGd, are involved in the pathogenesis of atopy. Both have serum and tissue half-lives. When allergen exposure stops, antibody synthesis should stop and the antibody concentrations should decrease. Halliwell and Kunkle (1978) reported that the radioallergosorbent test (RAST) reactivity of one ragweed allergic dog varied in excess of 300% when samples were taken at different times of the year. As expected, levels in the early summer were much lower than they were during the ragweed season. The variation in serum concentration could influence the results of skin testing.

Nesbitt *et al.* (1984) addressed the question of the seasonal variability of skin test results. His data are difficult to interpret, but he found some expected seasonal variations such as decreased reactivity to grasses during the winter. Unexpected reactions included a decreased reactivity to trees in spring and an increased reactivity to mixed ragweed in the summer before the peak ragweed season. The decreased reactivity to trees could be explained by anergy, but the ragweed reaction is hard to explain. Nesbitt *et al.* (1984) proposed that the high allergen load of the summer increases the dog's skin reactivity and thus lowers the allergic threshold to allergens. Accordingly, this phenomenon would increase the sensitivity of skin testing or increase the incidence of false-positive reactions.

When over 100 atopic dogs were tested three times at six-month intervals (Garfield, 1992), there was no difference in the overall results whether the testing was performed before, during, or after the allergy season. Since it appears that atopic dogs maintain allergen-specific IgE production long after the allergen has disappeared (Halliwell and Kunkle, 1978; Miller *et al.*, 1992), skin testing can be performed year round, as the above data suggest. However, testing too far away from the end of allergen exposure could decrease the skin test reactivity in some dogs, especially those with weaker (+2) reactions.

To maximize the reliability of a skin test, it may be best to test the animal within 60 days of the end of the allergy season. Tests done before the pollen period may be negative (false-negative) because the serum antibody concentration has dropped too low to be detected. Tests carried out during the peak pollen season may be false-negative. Such reactions could be due to pollen interference (anergy). During peak pollen periods, the animal can be exposed to such high concentrations of exogenous pollens that too few sensitized mast cells remain to be detected by skin testing. This anergy decreases as the number of sensitized mast cells increases.

The best time to test an animal intradermally depends on the seasonality of its problem. Animals with short well-defined pollen allergy periods should be tested at the end of the season. Animals with an allergy to indoor allergens only usually will react year round, but the early spring is the best time to test them. During the winter, the indoor allergen load increases because of the closed nature of the house and animals tend to spend more time inside. When the test is carried out in the spring, the animal's serum antibody concentration should be at its peak, but the antigen load should be decreasing so anergy will not be noted.

It is difficult if not impossible to define the best time to test a dog with long seasonal allergies (e.g. March through December) or the dog with perennial allergies. Valid results for all allergens can probably be obtained at any time, but testing in the fall or early winter is common. At this time, outdoor allergens should be significantly decreased while indoor allergens should not be high enough to cause anergy. Valid reactions to late summer, fall, and indoor allergens should be obtained, but spring and early summer allergens may be missed. A careful review of the history and skin test results will indicate if the animal's allergens have been well defined. If the spring and early summer reactions are questionable, the animal should be retested for those allergens in the late spring or early summer.

Some atopic animals will respond well to immunotherapy, but will start to scratch again at a later date. Provided the immunotherapy is not discontinued and the animal has no confounding pruritic disease, the most common reason for the return of pruritus is that the animal has become clinically allergic to new allergens. The original skin test results should be reviewed and the animal should be retested for those allergens that were not reactive on the first test.

Skin Test Site and Preparation

By convention, the skin over the lateral thorax is used for skin testing. If the animal is to be tested for only a few antigens, the abdominal skin can be used, but the testing is more difficult for several reasons: beyond restraint problems, the thinner abdominal skin is more difficult to test and the glabrous skin is more reactive then the skin elsewhere (August, 1982). The site should be clipped carefully with a number 40 blade or shaved. If the area is dirty, the site can be gently cleaned with a moist towel, but it should not be scrubbed. Inflamed or infected skin should not be used for testing. If a few pustules or papules are present, the site can be used, but these lesions should be avoided.

The skin test sites are marked with a waterproof marker. Typically, a dot is placed on the skin and the skin above or below the dot is tested. Occasionally, an axonal reflex from a strong positive reaction will enhance the reactivity of adjacent test sites. To avoid this, the test sites should be approximately 3–4 cm apart.

Skin Test Methods

Direct allergy skin testing can be done by the scratch, prick, or intradermal method. Minute amounts of allergen are used in the scratch and prick test and these tests are used in man to minimize the risk of severe systemic reactions. The prick test is performed by pricking the skin with a needle or lancet through a drop of allergen solution. With the scratch test, a scratch is made in the skin and the allergen is gently rubbed into the wound. With both methods, the patient must remain still for 15 minutes to prevent mixing of the antigens. Since animals rarely develop serious reactions to intradermal skin tests, have less sensitive skin than man, and will not remain still for 15 minutes, the scratch and prick tests are rarely used in animals. In addition, two authors (TW, WHM) have performed a pilot prick test study in dogs and found that extremely high concentrations of allergens were necessary in order to obtain results comparable to those of the intradermal test.

Intradermal, or more correctly intracutaneous, allergy testing is the method used in veterinary dermatology. The major advantages are that it is more sensitive, more accurate, and easier for the patient than the prick or scratch test. Since the method involves a larger allergenic challenge, false-positive reactions can occur and anaphylactic reactions, although very rare, have been reported (Scott *et al.*, 1995).

Technique

Most animals will tolerate a short skin test without sedation. Animals who struggle excessively may invalidate the skin test. Vicious animals or those who are expected to resent skin testing can be sedated or anesthetized. Potent hypotensive agents, morphine derivatives (because they are histamine liberators), and acepromazine should not be used. In the dog, xylazine, zolazepam, medetomidine, and tiletamine–zolazepam do not seem to block skin test reactivity, while ketamine is satisfactory for cats. Gas anesthesia can be used in either species. The animal is usually held or placed in lateral recumbency for testing.

Most veterinary dermatologists store their allergens in the refrigerator in tuberculin syringes with 26 or 27 gauge intradermal needles. The needles are not changed between dogs unless a needle becomes contaminated, bent, or dull. To the best of the authors' knowledge there are no reports in the veterinary literature documenting the transfer of an infectious disease from one patient to another during skin testing with the same needle. However, since cats can be asymptomatically infected with the leukemia or immunodeficiency virus, it seems to be prudent to change the needles between cats, especially if two or more are to be tested at the same time. Needle change when different species are tested should also be considered. After testing, the bevel of the needle will be coated with the patient's serum. If the next patient tested is allergic to the species tested previously (e.g. dog allergic to cats), the serum contaminating the needles might trigger mast cell degranulation, leading to false-positive skin test results or, far less likely, anaphylaxis. It is common practice to replace the needle before the syringe is refilled from the stock bottle. One author (TW) does not change the needle at each refill and has had no problems.

It is common practice to remove the skin testing syringes from the refrigerator 15–30 minutes before testing to prevent the patient struggling due to the injection of cold allergen. Depending on the number of animals tested each week, the length of time that the allergens are at room temperature can be considerable. As mentioned earlier, allergens can bind to the walls of plastic syringes and the rate of adherence is probably influenced by the frequency and length of time that the allergens are exposed to room temperature. Until detailed data are available on the influence of time and temperature, plastic syringes should be refilled frequently to avoid loss of potency. Refilling every seven days would seem to be optimal, but the available data suggest that a 14-day interval is probably satisfactory.

After the test site has been marked, the testing can be started. All air bubbles should be expelled from the syringe before testing. If air is injected with the allergen, a 'splash' reaction will occur and this reduces the precision and reliability of that test site. The skin at each test site should be held taut and the point of the needle is gently inserted in a forward lifting motion as if to pick up the skin with the tip of the needle. As the tip enters the skin, the pickup motion is gradually converted into a forward and downward pressure while the syringe barrel is lowered toward the skin. The bevel should lie completely within the epidermis. After the needle is placed, 0.02–0.05 ml of the allergen is forced into the skin to form a small bleb. Most clinicians use 0.05 ml as this is easier to measure on the syringe. It is imperative that the volume of each test antigen is exactly the same at each test site otherwise an accurate comparison of skin reactivity is impossible. Figures 4.2 and Plate 2 demonstrate the testing procedure.

If the needle is placed too deeply, the normal translucent bleb will not be seen. Hemorrhage also indicates poor needle placement. If a 'splash' reaction occurs or if the needle is placed too deeply, the test should be repeated at a new test site. Repeating the injection at the same test site can increase the incidence of false-positive reactions at that site and adjacent sites due to an axonal reflex.

After the testing has been completed, the anesthesia can be stopped. Manually restrained dogs are allowed to sit up, but must be prevented from scratching or licking the test site. Trauma to the test area will make reading the test difficult and can increase the incidence of false-positive reactions.

Interpretation of Skin Test Results

The allergy skin test reaction is a wheal, which reaches maximum size 12–17 minutes after the injection. The size of the reaction depends on the volume injected, the

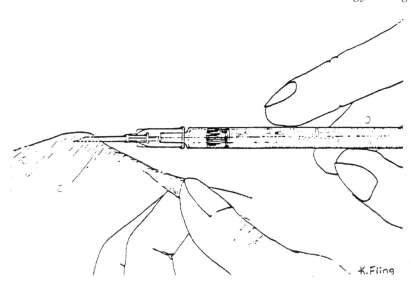

K.Fling

Figure 4.2 *Schematic of needle placement during intradermal testing.*

sensitivity of the mast cell system, and the sensitivity of the patient. Tests should be read 15 minutes after the injections have been completed. If a large number of allergens are used, the testing will take at least 15 minutes and the early injections will be ready to read at the end of the testing. In this case, the test is read at 15 and 30 minutes to make sure that no significant reactions are missed. Reading 15–20 minutes after performing the skin test is extremely important, since wheal size may be significantly reduced after 30 minutes. Cats' skin tests are difficult to read and should be checked at 10, 15, and 30 minutes. Two of the authors (LMR/WHM) skin test cats and believe that reliable results can be obtained. The remaining author (TW) does not. The reason for this is the difficulty or even inability to read the skin test. Skin reactions in cats are poorly circumscribed and weak on many occasions (Scott *et al.*, 1995). In some cases there are clearly defined wheals, but in others the results are inconsistent. Poor test results make it difficult, if not impossible to select allergens for immunotherapy.

Wheal size and quality are used to grade skin test reactions. The room should be darkened and the test site should be transilluminated with a bright light. This allows better visualization of the size and redness of the wheal.

Positive reactions can be defined by several different methods, each of which has its own advantages and disadvantages. If one is only interested in defining positive and negative reactions, any wheal significantly larger in diameter than the size of the negative control (i.e. 3 mm or greater) would be positive. Simply defining positivity or negativity makes the interpretation of false positive reactions difficult and potentially places the clinician at a disadvantage when antigens are selected for immunotherapy.

Most veterinary dermatologists use a grading system to classify the skin test reactions. Both objective and subjective considerations can be included. Objectively, wheal size is evaluated. A wheal the same size as the negative control is graded as a 0, while a wheal the size of the histamine reaction is a +4. Occasionally, a reaction larger than a +4 will be seen. A +1, +2, or +3 reaction is one which is one-quarter, one-half, or three-quarters the way between the size of the negative and positive controls. This gradation can be determined visually after some experience has been gained or the wheal diameters can be measured and the calculations can be made precisely. Instead of grading between 0 and +4, the diameter of the wheal can be expressed in mm. In other words each reaction to an allergen equal to or larger than the mean of the diameters of the negative and positive control, is judged as positive.

A permanent record of the skin test can be made as follows. Each wheal is circled with a dark marker and then the row is covered with clear transfer tape. As the tape is peeled from the animal's body, the marks around the wheals are lifted onto the tape. The tape is then transferred to the medical record and the wheal diameters can be measured accurately. Since reactions are usually oval or irregular (Figure 4.3), the average diameter is calculated by taking the sum of the greatest and smallest diameters and dividing by two.

Subjective considerations used include the induration, erythema, and steepness of the wall of the wheal. Flaring and pseudopods are common in human skin tests, but are rare in the dog. If two wheals are of identical size but one is more erythematous and indurated, it would be considered more reactive. Nesbitt *et al.* (1984) estimated that subjective considerations increase the incidence of positive reactions by 20–30%. An objective evaluation of these factors has not been performed so far. One author (TW) does not include induration, erythema, reflex erythema (which is erythema beyond the borders of the wheal), and pseudopods in his reading of the skin test. A skin test is shown in Plate 2.

After the results of the skin test have been recorded, the significance of the reactions, either positive or negative, must be evaluated in the light of the patient's exposure and clinical history. False-positive and false-negative reactions do occur. Positive reactions can be true or false-positives and true reactions only indicate that the patient has a skin sensitivity. The clinical significance of each reaction is based on the historical correlation.

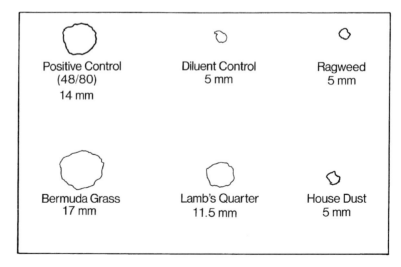

Figure 4.3   *Outline of allergy test reactions (actual size).*

False-positive reactions

Any positive reaction that occurs without a known history of exposure should be viewed as a false-positive. The question arises as to how this can occur. Most likely it is explained by the use of non-standardized allergens. Reactions that can be correlated with exposure, but do not fit the animal's clinical history, can be insignificant true reactions or false-positive reactions. A house dust skin test sensitivity in a dog with summer pruritus could be a true or a false-positive reaction. A true reaction could be a harbinger of a future or a remnant of a previous sensitivity. A false-positive reaction may be of no significance to the animal, but it is of significance to the clinician as the testing procedure needs to be reviewed.

The common reasons for the occurrence of false-positive reactions are shown in Table 4.17. Skin test reactions from all skin tested dogs should be kept in tabular form and reactions that do not fit the exposure or clinical history should be identified. If an allergen is apparently causing false-positive reactions in over 10% of the test population, the preparation of the allergen should be checked. House dust, house dust mite, sheep wool, and silk are known irritants and should be used at low concentrations. Epidermals (human, cat, horse), mold mixes, *Rhizopus nigricans*, insect mixes, red ant, tobacco, kapok, mixed feathers, and newsprint have also been reported to cause false-positive reactions. It is questionable whether some of these substances should be considered of any relevance for atopic dermatitis. Dogs who are skin tested repeatedly can develop skin sensitivities that are probably not of clinical significance. Reactions in these animals must be evaluated critically.

Dogs with very irritable skin (dermographism or traumatized skin test site) will often show many positive reactions. If the negative control reaction approaches the size of the positive control reaction or if the dog shows many positive reactions to allergens, that do not correlate with the exposure history, the results of the entire skin test are suspect and the test should be repeated at a later date.

False-negative reactions

False-negative skin test results are frustrating and difficult to evaluate. Common

Table 4.17 *Reasons for false-positive reactions.*

1. **Improper technique**
   A. Poor test site selection
   B. Poor test site preparation
   C. Injections too close together
   D. Excessive volume
   E. Traumatic needle placement

2. **Irritant test allergens**
   A. Excessive concentration
   B. Contamination
   C. Preservation with glycerin

3. **Irritable skin**
   A. Injections too close
   B. Dermographism

reasons for false-negative reactions are shown in Table 4.18. Not all classically atopic dogs will react to a skin test. Most publications report immediate skin test reactivity in 80–100% of dogs with clinical manifestations of atopic dermatitis (Scott, 1981; Carlotti and Costargent, 1994; Koch and Peters, 1994; Scott *et al.*, 1995; Sture *et al.*, 1995; Willemse, 1994).

The most common causes for a completely negative skin test are that the tentative diagnosis of atopy is incorrect, drug interference is occurring, or the causative allergens have not been tested. If the positive control reaction is not adequate, the test results are invalid. When drug interference is suspected, the patient should be tested with the positive and negative control weekly or bi-monthly until satisfactory reactions occur. A positive histamine reaction does not guarantee that the skin test will be valid. The histamine reaction tests the reactivity of the skin and not the reactivity of the IgE/mast cell system, which can be less reactive than the skin. If the patient is a strong atopic suspect, but does not react to any test antigens, the skin test can be repeated in 2–4 weeks. However, if the patient has been carefully screened, the likelihood of positive results at this second testing are low.

Table 4.18   *Reasons for false-negative reactions.*

1. **Improper technique**
    A. Wrong test site
    B. Insufficient volume
    C. Injection of air
    D. Subcutaneous injection
    E. Reading time after injection > 20 minutes

2. **Insufficient allergenic principle**
    A. Poorly manufactured allergen
    B. Old or outdated extract
    C. Solution too dilute
    D. Mixed antigen used
    E. Poorly prepared antigen

3. **Drug interference**
    A. Glucocorticoids
    B. Antihistamines
    C. Nonsteroidal anti-inflammatory drugs
    D. Immunosuppressive drugs
    E. Tranquilizers, sedatives
    F. Adrenergic compounds
    G. Progestational compounds
    H. Allergy immunotherapy

4. **Inherent host factors**
    A. Coat pigmentation
    B. Stress
    C. Estrus, pregnancy, or pseudocyesis
    D. Patient's age

5. **Incorrect antigen selection**

6. **Test done at the wrong time**

Failure to include the appropriate allergens in the test set can also cause false-negative allergy tests. Most patients presented for skin testing are nonseasonally pruritic and most skin test-positive dogs react to multiple antigens.

A more troublesome problem occurs when the dog is symptomatic during a certain period, but the reactions to the relevant allergens are negative; these reactions may be false-negatives. The historic correlation and the antigen selection should be reviewed and the skin test for the relevant allergens should be repeated. If the perennially pruritic dog shows no variation in the intensity of pruritus, it can be difficult if not impossible to detect false-negative reactions.

Other Methods of Allergy Testing

A wide variety of laboratory methods are available to assess allergic sensitivity, but these are practical only on a research basis. In clinical veterinary allergy, provocative exposure testing and serologic allergy tests can be used to try to document an animal's sensitivity to a substance.

Provocative testing

The basis of the provocative test is the purposeful exposure of an animal to a known or suspect allergen. In the clinical situation, a large dose of the allergen is given, so serious adverse reactions could occur. Provocative exposure testing is most applicable for food or contact sensitivity, but can also be used for other allergic conditions.

To obtain the most meaningful data, the test substance should be as pure as possible. The animal should be allowed to inhale, ingest, or contact the substance for a sufficient period of time to see the allergic reaction. If the animal reacts to a substance, it should be withdrawn and the animal should be given a sufficient period of time to return to normal before further testing.

In atopy, provocative exposure testing has limited applicability. The test can be used to determine the significance of some skin test or serologic test results. Since pollens and mold spores are not easily obtainable, provocative exposure testing is typically restricted to indoor allergens. For example, a dog reacts to feathers on the skin test, but the significance of this reaction is uncertain. The animal should be confined to a small clean room, typically a bathroom, and feathered products from the house should be put in the room. Shaking the objects would increase the concentration of 'allergen' in the room and should hasten the animal's response. If the animal is allergic to the objects, the signs should intensify almost immediately.

Aside from the difficulty in obtaining test antigens, provocative exposure testing for inhaled allergens is messy and the results can be unreliable. Most animals are not used to being confined to the bathroom and this can cause the animal to become mildly to markedly apprehensive. Very nervous animals may not scratch even if they are allergic to the substance, so negative results can be inconclusive. Positive results probably indicate a sensitivity, but the reaction may not be as specific as suspected. For example, old feathered products contain feathers, danders, dust, and house dust mites, so the animal could be reacting to one or more of these other allergens. Preliminary data have recently became available about aoroallergen contact sensitivity in atopic dogs (Frank and McEntee, 1995). Ten healthy control dogs and 18 dogs suspected of being atopic were intradermally and patch tested with yellow duck, timothy grass, and mixed house dust mite allergens. One asymptomatic control dog and one atopic dog developed reactions with both test methods to the house dust mite extract at 72 hours. The significance of these findings in clinical allergy should be elucidated.

Serologic tests

Serologic tests are used to measure or estimate the amount of allergen-specific antibody in a patient's serum. In veterinary medicine, two different methods are used commercially. The RAST uses radioactively labeled antisera while the enzyme-linked immunosorbent assay (ELISA) uses antibodies coupled to enzymes. Experimentally, relative amounts of canine allergen-specific IgE have been measured using the Western immunoblot test (Anderson *et al.*, 1996).

RAST and ELISA are mechanistically very similar. The patient's serum is added to wells containing different antigens in polystyrene titer plates. One ELISA test was a liquid-phase procedure instead of the classical plate-bound technique (Anderson *et al.*, 1996). After an appropriate incubation period, the titer plates are washed to remove any residual traces of the patient's serum. Next, radioactive or enzyme-linked anti-immunoglobulin antisera is added to the wells and allowed to incubate. After incubation, the plates are washed again to remove any unbound anti-immunoglobulin antisera. In the RAST test, the radioactivity of each well is then measured. In the ELISA test, chemicals are added to the wells to cause a color change, which can be visualized or measured. The higher the radioactivity count or the more intense the color change, the higher the concentration of anti-immunoglobulin in the well. Since the anti-immunoglobulin binds only to immunoglobulins, the radioactivity or intensity of the color change correlates with the concentration of allergen-specific antibody in the patient's serum. Both ELISA and RAST tests are commercially available for dogs and cats, but their diagnostic value is still not clear. This conclusion is based on the data where the agreement between *in vivo* and *in vitro* tests was seen to be variable and dependent upon the allergens involved, and on data where the sensitivity and specificity of tests were calculated.

Species-specific anti-immunoglobulin antisera must be used. In a study in dogs with experimentally-induced ragweed hypersensitivity, Peng *et al.* (1993) found a higher correlation between serum ragweed-specific IgE values (measured by ELISA) and passive cutaneous anaphylaxis (PCA) titers using a polyclonal IgE antibody rather than a monoclonal antibody. On a per antigen basis, serologic tests are more expensive than intradermal tests. To minimize the cost of these serologic tests, antigen groups rather than individual allergens are evaluated. Different allergens from similar groups are mixed in one well. Grasses are mixed with grasses, weeds are mixed with weeds, and so forth. The number of wells or groups tested as well as the number of allergens per group is variable.

In the original investigatory work on IgE RAST testing in dogs, Halliwell and Kunkle (1978) found extreme variability in the test results depending upon which allergen was used. For ragweed, there was an 82% agreement between positive skin results and positive RAST results. The positive correlation for house dust mite was 42%; for timothy grass, 64%; for English plantain, 39%; for lamb's quarter, 27%; and for dandelion, 12.5%. There was no consistent tendency for dogs with stronger skin test reactions to give higher RAST values. He found excellent correlation (100%) between negative RAST and negative skin test results.

Using an ELISA method, Willemse *et al.* (1985) found measurable allergen-specific IgGd antibody levels in 89% of his skin test-positive allergic dogs, while 55% of his skin test-negative but clinically allergic dogs had elevated titers. Similar to Halliwell and Kunkle (1978), he found that the correlation between postive skin test results and positive ELISA test results varied with the test antigen, ranging from 7% for cat dander to 65% for house dust. Recent evaluation of this ELISA (Willemse, 1994) has shown the following agreement between the IgGd ELISA and immediate skin test reactivity: for house dust mites (*D. farinae* and *D. pteronyssinus*), 62.5–84%; for storage mites (*Tyrophagus putrescentiae, Acarus siro,* and *Glycyphagus domesticus*) 50–84.6%; for epidermals (dog dander, cat dander, human dander), 25–60%; and for pollens (grasses, weeds, and trees) 33.3–75%.

The results of Halliwell and Kunkle (1978) and Willemse (Willemse *et al.*, 1985; Willemse, 1994) are not directly comparable since they used different methods, antibodies (IgE and IgGd respectively), allergens, and patients. Willemse's group of skin test-negative, but ELISA-positive dogs (Willemse *et al.*, 1994) can be explained in several different ways. These dogs could truly be allergic to the allergens, but showed false-negative skin test reactions or, alternatively, the ELISA reactions could be false-positives.

The RAST and ELISA tests available on a commercial basis measure IgE antibodies and most use allergen groups instead of individual antigens for testing. If IgGd is important in the pathogenesis of canine atopy, the measurement of just IgE would cause an increased incidence of false-negative serologic test results. The low sensitivity of Halliwell's IgE RAST would support this contention. Another common problem with both tests is that group allergens are used. Positive reactions can be difficult to evaluate. A group positive could be due to positive reactions to each component or a strong reaction to only one antigen. Accordingly, antigen selection for immunotherapy can be difficult. Another problem is that serologic tests can show positive results while the skin test for the same antigens is negative. The serologic test could be detecting a low level of sensitivity on the animal's part or the reactions could be false-positives. The authors have seen serologic data where the dogs are supposedly sensitive to allergens to which they have never been exposed. Completely irrelevant results can also be seen with skin testing, but the incidence appears to be very low. These false-positive reactions could have been due to technical problems encountered during the testing or could point out shortcomings of serologic testing.

Fortunately there is an increasing number of reports on the reliability of commercial serologic allergy tests on allergen-specific IgE in animals. Kleinbeck *et al.* (1989) reported an agreement between ELISA and skin test results ranging from 43–64% for pollens. With respect to these extracts the greatest degree of correlation was seen with individual components that included Bermuda grass, carelessweed, English plantain, and olive tree pollen. The lowest degree of correlation was evident with June grass, rye grass, giant ragweed, and birch tree pollen. The correlation for mite antigens was 43%. Bond *et al.* (1994) concluded that the poor specificity and the low positive predictive value of two commercial tests were reason enough to state that positive results using these IgE ELISAs were of no diagnostic value in canine atopy.

Similar conclusions were made by Codner and Griffin (1996) and Paradis and Lecuyer (1993) evaluating other commercial IgE ELISA or RAST tests. Anderson *et al.* (1996) determined the sensitivity and specificity of an IgE ELISA and total-IgG ELISA compared with the intradermal test. It should be emphasized that total IgG other than IgGd has been studied. The median sensitivity (%) and specificity (%) of the IgE test for grasses were 45% and 49%; for weeds, 30% and 70%; for molds, 36% and 63.5%; for trees, 22% and 74%; and for house dust, 30% and 42%. Similar data for the IgG ELISA for grasses were 81.5% and 17%; for weeds, 57% and 48%; for molds, 52.5% and 45.5%; for trees, 22% and 58%; and for house dust, 75% and 0%. Combining these data did not clearly differentiate in favor of one test.

Although several commercial laboratories offer *in vitro* assays for the diagnosis of atopy and food hypersensitivity in cats, the performance of these tests is largely unknown. In one study of 36 cats with allergic skin disease (Foster and O'Dair, 1993), the IgE ELISA test showed low predictive value for flea bite hypersensitivity and atopy and was not considered to be a useful diagnostic test. The authors' limited experience with these feline serologic tests also casts doubts on their reliability.

In human medicine, the rates of correlation between RAST and skin test results vary widely depending upon the study, method of skin testing used, and the allergen investigated. The original report on RAST testing in man showed a 68% correlation between RAST and intradermal test results. The discrepancies were mostly due to weakly positive skin tests combined with negative RAST results. Less sensitive skin test methods such as the prick or scratch test give better correlations with RAST results. It is generally agreed that there is good correlation between negative RAST results and negative skin test results so RAST testing is useful in distinguishing between true- and false-positive intradermal test results.

In man, the rate of correlation between RAST results and provocative challenge testing is better than the rate of correlation with intradermal testing. When RAST results are evaluated in the light of the patient's history coupled with intradermal and/or provocative testing, a correlation rate of 90–95% can be achieved. Thus it would appear that RAST testing can be very useful in identifying clinically significant allergens.

Assuming that serologic tests are or could be made reliable, they have several advantages. The office testing is quick and painless for the patient and the veterinarian does not have to invest in dated biologic materials. The cost to the client will be at least as expensive if not more so, than a skin test, but since all veterinarians will be able to do the testing, the dollar value associated with a trip to the veterinary dermatologist will be eliminated. Most of the factors causing false skin test reactions have limited applicability here. In man, samples can be taken while the patient is taking anti-inflammatory drugs. In dogs, 21 days of corticosteroid therapy does not seem to influence serologic test results. In addition antibody titers seem to persist for at least 60 days after allergen exposure (Miller *et al.*, 1992). Whether long-term administration of corticosteroids has any impact on test results needs to be investigated. Hence, steroids should not be administered for more than three weeks before *in vitro* allergy testing. The effects of conditions such as pregnancy and serious metabolic diseases have not been studied. Until information is available about the effects of these conditions, allergy testing should be postponed until the animal is healthy.

Although the timing of allergy testing can affect the results (Halliwell and Kunkle, 1978) it should be realized that serologic tests can detect very low antibody concentrations. Therefore the timing of sample collection may not be as critical as it can be in skin testing. Except for seasonal allergies or perennial allergies with seasonal exacerbations, *in vitro* tests could be performed at the beginning or at the end of the season.

When there are discrepancies between serologic and intradermal results, one must decide which is correct. As skin testing has been used for years, most dermatologists feel that this test is more reliable. The animal's response to immunotherapy can help determine the accuracy of the serologic test results. The efficacy of immunotherapy based on IgE RAST and ELISA results and/or intradermal testing commonly range from 60–80% (Scott *et al.*, 1995). Combining the results of *in vitro* testing and intradermal testing has been shown to increase the efficacy of hyposensitization. In a double-blind placebo-controlled study on the efficacy of hyposensitization at least 50% improvement was noticed in 60% of the dogs treated with vaccine based on skin test results (Willemse *et al.*, 1984). This percentage rose to 80% if the animals were hyposensitized on the basis of the cumulative results of the intradermal test and the IgGd ELISA (Willemse, 1994).

At the moment it is still not clear what the diagnostic, and therefore therapeutic value of *in vitro* allergy tests is in comparison to that of the intradermal test. With the currently available commercial tests, it is clear that the intradermal test is superior to the *in vitro* tests and should be considered the gold standard. Future refinements in the *in vitro* tests may make the two tests more equal. Despite their shortcomings, the current *in vitro* tests for dogs do have a place in veterinary allergy. The same cannot be said for the cat test. Since intradermal testing is not available to all clients, the *in vitro* test offers the option of immunotherapy to many dogs that would otherwise have to be managed with various medications. If the test results are evaluated critically in the light of the patient's history and not just accepted at face value, the response rate to immunotherapy approaches that seen with the intradermal test (Anderson and Sousa, 1993). As mentioned earlier, the combination of *in vitro* and intradermal results may describe a dog's allergies more completely and therefore increase the efficacy of immunotherapy (Willemse, 1994). Large double-blind placebo-controlled studies with standardized case selection (Willemse, 1986) are needed to support or refute the preliminary data which now exist. The results of these studies are eagerly awaited.

References

Anderson RK, Sousa CE. *In vivo* vs *in vitro* testing for canine atopy. In Ihrke PJ, Mason IS, White SD (eds) *Advances in Veterinary Dermatology*, Volume 2, Workshop Report 7. Pergamon Press, Oxford, UK, pp. 425–427, 1993.

Anderson R, Griffin C, Miller W, *et al. In vivo* vs. *in vitro* testing for atopy. *12th Proc Ann Members' Meeting Am Acad Vet Derm & Am Coll Vet Derm.* Congress Organisation, Las Vegas, Nevada, 1996, pp. 14.

August JR. The reaction of canine skin to the intradermal injection of allergenic extracts. *J. Am. Anim. Hosp. Assoc.* **18:** 157–171, 1982.

Bessot JC, de Blay F, Pauli G. From allergen sources to reduction of allergen exposure. *Eur. Resp. J.* **7:** 392–397, 1994.

Bevier DE. The reaction of feline skin to intradermal injection of allergenic extracts and passive cutaneous anaphylaxis using serum from skin test positive cats. In

Von Tscharner C, Halliwell REW (eds) *Advances in Veterinary Dermatology*, Volume 1. Baillière Tindall, London, pp. 126–136, 1990.

Bond R, Thorogood SC, Lloyd DL. Evaluation of two enzyme-linked immunosorbent assays for the diagnosis of canine atopy. *Vet. Record* **135**: 130–133, 1994.

Campbell KL, Hall IA. Effect of storage of allergens in plastic and glass syringes on the results of intradermal skin testing in dogs. *Proc. Am. Acad. Vet. Dermatol. & Am. Coll. Vet. Derm.* **9**: 48, 1993.

Carlotti DN, Costargent F. Analysis of positive skin tests in 449 dogs with allergic dermatitis. *Eur. J. Comp. Anim. Pract.* **4**: 42–59, 1994.

Codner EC, Tinker MK. Reactivity to intradermal injections of extracts of house dust and house dust mite in healthy dogs and dogs suspected of being atopic. *J. Am. Vet. Med. Assoc.* **206**: 812–816, 1995.

Codner EC. Reactivity to intradermal injections of extracts of house dust mite and flea antigen in normal cats and cats suspected of being allergic. *Proc. 12th Ann. Members' Meeting Am. Acad. Vet. Derm. & Am. Coll. Vet. Derm.* Congress Organisation, Las Vegas, Nevada, pp. 26–27, 1996.

Codner EC, Griffin CE. Serologic allergy testing for dogs. *Comp. Cont. Ed.* **18**: 237–247, 1996.

D'Ammato G, Spieksma FTM, Bonini S. *Allergenic Pollen and Pollinosis in Europe.* Blackwell Science, Oxford, 1991.

Driessen MNBM, Derksen JWM, Spieksma FTM, *et al. Pollenatlas van de Nederlandse Atmosfeer.* Onkenhout Publ, Hilversum (the Netherlands), 1988.

Foster AP, O'Dair H. Allergy testing for skin disease in the cat *in vivo* vs *in vitro* tests. *Vet. Dermatol.* **4**: 111–115, 1993.

Frank LA, McEntee MF. Demonstration of aeroallergen contact sensitivity in dogs. *Vet. All. Clin. Immunol.* **3**: 75–80, 1995.

Frank LA, Kunkle GA, Beale KM, *et al.* Comparison of serum cortisol concentration before and after intradermal testing in sedated and nonsedated dogs. *J. Am. Vet. Med. Assoc.* **200**: 507–510, 1992.

Garfield RA. Injection immunotherapy in the treatment of canine atopic dermatitis: comparison of 3 hyposensitization protocols. Presented at the Annual Members Meeting of the American Academy of the Veterinary Dermatologists and the American College of Veterinary Dermatology, **8**: 7–8, 1992.

Halliwell REW, Kunkle GA. The radioallergosorbent test in the diagnosis of canine atopic dermatitis. *J. All. Clin. Immunol.* **62**: 236–242, 1978.

Johnson CA. The effects of constant and variable temperature on the biological activity of allergens stored in plastic and glass syringes. *Proc. Am. Acad. Vet. Dermatol. & Am. Coll. Vet. Derm.* **11**: 18–19, 1995.

Kleinbeck ML, Hites MJ, Loker JL, *et al.* Enzyme-linked immunosorbent assay for measurement of allergen-specific IgE antibodies in canine serum. *Am. J. Vet. Res.* **50**: 1831–1839, 1989.

Koch HJ, Peters S. 207 Intrakutantests bei Hunden mit Verdacht auf atopische Dermatitis. *Kleintierpraxis* **39**: 25–36, 1994.

Lee RD. Allergy to storage mites. *Clin. Exp. Allergy* **24**: 636–640, 1994.

Mason IS, Lloyd DH. Evaluation of compound 48/80 as a model of immediate hypersensitivity in the skin of dogs. *Vet. Dermatol.* **7**: 81–83, 1996.

Miller WH Jr, Scott DW, Cayette SM, *et al.* The influence of oral corticosteroids or declining allergen exposure on serologic allergy test results. *Vet. Dermatol.* **3**: 237–244, 1992.

Nesbitt GH, Kedan GS, Caciolo P. Canine atopy. Part I: Etiology and diagnosis. *Comp. Cont. Ed.* **6:** 75–84, 1984.

Noli C, Bernadina WE, Willemse T. The significance of reactions to purified fractions of *Dermatophagoides pteronyssinus* and *Dermatophagoides farinae* in canine atopic dermatitis. *Vet. Immunol. Immunopathol.* **52:** 147–157, 1996.

Paradis M, Lecuyer M. Evaluation of an in-office allergy screening test in nonatopic dogs having various intestinal parasites. *Can. Vet. J.* **34:** 293–295, 1993.

Peng Z, Simons FER, Becker AB. Measurement of ragweed-specific IgE in canine serum by use of enzyme-linked immunosorbent assays containing polyclonal and monoclonal antibodies. *Am. J. Vet. Res.* **54:** 239–243, 1993.

Rosenbaum MR. The effects of mold proteases on the biological activity of pollen allergenic extracts in atopic dogs. *Proc. 12th Ann. Members' Meeting Am. Acad. Vet. Derm. & Am. Coll. Vet. Derm.* Congress Organisation, Las Vegas, Nevada, 1996, pp. 20–21.

Schwartzman RM. Immunologic studies of progeny of atopic dogs. *Am. J. Vet. Res.* **45:** 375–378, 1984.

Scott DW. Observations on canine atopy. *J. Am. Anim. Hosp. Assoc.* **17:** 91–101, 1981.

Scott DW, Miller WH, Griffin CE. *Small Animal Dermatology*, 5th edition Philadelphia, Saunders Co., 1995.

Sture GR, Halliwell REW, Thoday KL, *et al.* Canine atopic dermatitis: the prevalence of positive intradermal skin tests at two sites in the north and south of Great Britain. *Vet. Immun. Immunopathol.* **44:** 293–308, 1995.

Vollset I. Immediate type hypersensitivity in dogs induced by storage mites. *Res. Vet. Sci.* **40:** 123–127, 1986.

Willemse T, Van den Brom WE. Evaluation of the intradermal allergy test in normal dogs. *Res. Vet. Sci.* **32:** 57–61, 1982.

Willemse T, Van den Brom WE. Investigations of the symptomatology and the significance of immediate skin test reactivity in canine atopic dermatitis. *Res. Vet. Sci.* **34:** 261–265, 1983.

Willemse T, Van den Brom WE, Rijnberk A. Effect of hyposensitization on atopic dermatitis in dogs: a double blind, placebo-controlled study. *J. Am. Vet. Med. Assoc.* **184:** 1277–1280, 1984.

Willemse T, Noordzij A, Van den Brom WE, *et al.* Allergen-specific IgGd antibodies in dogs with atopic dermatitis as determined by the enzyme-linked immunosorbent assay (ELISA). *Clin. Exp. Immunol.* **59:** 359–363, 1985.

Willemse T. Atopic skin disease: a review and a reconsideration of diagnostic criteria. *J. Small Anim. Pract.* **27:** 771–778, 1986.

Willemse T. Hyposensitization of dogs with atopic dermatitis based on the results of *in vivo* and *in vitro* (IgGd ELISA) diagnostic tests. *10th Proc Am Coll Vet Derm*, Congress Organisation, Charleston (USA), April 14–17, 1994, pp. 61.

World Health Organization. Allergen nomeclature. WHO/IUS Allergen Nomenclature Subcommittee World Health Organization, Geneva, Switzerland. *Clin. Exp. Allergy* **25:** 27–37, 1995.

$$5$$

Immunotherapy

Introduction

The three management options available for allergy are avoidance, symptomatic therapy, or immunotherapy. Avoidance is ideal since in the absence of antigen there are no symptoms and therefore no treatment is needed, but total avoidance of the causative allergen is only possible or practical for food, drug, or contact allergies and rarely achievable for inhalant allergies. At best, avoidance in atopy can decrease exposure, which may lessen symptoms. Symptomatic treatment is limited to counteracting or diminishing the symptoms. No studies have shown that pharmacologic treatment of atopy modifies the spontaneous long-term and usually progressive course of the disease. Symptomatic or pharmacologic therapy is discussed in Chapter 6.

The purpose of establishing a specific diagnosis in allergic disease is the institution of specific treatment. Allergen avoidance and immunotherapy are the only specific treatments available to allergic patients. The most promising aspect of immunotherapy is that it has the potential to induce a prolonged clinical remission in selected patients (Creticos, 1992). The normal course of atopy, especially in dogs, is progressive, with the condition worsening each year. In addition to altering the spontaneous course of atopy, immunotherapy may also prevent the onset of new sensitizations (Des Roches, 1995). In other words, immunotherapy may be a causal treatment (treating the cause of the disease rather than the symptoms).

History

The first published report of immunotherapy was by Noon in 1911, who treated human seasonal rhinitis with a series of injections of pollen extracts. He theorized that the excellent results he obtained was caused by antitoxin immunity. Besredka (cited in Patterson *et al.*, 1983; Nelson *et al.*, 1993) later coined the term 'desensitization' to refer to repeated injections of gradually increasing sublethal doses of antigen into previously sensitized animals. He believed that this process slowly depleted or neutralized anaphylactic antibodies (or depleted mediators), thus protecting against anaphylaxis. Cooke (1915) was unable to observe any change in skin test reactivity in a group of human atopics following a series of pollen injections. He attributed this to unneutralized antibody and suggested that the term 'hyposensitization' be substituted for 'desensitization'. Cooke called the serum factor found in high titers in treated hay fever patients 'blocking antibody'. He theorized that the relief afforded by hyposensitization was caused by the competition between circulating blocking antibody and cell-fixed reagin, now known as IgE.

In 1941, Wittich described a four-year-old female fox terrier with seasonal (fall) pruritus, rhinitis, and hives of three years' duration. He found strong positive skin test reactions to fall weeds, especially ragweed, and the dog was successfully hyposensitized with injections of these specific antigens. This was the first published clinical description, as well as the first report of successful immunotherapy, in canine atopy. In 1982, Reedy described a group of feline skin diseases with positive skin tests to inhalant allergens that responded to injection immunotherapy.

Definition

Immunotherapy in the field of allergy consists of giving gradually increasing doses of specific causative allergen(s) to allergic patients in an attempt to increase their tolerance for and reduce their sensitivity to these allergens. Immunotherapy entails manipulation of the patient's immune system and when effective may be considered as 'immunomodulation'. Desensitization and hyposensitization are not appropriate terms in atopy since they imply mechanisms that are not completely accurate. Although all three terms will be used interchangeably in this chapter, immunotherapy, which does not imply the type of immunologic mechanism involved in the therapeutic effect obtained, is a neutral and therefore preferred term for desensitization or hyposensitization.

In certain clinical situations, such as drug-induced or serum-induced anaphylaxis, antigens can be administered with sufficient rapidity and in sufficient quantity to rapidly neutralize the IgE antibody available (Sullivan, 1993). Skin tests may become negative and the patient is briefly clinically tolerant to the drug or serum proteins. This can be considered to be true desensitization and is used primarily in human patients with allergy to penicillin, horse serum, or insulin. Although immunotherapy is used for unrelated therapeutic approaches, particularly in oncology, in this chapter it will primarily apply to the type of injection therapy used to modify the IgE antibody-mediated immediate-type reactions to aeroallergens.

Mechanism of Action

A wide variety of immunologic events occur during immunotherapy. Although a great deal is known about the process in man, the exact mechanism for its clinical effectiveness is not completely understood. Little work has been done in animals to explain the mode of action. The following discussion is based on data from humans. The first change seen is an increase in the serum concentration of allergen-specific IgG. These IgG antibodies are thought to act as blocking antibodies by combining with circulating allergen to form immune complexes incapable of causing mast cell degranulation. These changes can be seen after only a few months of therapy and may explain some of the early improvement seen with immunotherapy. Although the concentration of IgG correlates with the quantity of antigen administered, the beneficial effects are variable. In some studies (Connell and Klein, 1970), the increase in blocking antibody concentration correlates well with clinical improvement while poor correlation has been seen in other studies. Measurement of allergen-specific IgG concentration does not predict accurately how a patient will respond to immunotherapy as the highest titers are not necessarily found in the patients with the mildest symptoms. The IgG concentration will eventually plateau despite the continuation of immunotherapy.

A second change seen during the initial phase of immunotherapy is an increase in the concentration of both circulating and bound allergen-specific IgE. These early increases in specific IgE do not seem to be pathogenic, probably as a result of a reduced binding affinity of the Fc receptor on the molecule, or a switch in production from IgE+ to IgE– (Malling and Weeke, 1993). Lichtenstein (1988) described a heterogeneity for IgE and designated IgE molecules that interact with histamine-releasing factor (HRF) as IgE+ and the remaining IgE molecules as IgE–. After long-term successful immunotherapy a decrease in allergen-specific IgE can be demonstrated in some allergic patients, but it is rarely eliminated entirely, so a state of true desensitization is not reached. In these patients, the normal post-seasonal rise in IgE antibody levels is abolished, suggesting the development of an immunologic tolerance. This modulation of IgE production is thought to be an effect of immunotherapy on the T lymphocyte population, which regulates antibody production (deVries, 1994). Even though the concentration of serum IgE antibody to ragweed in highly sensitive untreated patients correlates with their symptom scores, the decrease in allergen-specific IgE alone is not sufficient to account for the clinical improvement seen with successful immunotherapy. In one study (Nish *et al.*, 1994), antigen–specific IgE was decreased from baseline in only two of nine atopic subjects after six months, while antigen-specific IgG increased in eight of nine subjects. This is consistent with the observation that decreases in the seasonal rise in IgE antibody concentration may not correlate with clinical improvement; in any one patient, clinical efficacy may be achieved with a decrease, no change, or an increase in the concentration of IgE.

In some human patients, elevations in IgA and IgG concentration can be demonstrated in nasal secretions following immunotherapy (Platt-Mills *et al.*, 1976). This is particularly interesting since allergens in atopy are airborne. As such, they are introduced to the immune system through the mucosal surfaces in the airways or gut. From this point of view, secretory IgA is likely to be involved. The elevated IgA concentration following immunotherapy could indicate a local trapping of the allergen at the mucous membranes.

A growing body of evidence supports T cell modulation as the basis for effective immunotherapy. Allergen-specific T lymphocyte suppressor cells cannot be found in the blood of untreated atopic patients (Rocklin, 1983). However, with immunotherapy, allergen-specific suppressor cells can be found. With all these findings, it would appear that immunotherapy is affecting the control mechanisms of the immune response and not just antibody production. In venom allergy, immunotherapy has been shown to reduce the expression of the low-affinity IgE receptor on T and B cells (Prinz *et al.*, 1991). Additionally, some patients show decreased sensitivity of their mast cells (Malling and Weeke, 1993). Degranulation of these cells requires a greater insult and there may be a reduction in chemical mediator release. Hypothetically, the mechanism of immunotherapy could 'turn-off' the allergic reaction, thereby interrupting the chain of events characterizing the allergic disease. First, immunotherapy induces a switch of the preferential differentiation from T helper (TH) 2 type effectors to the TH1 type cells. The switch of cytokine profile to a primary interleukin-2 (IL-2) and interferon (IFN) γ response results in inhibition of the IL-4-dependent IgE production, reinforced by a decrease in the production of IL-4 from TH2 cells. Secondly, the activity of mast cells is reduced because of a lack of IL-3-dependent activation, a reduced local production of IgE, and a decreased production of histamine-releasing factors. A cytokine-independent decrease in mediator release from mast cells could concurrently be present, as well as a switch from IgE+ to IgE–. In combination with a reduced production of IL-5, the activity of eosinophils is decreased, resulting in less inflammation and destruction.

Allergic reactions tend to be biphasic. After the initial mast cell activation, there is a second reaction 2–8 hours later referred to as the late phase reaction (LPR). This is characterized by an influx of inflammatory cells, predominantly neutrophils and eosinophils (Georgitis, 1995). There is also further leukotriene and histamine release during the LPR indicating alternative sources of these inflammatory mediators other than the mast cell. In terms of reactivity, the tissues during the LPR also respond to lower doses of allergen than the initial exposure (Becker *et al.*, 1989).

Immunotherapy decreases the size of the cutaneous LPR more than the cutaneous early response, but the mechanisms remain obscure (Iliopoulos *et al.*, 1991). IL-12 may promote TH1 responses and inhibition of LPR following successful immunotherapy (Durham, 1995). A decrease in allergen-induced histamine-releasing factor production is one possible explanation for the decrease in cutaneous LPR histamine production. It is postulated that suppression of the immediate skin response may occur as a consequence of a reduction in mast cell numbers, whereas suppression of the LPR results from modification of the T lymphocyte response to allergen after successful immunotherapy (Walker *et al.*, 1995). The LPR is apparently more relevant to clinical disease with a progressive decline in symptoms being accompanied by a similar decline in the cutaneous LPR to grasses. Although the decrease in LPR paralleled clinical improvement, there was no significant correlation between the size of the LPR or magnitude of change in the late response and seasonal symptoms or medication requirements. This raises the possibility that inhibition of the LPR may represent an early clinical marker of response to immunotherapy. Even more relevant are the concomitant effects of immunotherapy on the various lymphokines and cytokines that direct cellular responses. This supports the hypothesis that immunotherapy alters the allergic inflammatory response through T cell tolerance (VanMetre and Adkinson, 1993).

Immunotherapy significantly decreases both early and late histamine release (Kuna *et al.*, 1989). This suggests that immunotherapy might be exerting a down-regulating effect on both the mast cell, presumably the source of early histamine, and the basophil, which may contribute to the late histamine release. Immunotherapy may suppress the function of TH2 cells and their cytokine production rather than having a direct quantitative effect on the nonlymphocytic inflammatory cells. Immunotherapy can suppress the production of histamine-releasing factor and augment the production of histamine-releasing inhibitory factor (IL-8) (Hsieh, 1995). This mechanism may account partly for its clinical efficacy. Immunotherapy decreases the enhanced proliferation of peripheral blood lymphocytes and suppresses cytokine production (mitogenic factor, macrophage inhibiting factor) to allergen (Evans *et al.*, 1976). Other proposed mechanisms responsible for these changes include specific or nonspecific diminished cellular responsiveness, or a combination of these antibody and cellular changes (VanMetre and Adkinson,

1993). No single factor is likely to be responsible for the improvement seen with immunotherapy.

Selection of Candidates for Immunotherapy

In order for a patient to be a candidate for immunotherapy:

- the patient must have a history and symptoms characteristic of atopy;
- other possible causes should be ruled out;
- the symptoms should be severe enough and last long enough to justify allergy testing and immunotherapy;
- the patient must have demonstrable *in vivo* or *in vitro* evidence of specific IgE or IgGd sensitivity to relevant allergen(s);
- the allergens cannot be sufficiently avoided or eliminated and are known to be effective in immunotherapy;
- the patient is not responding adequately to non-steroidal drug treatment, is having undesirable side effects, or requires frequent use of glucocorticoids;
- the wishes, patience, and intelligence of the owner have been considered.

The classical and nonclassical signs and symptoms of atopy are discussed in Chapter 2, as are the important differential diagnoses. Even though atopy may begin with relatively mild seasonal symptoms, it is usually a progressive disease that worsens each year. Veterinarians are advised to discuss this possibility with the owners early in the course of the disease to avoid misunderstandings about treatment options and relapses. This is especially true if glucocorticoids are to be used in the symptomatic treatment (see Chapter 6).

A critical issue is whether a given positive allergy test is clinically relevant. Not all patients with positive skin or serum test reactions to a specific allergen are clinically sensitive to that allergen (Norman *et al.*, 1973). Unless the significance of the reaction can be proved by provocative exposure, the significance can only be estimated by the veterinarian after a careful review of the symptoms, history, and allergy test results.

The animal's age and degree of sensitivity are used by some clinicians to select candidates for immunotherapy. Although there have been reports to suggest that younger patients respond better and quicker (Nesbitt, 1978), older patients with a long history of allergies can also respond to immunotherapy (Scott, 1981). The degree of sensitivity should not be used to select candidates for immunotherapy. In retrospective studies (Reedy, 1979), patients with weak but significant positive allergy tests respond as well to immunotherapy as patients with strong positive allergy tests. Therefore age and degree of sensitivity alone should not be used to exclude animals from immunotherapy.

Although the clinician may consider a given patient an ideal candidate for immunotherapy, the final decision rests with the owner. Allergy tests should not be performed unless the owner understands that the main purpose will be to select allergens for long-term immunotherapy. No owner should ever be encouraged to begin immunotherapy unless all factors such as cost, chances of success, lag time, concomitant therapy, length of treatment, risk, dedication, and patience have been

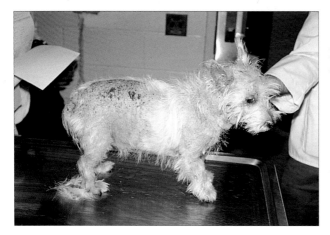

Plate 1 *Generalized self-trauma in a chronically atopic dog.*

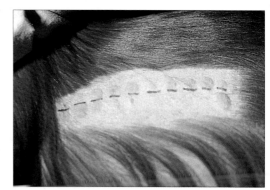

Plate 2 *Intradermal skin testing.*

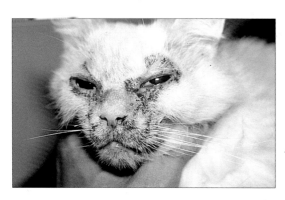

Plate 3 *Facial pruritus induced by a food hypersensitivity to milk.*

Plate 4 *The ventral abdomen of the dog in Figure 8.1 (page 194).*

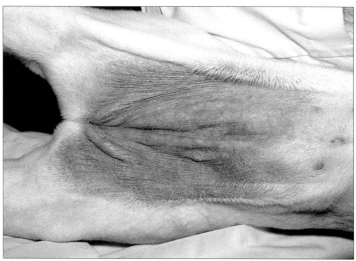

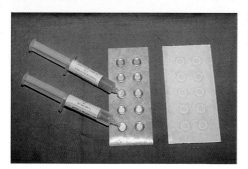

Plate 5 *Patch testing kit for allergic contact dermatitis. (Courtesy of Dr Thierry Olivry.)*

Plate 6 *3+ reaction to nickel in a dog allergic to cement.*

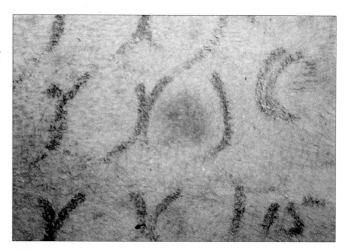

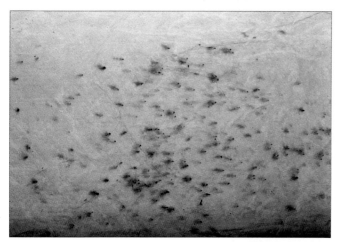

Plate 7 *A moistened paper towel turning reddish-brown near the flea feces.*

Plate 8 *Swelling, ulceration, and depigmentation of the bridge of the nose and nasal planum in a cat with mosquito bite hypersensitivity.*

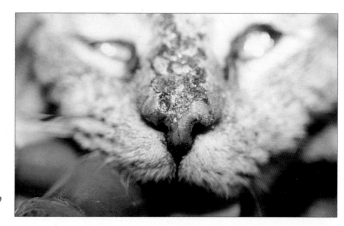

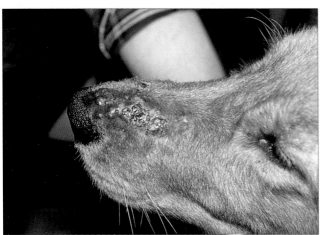

Plate 9 *Multiple papules and ulcers on the bridge of the nose and upper eyelid in a dog with eosinophilic furunculosis.*

Plate 10 *A hemorrhagic bulla in the interdigital space.*

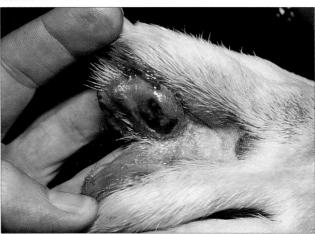

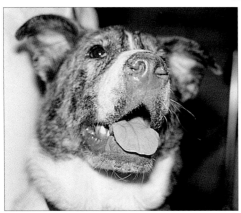

Plate 11 *Nasal and mucocutaneous depigmentation and erosion due to a trimethoprim–sulfadiazine drug reaction. The dog was also febrile, lame, and thrombocytopenic.*

Plate 12 *Diffuse nonblanching hemorrhage due to an amoxicillin drug reaction*

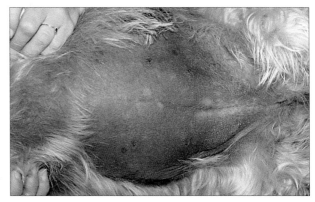

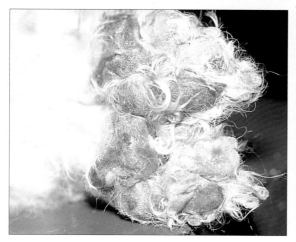

Plate 13 *Full-thickness ulceration of all pads in a dog with toxic epidermal necrolysis.*

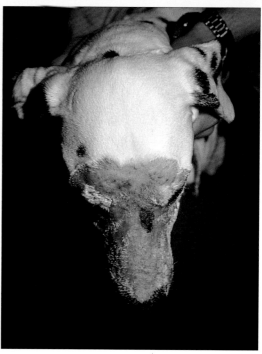

Plate 14 *Sharply demarcated erythema and hair loss in a dog with* Trichophyton mentagrophytes *infection. (Courtesy of DW Scott.)*

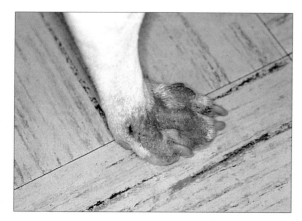

Plate 15 *Pedal alopecia and erythema in a dog with a Malassezia pododermatitis.*

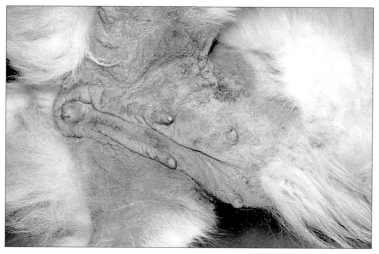

Plate 16 *Alopecia, erythema, and lichenification of the ventral abdomen, medial thighs, and vulvar area.*

fully explained and understood. For the best results, the owner should consider the long-term advantages of instituting immunotherapy early in the course of allergic diseases in combination with pharmacologic treatment.

Contraindications

Immunotherapy is not appropriate for every atopic patient. There have been no reports demonstrating a therapeutic role for immunotherapy for food hypersensitivities in man (Sampson, 1993) or animals (see Chapter 7). Although hyposensitization to certain contactants has been shown to be possible in humans (Maibach *et al.*, 1993), no studies have been reported on its effectiveness in animals (see Chapter 8). Some questions remain about the appropriateness of immunotherapy with allergens such as house dust, flea extracts, mixed insects, wool, cotton linters, and tobacco (see 'Allergen Selection' below). Also, it is probably best to advise against undertaking immunotherapy in patients with immunopathologic conditions or malignancies (VanMetre and Adkinson, 1993).

Practical Aspects of Immunotherapy

Selection of Allergens

Although positive skin or serum allergy tests are necessary for initiating immunotherapy, they should not be the sole determinant in antigen selection. Some allergy test results can be false clinically insignificant positives and indicate immunologic sensitivity with no clinical relevance. Ideally, only allergens causing the patient's symptoms should be used for immunotherapy. The aeroallergens proven to be most effective in immunotherapy are weeds, grasses, and trees (Reedy, 1979; Patterson *et al.*, 1983). Other aeroallergens may also be useful. One author (TW) has observed that no particular allergen nor combination of allergens has proved to be better in immunotherapy than others (Willemse, 1994). Since each pollen has a distinct regional pollinating season, a knowledge of these patterns (see Chapter 3) is helpful to correlate the symptoms, history, and allergy test results. For example, if a patient's symptom history and allergy test correlate with the pollen count or season for a particular allergen or group of allergens, then those allergens are probably significant. Some clinicians feel that only 'selective' allergens that correlate with both the symptom history and the allergy test results should be used in immunotherapy, but often the symptom history and allergy test do not correlate, making selection of appropriate allergens for immunotherapy more difficult. Because of the long tedious and expensive nature of immunotherapy, it may be best to err somewhat on the side of inclusion of an antigen.

While history should always be considered, it is not wise to select allergens for immunotherapy based on historic information alone. The chance of selecting the correct allergens will be low. However, unless the order of significance can be modified by some historic information, most clinicians will view the stronger reactions as the most significant and these allergens are selected first, followed by the less reactive allergens. However, since allergy test results may be influenced by the time of the year they are performed, reaction strength is not an absolutely foolproof method of selecting important allergens. This may be especially true with serum tests measuring circulating IgE, which has a shorter half-life than cell-fixed IgE (Ishizaka and Ishizaka, 1975). For example, if the patient's symptoms are distinctly seasonal, the ideal time to allergy test would be shortly after the season to ensure maximum reactivity. This may be less important in patients with perennial symptoms, but should still be considered.

Immunotherapy is allergen-specific. If a response is seen, it will be to that allergen or those cross-reacting with it and not to all allergens. Some allergens cross-react. For example, most grasses (except Bermuda) are reported to cross-react, weeds less so, and trees the least (VanMetre and Adkinson, 1993). A patient that is both grass and ragweed sensitive may improve with ragweed immunotherapy during the ragweed season, but the grass allergies will not be affected. Allergy testing (both skin and serum) with individual allergens is highly recommended because it is more precise and leads to more specific immunotherapy. Allergy testing with allergen mixtures (e.g. grass mixes, weed mixes) may lead to either exclusion of some important allergens (false-negatives) or inclusion of some allergens in the treatment vial to which the patient is not allergic (so-called irrelevant allergens). Immunotherapy with allergen mixtures has been reported to be as efficacious in humans as allergen-specific therapy, but may be associated with skin sensitization in some patients (Marsh *et al.*, 1972). In one study, multiple intradermal allergy tests induced positive skin tests in a group of dogs (Schmeitzel, 1968), but clinical sensitization accompanying these newly acquired skin reactivities was not demonstrated. In another study, no significant increase in intradermal reactions was found in normal nonallergic dogs after six months of immunotherapy with irrelevant antigens and all dogs remained asymptomatic (Codner and Lessard, 1992). Although immunotherapy with an irrelevant allergen probably does not induce new clinical allergies, it is more costly and wasteful and may not be beneficial.

In the past, house dust extract has been the allergen most commonly used in immunotherapy, but evidence is emerging to suggest that house dust extracts should no longer be used for immunotherapy (FDA Allergenic Products Advisory Committee, 1986). House dust extracts, which are made from pooled sweepings from homes, contain multiple common allergens that would be expected in the home environment including human dander, house dust mite, animal danders from cats, dogs, other domestic animals, and various rodents, molds, pollens, algae, and insect debris. The amounts of some of these allergens in house dust is variable, but can be considerable. House dust may also contain various amounts of toxic chemicals such as insecticides, detergents, and mycotoxins. Since house dust is highly heterogeneous, it cannot be standardized. In many countries house dust extracts have been withdrawn from the market. On the other hand, house dust mite is very specific and highly effective in immunotherapy (see 'Standardized Allergens' below).

Flea bites are reported to be the most common cause of pruritus in dogs and cats. The incidence of flea bite hypersensitivity based on skin testing in dogs varies in different parts of the USA and Europe from 15–80% (Halliwell, 1981; Schick and Fadok, 1986). Effective hyposensitization to flea bites would be a great aid to preventing or reducing pruritus in both dogs and cats. However, double-blind immunotherapy studies with currently available commercial flea extracts have proved no more effective than placebo (Halliwell, 1981). It is hoped that improved and more effective flea allergens will be available in the future. Immunotherapy with aqueous insect extracts such as cockroach has been advocated by some investigators (Griffin, 1993a), but again further studies are needed to clarify this form of therapy. There is also little evidence to support the inclusion of substances such as wool, kapok, feathers, cotton linters, and tobacco, in allergic extracts.

Types of extracts used in immunotherapy

In the USA, aqueous extracts are most commonly used in injection immunotherapy. They are absorbed quickly, so frequent injections must be given, and therefore adverse reactions are more common. Aqueous extracts may be preserved with either phenol or glycerin. Phenolization can cause the extract to lose potency, especially at high storage temperatures with weaker dilutions. Cats are very sensitive to phenol, but to date, no reports of toxicosis have been reported with the use of phenolized extracts in the cat. Glycerin-preserved extracts retain their potency better than phenol-preserved extracts, but can cause local reactions, both at skin test and immunotherapy injection sites and are not therefore commonly used.

Alum-precipitated extracts were developed to delay absorption of allergen, which would allow lengthening of the interval between injections, decrease the number of injections, and decrease the probability of adverse reactions. These extracts are commonly used in Europe and have proved to be effective (Reedy, 1979; Scott, 1981; Willemse *et al.*, 1984; Baker, 1990; Willemse, 1994). As not all allergens are available in the alum formulation and persistent cutaneous nodules or sterile abscesses can occur in humans, alum-precipitated extracts are not frequently used in the USA. One author (TW) routinely uses a European alum-precipitated extract in dogs and does not see nodules or abscesses. Efficacy with alum-precipitated allergens is discussed below.

Another form of repository immunotherapy, which is rarely used today, is an antigen–mineral oil emulsion. Advantages include the need for fewer injections, slower absorption, fewer systemic reactions, and possibly better results due to increased lymphoid processing (see below). Persistent nodules, sterile abscesses, and granulomas are, however, fairly common, but when myelomas and sarcomas were reported in mice following the use of these products, their use was discontinued in the USA.

A variety of modified or purified allergens are being investigated in man to see if the incidence of adverse reactions can be decreased while the ease and effectiveness of immunotherapy are improved. The principle of using modified extracts is to reduce or remove allergenicity (i.e. the ability to induce IgE-mediated reactions) and at the same time preserve or increase immunogenicity (i.e. the ability to stimulate the immune system) so that the extracts remain clinically effective. It is currently not known whether it is possible to modify the IgE-binding epitopes totally and retain the immunologic activity of the extract. These allergens have not been evaluated in veterinary medicine. Allergoids are produced by treating allergens with formalin to alter the antigenic determinants, detoxify pollen extracts, and destroy immediate-type reactivity, but retain the ability to induce antibody formation. Allergoids are licensed and manufactured for general distribution in Europe, but are not yet available in the USA. Polymerized allergens are made by treating purified allergens with glutaraldehyde, which produces an allergen with a higher molecular weight. Photoinactivated allergens are made by using ultraviolet light to break the lysine–sugar bond, a possible site of the allergenic determinant. Coupling allergens to tolerogenic carriers such as the cell wall of brown algae produces alginates. Modification of purified allergen with urea has been shown to stimulate suppression of IgE synthesis in mice without altering the IgE response (Ishizaka *et al.*, 1975). Another experimental and potentially improved method of immunotherapy is the use of antibodies against IgE receptors. The clinical effectiveness of these modified allergens is currently unknown, but studies continue. Although immunomanipulation is still in the experimental stage, it opens up exciting prospects.

Concentration of allergenic extracts

In addition to protein nitrogen units (PNU), weight/volume (W/V) and nitrogen units discussed in Chapter 3, the concentration of allergenic extracts can also be expressed as Freeman–Noon units, mg total nitrogen, allergy units (AU), and bio-equivalent allergy units (BAU). Currently, PNUs are most commonly used for immunotherapy in veterinary practice in the USA and depending upon the allergen company and type of allergen involved, PNU, W/V, and Noon units are mainly used in Europe. For simplification, PNU is the allergen concentration system that will be used in this chapter.

Most currently available commercial allergenic products are unstandardized and there may be no association between the units on the label and the potency of the product. Some allergenic extracts have been shown to vary nearly 1000-fold (Gleich *et al.*, 1974). The US Food and Drug Administration (FDA) has initiated a program to ensure that extracts are of consistent allergenic potency. Standardized allergenic extracts have defined potency and are labeled with a common unit, BAU, which reflects the clinical potency of the product. Extracts currently labeled AU are intended to be gradually converted to BAU. The dose in BAUs provides guidance in diagnosis and treatment, since doses associated with safety and efficacy with one standardized product may be applicable to other standardized products.

Several purified allergens have been isolated and characterized including those from short ragweed pollen, grass pollen, Hymenoptera venom, cat, and house dust mite. The availability of purified allergens has made it possible to determine minimally effective immunotherapy maintenance doses for humans. For example, maintenance ragweed immunotherapy doses should contain 6–24 μg *Amb a I*, while optimal maintenance immunotherapy doses for house dust mite-induced allergy contain approximately 7 μg *Der p I* (Yuninger, 1995). Standardized allergenic extracts have not been studied in immunotherapy in veterinary medicine.

Once the list of significant allergens for immunotherapy has been developed, several options are available. Treatment sets can be ordered from the commercial laboratory that performed the serologic tests or supplied the skin testing antigens. The clinician selects specific allergens from the allergy test to be included. Most laboratories recommend limiting the number of allergens to 10–12 per vial, but more can be included on request. In the USA, two vials are usually sent, one 5 ml containing 1000–2000 PNU/ml, and a second 10 ml vial containing 10000–20000 PNU/ml (see 'Immunotherapy Protocols' below). If a more dilute vial is desired, it can be made by the clinician. In the USA, it may take up to five weeks to receive prescription treatment vials since they must be compounded, standardized, and tested for sterility before shipping. In Europe, usually one vial containing 10000 PNU or its equivalent is used for immunotherapy. It can be ordered and received within one week. Another option is ordering regionalized allergen mixtures, which contain all the pollens believed to be important in that region regardless of allergy test results. The pros and cons of this approach have been discussed.

If the clinician performs large numbers of allergy tests each year, treatment vials can be mixed in-house. The advantages are the lower cost and immediate availability, and the clinician can prepare any strength or variation considered appropriate for the individual patient. The disadvantages include the cost of the allergen inventory and technician time necessary to mix the treatment vials. Mixing in-house allergens is uncommon in Europe. Regardless of the source, treatment vials should only include those significant allergens to which the patient is sensitive.

Immunotherapy treatment sets can be produced as single vial mixtures or each allergen can be kept in its own vial. Clinicians who use immunotherapy protocols with each allergen in its own vial typically restrict the number of allergens to approximately ten. If a larger number is used, it becomes very expensive and cumbersome to administer. Most clinicians use single vial mixtures in which multiple different allergens are all mixed in one vial. The greater the number of allergens included, the lower the concentration of each individual allergen. By convention, most clinicians include a maximum of 10–12 allergens/vial. Mixtures (e.g. grass mix, weed mix) count as one allergen. When only a portion of the patient's allergens are used for immunotherapy, the hope is that successful immunotherapy to these allergens will take the animal below its allergic threshold. When large numbers of allergens are included, most clinicians will use two or three multiple vials, each containing 10–12 allergens. In this case, it is wise to separate pollens from for example molds, house dust, and epidermals. Proteases in mold, house dust, epidermal, and insect extracts have been reported to increase and cause degradation of mixtures stored for up to three months (Esch, 1990; Rosenbaum, 1996). Some clinicians include all significant allergens in one vial (15–20 or more). There are few published reports indicating that including large numbers of allergens in a treatment vial is less effective than limiting the number of allergens (Scott, 1981). Very large numbers of allergens might dilute each allergen so much that it is difficult to give an effective dose of allergen. The minimal effective dose of an allergen for injection immunotherapy is at present unknown in veterinary medicine.

To make a treatment set, the volume of each allergen is determined by dividing the volume of the most concentrated vial by the number of ingredients. Usually, equal volumes of all allergens are added, but if certain allergens are considered to be more significant, a larger volume of those allergens can be used. For a 10 ml treatment vial with ten ingredients, 1 ml of each allergen would be added to the sterile vial. Mixtures count as one antigen so the vial may actually contain more than 12 allergens. Typically, treatment vials contain 10 000–20 000 PNU/ml. Some clinicians purchase antigens in 40 000 PNU/ml strengths because of the cost savings. Not all allergens are available in this strength, so treatment vial preparation can be confusing when different strengths are used. Confusion is minimized if the concentrated allergens are diluted down to the strength of the other allergens before treatment sets are made. The entire vial of the 40 000 PNU/ml antigen should not be diluted at one time to ensure potency.

Since all immunotherapy protocols use a gradually increasing dose schedule, at least two vials will be necessary. Once the full-strength maintenance vial (vial #3) is made, the diluted vial or vials are made by tenfold dilutions of vial #3. One can take 0.4 ml of vial #3 and mix that with 3.6 ml of sterile diluent to make vial #2. Vial #1 is made by taking 0.4 ml of vial #2 ,which is added to 3.6 ml of sterile diluent. Further dilutions can be made in a similar fashion based on the sensitivity of the patient. Only phenolized sterile diluent should be used for making dilutions. All allergenic extracts should be kept under refrigeration and never allowed to freeze, as this destroys their potency and stability.

Routes of administration

The subcutaneous route of injection is most commonly used in immunotherapy since it is safe, simple, and easy to administer. Intradermal injections have the advantage of slower allergen absorption, but smaller doses must be given and the injections are painful and technically more difficult to give. Other routes of administration include oral, inhalation, and intralymphatic. The major advantages of oral immunotherapy are safety and ease of administration. The allergen must be enteric coated to protect it from digestive fluids. The recommended oral dosage studied in humans is approximately 80–200 times higher than that used for conventional subcutaneous immunotherapy, reducing the practicability of this form of treatment (Creticos, 1995). Gastrointestinal discomfort has been reported in some human patients receiving high oral doses. Oral immunotherapy may be an alternative to injection immunotherapy, but further studies are needed to characterize the most appropriate mode of delivery, the optimal therapeutic dose, and the degree of effectiveness compared to that of conventional parenteral immunotherapy. Oral immunotherapy has not been studied in veterinary medicine. Sublingual immunotherapy was no more effective than placebo in reducing symptoms or affecting immunologic measures of sensitivity in atopic humans (Nelson et al., 1993). Inhalation of high concentrations of pollens can lead to natural hyposensitization. Local intranasal immunotherapy given once every other day for 8–10 weeks before the ragweed pollen season caused a significant reduction in human rhinitis symptoms during the pollen season, but was not as effective as high-dose injection immunotherapy (Georgitis, 1995).

Within limits, the concentration of the allergen reaching the lymphoid tissue is important in the development of an immune response. A portion of administered intravenous, intramuscular, subcutaneous, or intradermal injection is lost before it reaches the lymphoid system. A larger dose is administered to compensate, but as previously mentioned, this can increase the potential for side effects. Intralymphatic injections should theoretically result in maximum lymphoid exposure with smaller doses. This route of administration is currently used in the immunotherapy of cancer, but will probably never be practical for treating allergies. In unpublished studies (Austin, 1977), intralymphatic administration of allergen to allergic dogs produced results superior to those of conventional subcutaneous injections. Vehicles carrying the antigen directly to the lymphatics have not been developed, but offer interesting possibilities.

Immunotherapy protocols

In veterinary medicine, there is no standard schedule for immunotherapy. Several basic protocols are used, but each has been modified by various clinicians. Most clinicians report very similar success rates with different protocols, so one would not appear to be better than another. What is unknown is whether a patient who fails to respond to one protocol would respond to another. Until data are available indicating that one protocol is superior, one should select a schedule and gain experience with it. The injection immunotherapy schedules used by the authors are included in the Appendices B–D at the end of this chapter.

All immunotherapy protocols consist of a starting dose, a loading or increasing period, and a maintenance dose. The initial dilution of allergen extract, starting dose, and progression of loading dosage may be estimated on the basis of the patient's history and allergy test results. For example, a patient with a history of severe sensitivity, markedly strong allergy tests, or previous systemic allergic reactions, should be started with lower doses of more highly diluted extract. The starting dose is usually 0.1 ml of the most dilute treatment vial and should be tolerated by most sensitive patients. If the initial dose is tolerated without a significant local reaction, increasing doses of that dilution may be administered according to a schedule similar to that shown in Table 5.1. During the loading period, the amount of allergen is gradually increased at weekly or twice-weekly intervals. If twice-weekly injections are given, they should be given at least two or more days apart.

This schedule is intended only as a guide and must be modified according to the reactivity of the individual patient. Needless to say, you must proceed cautiously in the treatment of the highly sensitive patient who has a history of or develops large local or systemic reactions (see below).

This protocol allows the use of large numbers of allergens. If all of the allergens are mixed in one vial, the protocol is followed exactly. If two or more vials are used, it is probably best not to give injections from multiple vials on the same day, but to space them by at least two days. That way, if a reaction occurs, the causative extract can be identified. If no problems occur during loading, the schedules can be merged

Table 5.1 *Leisurely low-dose schedule.*

Injection number	Week	Vial #1 (200 PNU/ml)	Vial #2 (2000 PNU/ml)	Vial #3 (20 000 PNU/ml)	Total dose (PNU)
1	1	0.1			20
2	2	0.2			40
3	3	0.4			80
4	4	0.8			160
5	5	1.0			200
6	6		0.1		200
7	7		0.2		400
8	8		0.4		800
9	9		0.8		1600
10	10		1.0		2000
11	11			0.1	2000
12	12			0.2	4000
13	13			0.4	8000
14	14			0.8	16 000
15	15			1.0	20 000

during the maintenance phase. Injection number 15 on this schedule is then continued as maintenance (see below).

Intense rush immunotherapy

Intense rush immunotherapy was developed to get the patient to maintenance therapy as quickly as possible, but because of the nature of atopic disease in animals, this protocol has not been extensively studied and is rarely used. The intense rush schedule (Table 5.2) requires very careful monitoring in the hospital. At the first sign of any problem, the protocol should be discontinued. This protocol cannot and should not be used for large numbers of allergens. In one human study (Sharkey, 1995), subjects were premedicated with astemizole, ranitidine, and prednisone for three days including the day of rush immunotherapy. Eight injections were given over six hours followed by a two-hour observation period. Apparently, there were no more systemic reactions than with more leisurely schedules. All patients were able to reach maintenance dose months sooner than with weekly or biweekly schedules. However, evidence is lacking that symptoms are relieved sooner with rush immunotherapy. Once maintenance is reached, the injections are administered according to the maintenance schedule used in the intense low-dose schedule.

Maintenance dose

The optimal maintenance therapeutic dose range depends on several factors. It should be both clinically effective (i.e. reduce symptoms) and safe (i.e. produce no systemic reactions). Too low a dose is ineffective, although safe; too high a dose may be effective, but can be associated with a higher incidence of systemic reactions. Some clinicians will continue increasing the maintenance dose to a 'maximally tolerated' dose (i.e. the largest volume of the most concentrated extract that does not result in a systemic or large local reaction). Recent human data (Creticos, 1994), however, indicate that it is not necessary to push to a 'maximally tolerated' dose for

Table 5.2 *Intense rush schedule.*

Injection number	Hour	Vial #1 (200 PNU/ml)	Vial #2 (2000 PNU/ml)	Vial #3 (20 000 PNU/ml)	Total dose (PNU)
1	0	0.1			20
2	4	0.2			40
3	8	0.4			80
4	12	0.8			160
5	16		0.1		200
6	20		0.2		400
7	24		0.4		800
8	28		0.8		1600
9	32			0.1	2000
10	36			0.2	4000
11	40			0.4	8000
12	44			0.8	16 000
13	48			1.0	20 000

immunotherapy to be effective. Rather, an 'optimal' maintenance dose, which is defined as the minimum dose of allergen extract required to provide subjective relief of symptoms without systemic or local reactions, is most likely to result consistently in clinical improvement. Further studies are needed to define more accurately the optimal maintenance dose for a variety of allergenic extracts and to determine whether the optimal dose is dependent upon an individual patient's sensitivity. For most animals, 1 ml of 20 000 PNU/ml should be an adequate maintenance dose. Small dogs and cats, as well as extremely sensitive patients, may require smaller doses (0.5 ml of 20 000 PNU/ml or 1.0 ml of 10 000 PNU/ml).

Once the maintenance dose has been reached, some clinicians will continue at intervals of 7–14 days until a clinical improvement is observed. Once a response is seen, the interval between injections can then be extended. Ultimately, a 2–4 week interval between maintenance doses is permissible, provided that the patient continues to have symptom relief. Since summer–fall are usually the worst seasons for most atopic animals, one author (LMR) does not increase the interval between maintenance doses until after the patient has experienced a symptom-free and drug-free summer–fall. Extracts should be replaced with fresh allergens every 9–12 months to preserve potency. As allergens deteriorate over time and may not be standardized, it is wise to reduce the first dose of a new batch of extract by 50% and then increase the dose back to the maintenance level.

Timing of immunotherapy

Allergen immunotherapy can be given on a co-seasonal, pre-seasonal, or perennial basis. The co-seasonal approach involves the administration of the allergens during the patient's allergy season only. In the pre-seasonal method, the injections are started 3–6 months before the allergy season and then discontinued during the allergy season. Since most animals do not respond to immunotherapy for at least 2–3 months, the co-seasonal or pre-seasonal methods do not allow a sufficient time for response and are not recommended for long-range ongoing treatment. Perennial therapy involves the year round administration of extract and permits the administration of the largest cumulative dose of antigen. Since this mode of therapy appears to be associated with the greatest clinical improvement, it is the one most commonly used and recommended.

The success rate of immunotherapy is not influenced by the time of the year that treatment is started (Nesbitt, 1984). However, in the patient with seasonal allergies, it may be best to begin immunotherapy post-seasonally since this allows sufficient time for the patient to reach maintenance therapy before the next allergy season. In the perennially allergic patient, injections can be started at any time of the year and the intensity of the treatment protocol is constant throughout the year.

Injection administration

Allergy injections must be given correctly, the schedule followed, and the patient observed for possible adverse reactions. Some clients are quite capable and comfortable with giving injections to their pets at home. Others are less so. If the client wants to learn to administer allergy injections, the technique is best taught by first observing an injection, usually by a veterinarian or veterinary technician, and then administering one or more to their pet in the veterinarian's office under supervision. If the client is still uncomfortable and lacks minimal proficiency, they probably should not be encouraged to administer allergy injections to their pet at home.

A disposable 1 ml allergen- or tuberculin-type syringe (0.01 ml gradations) with a short fine (1/2–5/8 inch, 25–28 gauge) needle should be used for each injection. With multiple single vials the allergens can be loaded into one syringe or multiple injections can be given. Special care must be taken to select the correct antigen vial, to draw the correct dose into the syringe, and not to mix antigens while they are loading a common syringe. Injections may be given anywhere on the body, but for convenience most injections are given in the dorsocervical or dorsosacral areas. It is a good idea to rotate injection sites to avoid injecting into the same site repeatedly. The area of the injection site should first be cleaned with alcohol and the injection made into subcutaneous tissue at an oblique angle. The plunger of the syringe should be withdrawn before the extract is injected. If blood is withdrawn, do not inject at that site; instead withdraw the needle and select another site for injection. If antigen is injected directly into the bloodstream, there is the possibility of an anaphylactic reaction. Air in the syringe should not be harmful if injected only subcutaneously, but since it displaces antigen, it can lead to underdosage. However, intravenous injection of air is dangerous and is not recommended. After the injection, press an alcohol sponge to the injection site, but do not rub as this can increase the rate of absorption and possible adverse reactions. Allergy injections should only be given when the animal can be observed for at least 30 minutes.

Injections do not have to be given the same time every day, but should not be given immediately before or after a full meal or heavy exercise (see below). The owner should be sent home with a complete list of instructions on allergen administration (see Appendix A at the end of this chapter). These instructions should be thoroughly reviewed with the client by the veterinarian or the veterinary technician before injections are given at home. It must be stressed that if any problems arise, the client should contact the veterinarian's office for instructions and before further injections are given.

Administration problems

One problem frequently reported by clients administering allergy injections at home is pain felt by their pet either during the injection or immediately afterwards. This is usually due to using a larger than recommended needle, injecting cold extract, or giving the injection intradermally. It is usually best in these cases for the client to administer the next injection in the veterinarian's office so that the cause can be determined and corrected. Accurate injection technique should minimize most of the pain of injection and local discomfort. If the problem persists when the injections are given at home, future injections should be given in the veterinarian's office. Since injections of cold extracts can be painful, after loading the syringe can be held in the hand or allowed to come to room temperature before injecting. The entire allergen vial should not be warmed to room temperature as repeated warming and cooling decreases the potency of the extract.

If the owner reports that their pet did not receive a full dose, either because of struggling, the needle pulling out, or going through the skin, it is best to assume that a full dose was given. If this occurred during the loading phase, the next injection should be a repeat of the questionable injection and given on schedule. If a partial dose was given during maintenance, no adjustments are necessary; the next injection should be a full dose and continued on schedule. If an injection is off schedule by only a few days, no adjustments are needed and the injections are continued on schedule. If an injection is missed or skipped during the loading phase, the previously administered dose is repeated. If the interval is longer than four weeks, the next injection should be reduced, working back on the schedule one step for each week missed beyond four weeks. If a maintenance injection is missed by one or two months, the next injection is reduced by 50% and the schedule resumed. If a maintenance dose is missed by more than two months, the schedule is restarted from the beginning of the maintenance vial. In summary, the longer the interval between injections, the more care must be exercised with resumption.

Reactions to immunotherapy injections

Local reactions

Small areas of redness and swelling at the injection site that produce little discomfort are fairly common and should cause no concern. Large local reactions, 5 cm or more in diameter, that cause considerable discomfort, occur within 30 minutes, and persist for 24 hours or longer, should be considered more serious since they may precede systemic reactions, especially if ignored and further increased doses are given. Local discomfort may be relieved by applying cold compresses and administering an oral antihistamine (see Chapter 6). All future injections should be preceded by an antihistamine and reduced by 50%. Subsequent increases in dosage should be made with caution. Delayed reactions (i.e. after 24–48 hours) do not usually precede systemic reactions, but may cause discomfort to the patient. Local subcutaneous nodules at the site of injection, especially with the use of alum-containing extracts, may itch, but usually disappear with time and do not indicate that immunotherapy should be discontinued.

Systemic reactions

Adverse reactions to allergy injections are rare (Halliwell, 1981). In one study (Angarano and MacDonald, 1991), the incidence was reported as 5% of patients. Manifestations range in severity from a few hives to generalized urticaria, angioedema, and severe anaphylaxis. The annual fatality rate from immunotherapy in humans has been estimated at 1 in 2.8 million injections (Lockey *et al.*, 1987). The incidence of fatalities in small animals is unknown, but probably even rarer. Adverse reactions usually occur within 30 minutes of injection and are often preceded by early warning signs. Pre-treatment with antihistamines reduces immunotherapy-induced side effects (Nielsen, 1995). The owner should be instructed to observe their pet for personality changes (anxiousness), changes in activity (lethargy, hyperactivity), panting, gastrointestinal signs (increased bowel sounds, frequent swallowing, retching, vomiting, diarrhea), changes in urinary habits, or muscular weakness. If any of these signs is seen, the patient should be checked by a veterinarian immediately, treated as needed, and further injections suspended until the cause has been determined and corrected. Anaphylaxis and shock are very rare, but obviously very serious problems since they may be fatal. A patient who has a systemic reaction after an injection of allergen extract requires immediate emergency treatment for anaphylaxis. Glucocorticoids do not usually have a place in the immediate steps taken during an anaphylactic reaction because of their slow onset of therapeutic effect. However, the anti-inflammatory effect of glucocorticoids is helpful for the prolonged systemic reactions.

Anaphylaxis

Signs
Restlessness, diarrhea, vomiting, circulatory collapse, epileptiform seizures, coma, and death.

Treatment
1. Intravenous epinephrine hydrochloride (adrenaline), 0.5–1.0 ml diluted 1:1000. If indicated, repeat in 10–30 minutes. Infiltrate the injection site subcutaneously with epinephrine, 0.3 ml diluted 1:10 000.
2. Ensure a clear air passage and administer oxygen by endotracheal tube or face mask.
3. Administer an intravenous injection of a rapidly acting glucocorticoid such as hydrocortisone sodium succinate, 100–500 mg or prednisolone sodium hemisuccinate, 50–200 mg. Repeat the injection in 3–4 hours, if necessary.
4. Give an intravenous injection of an antihistamine such as diphenhydramine hydrochloride, 0.5–1.0 mg/lb body weight.
5. Hospitalize and observe the patient closely, following the above procedures. If recovery occurs within 5–10 minutes following this intensive treatment the prognosis is good.

Causes.   The major causes of anaphylaxis are high skin or serum sensitivity, undergoing loading or build-up therapy, and previous systemic reactions. Other causes include changing to a new vial of extract, a dosing error, inappropriate dose adjustments, height of the allergen season, symptomatic before injection, not observing the patient for 30 minutes after injection, and a partial accidental intravenous injection. The high frequency of pollen extracts in anaphylaxis in humans following immunotherapy injections probably reflects the high prevalence of reactivity to these allergens and their high biologic potency (Gergen *et al.*, 1987). Systemic reactions are more common where injection schedules use an aggressive increase in dosage. Nevertheless, severe systemic reactions may occur with any schedule that increases allergen doses to the high levels that have been shown to be effective by controlled trials. Although rare, systemic reactions may occur with a previously tolerated maintenance dose. Some of these can be explained by unforeseen circumstances that modify the potency, delivery, or absorption of the dose.

Errors in the magnitude of dose are an important and preventable cause of systemic reactions, while serious allergic reactions can readily occur if a patient receives another patient's extract. Intravenous administration of an allergenic extract may cause a systemic reaction, and careful attention to technique will ensure an appropriate subcutaneous injection. The risk of systemic reactions is increased in patients that have previously had systemic reactions. Such high-risk patients should be immunized with considerable caution with regard to both the initial dose and subsequent dose advancement. As a precaution, they should be pre-treated with an antihistamine and all injections should be given in the veterinarian's office where emergency treatment is instantly available. Highly sensitive patients (e.g. with many numbers of strong reactions) also have an increased risk of a systemic reaction. Therefore their immunotherapy should begin with an appropriately lowered dose of the magnitude previously described. Also, as previously mentioned, vigorous exercise or a heavy meal just before the allergen injection may increase the risk of systemic reactions. The patient should be well recovered from the stimulating effects of exercise or food before the injection is given.

Systemic reactions occur with increased frequency during immunotherapy when a new vial of allergenic extract is substituted for the old (Tinkelman *et al.*, 1995a). Even if the prescription is unchanged, a new extract is more potent than the old one it replaces because of gradual loss of potency over time. Another cause is the variability in potency between batches of the same extract. Injection of the same volume of the new and more potent solution may introduce a dose that exceeds the tolerance of the patient and cause a systemic reaction. Such reactions can be reduced in frequency by reducing the first dose of the new extract. Immunotherapy injections should not be given when the patient has a fever or an illness.

Continuing immunotherapy following anaphylaxis. A careful review of the history around the time of injection may indicate a cause for the anaphylactic reaction. If no error or cause is identified, the next 2–4 injections should be given in the veterinarian's office, preceded by an antihistamine, and the dose reduced by 50–90%. If a reaction occurs, it can be treated immediately. If no signs occur in the office, the owner can return to administering the injections at home if desired, but antihistamines should thereafter always be given before every injection. If reactions only occur when the injections are given at home and not in the veterinarian's office, perhaps all future injections should be given under veterinary supervision. If a local reaction occurs despite a good injection technique, the dose may be too large or too concentrated. Local reactions usually subside within 24 hours and do not require treatment. If the reaction persists or bothers the patient, topical glucocorticoids with or without systemic medication will help.

Onset of improvement

The speed with which a patient responds to immunotherapy is variable. The exact time when the owner will see a response depends upon the severity of the disease, the immunocompetence of the animal, and many other factors. In one study (Willemse *et al.*, 1984), 41% improved in less than two months while 71% improved in less than six months. Most dogs will respond within the first 9–12 months if they are going to respond. In a survey of canine allergy practices in the USA, immunotherapy was considered ineffective if a dog did not respond by 8.7 months (De Boer, 1989). Approximately 25% of those patients that respond will do so within the first three months, 50% in 3–6 months, and the remaining 25% in 6–12 months (Reedy and Miller, 1989). All cases not responding by six months should be re-evaluated (Kunkle, 1980).

Concomitant therapy

Since the response to immunotherapy is usually not immediate, concurrent sympto-matic treatment may be necessary in the early stages to control symptoms (see Chapter 6). However, if the symptoms are completely controlled with medication, it would be impossible to tell if and when immunotherapy becomes effective. The aim of symptomatic therapy should be to decrease, but not completely eliminate, the symptoms. As immunotherapy starts to become effective, the owners will notice a decrease in their pet's symptoms, allowing a decrease in the amount of medication being given. Hopefully, all medications can eventually be discontinued.

In one retrospective study (Scott *et al.*, 1992), 65% of patients on immunotherapy required additional medication (antihistamines, fatty acids, and/or glucocorticoids) to control allergic signs during part or all of the year. Approximately 75% of atopic dogs can avoid systemic glucocorticoids if immunotherapy is combined with other nonsteroidal treatments (Griffin, 1993b). Some veterinarians report that dogs who do not receive glucocorticoid steroids during immunotherapy respond better (Shirk, 1986), but others do not support this observation (Griffin, 1993b). There have been no controlled studies indicating that glucocorticoids adversely affect the response to immunotherapy, but nor has the opposite been proven. However, it is best to avoid the use of glucocorticoids during immunotherapy if possible. In most cases, immunotherapy should be but a part of the necessary therapeutic program. The patient should continue to avoid the specific allergen as much as possible, because even the well hyposensitized patient with a demonstrated reduction in symptom–medication score has more symptoms when exposed to a high concentra-tion of a specific allergen than when exposed to a low concentration (VanMetre and Adkinson, 1993).

Schedule adjustments

Schedule adjustments are often made in response to adverse reactions. Some patients simply cannot tolerate the calculated maintenance doses. If the symptoms are controlled, remain at the highest dose not causing reactions as though it were maintenance. A common reason for owner-requested schedule adjustment is severe pruritus, especially during the loading phase. Unless the pruritus is intense, the patient should be treated symptomatically and no schedule adjustments made dur-ing the first six months of immunotherapy as the increase in pruritus may be tran-sient. With intense pruritus during the loading phase, a lower dosage and slower increase may be indicated. Once the symptoms subside, the dosage can be gradu-ally increased. Most patients will become less symptomatic as the maintenance dose is reached. In the rare cases that develop severe pruritus following each mainte-nance injection, the maintenance dose may need to be lowered to the point where the post-injection pruritus does not occur. At very low dosages, the frequency of injections may have to be increased. One author (LMR) has observed that dogs with maintenance injection reactions are usually responding well to immunotherapy and often simply need a slight temporary reduction in their dosage.

During maintenance, some animals may experience severe pruritus immediately following the first injection of a new vial. As previously discussed, this can usually be prevented if the first dose of a new vial is decreased by 50%. If severe pruritus continues in spite of this precautionary step or persists with the new vial, the dose may be gradually decreased to one that does not cause these symptoms. Some owners will report that the pruritus stops following the maintenance injection, but returns before the next one is due. A larger volume of allergen can be given or, more preferably, the frequency of injections can be increased. If, for example, the patient's pruritus starts to increase at day 10, the injections should be given every seven days. If the symptoms worsen during a patient's peak allergy season, it is usually better to treat this symptomatically than to adjust injection dosage. It should become less of a problem as hyposensitization is achieved. The authors stress that no injection protocol should be followed rigidly and the patient's symptoms totally ignored: sometimes individualization of an injection protocol is essential. Unless signs of an impending anaphylactic reaction are present, it is usually best not to make schedule adjustments before six months of treatment since peak effectiveness may not have been reached. After this time, if there is an improvement, the interval between maintenance injections can be increased.

Flares during immunotherapy

Some patients that are successfully managed with injection immunotherapy occasionally experience a flare in their symptoms. If the signs are severe or start suddenly, the patient should first be examined for external parasites and skin infections. Flares due to inhalant allergens are usually more gradual in onset and can be due to heavy pollen counts. Usually, after brief medical treatment, the symptoms will subside. Rarely a worsening of symptoms in a patient that has previously been responding to injection immunotherapy indicates that the patient has developed new sensitivities. If the symptoms are severe and persist, the possibility of other allergies such as food or contact allergy should not be overlooked. Although new allergies can develop, this is uncommon. Most patients that need re-allergy testing usually respond well for one year or more, and then suddenly worsen. Common causes of flares, such as fleas, infections, and other allergies (e.g. food, contact) should be ruled out before allergy testing is repeated.

Efficacy

Clinical efficacy is defined as a reduction in symptoms and, therefore, in the need for symptomatic treatment. Usually the owner is the sole source for this information. To help owners with their evaluation, one author (LMR) uses a symptom-number grading system where the client objectively grades the severity of the patient's symptoms between injections on a scale of 1–10. 0–1 are normal or nonpathologic symptoms, while severe unremitting symptoms are graded 9–10, and lesser symptoms a lower number. This symptom-number grade is independent of the benefit of drugs; in other words, if symptoms are present, their severity is graded, not the benefit from symptomatic drugs. Most owners can be taught to make critical observations on symptom-scores and results of treatment. Combining the owner's and the clinician's evaluation of the patient's response is the best way of judging the effects of immunotherapy in individual patients. There are no convincing data to support the view that *in vitro* or

in vivo parameters can replace clinical evaluation of efficacy or predict clinical outcome. Therefore neither skin nor serum testing can be recommended at present for
evaluating the efficacy of immunotherapy.

In the veterinary literature (Halliwell, 1989; Reedy and Miller, 1989; Baker, 1990;
Griffin, 1993b; Scott *et al.*, 1995), a response to immunotherapy is often described in
the vague category of improvement and the reported response rates range from
50–100%. Some investigators consider that immunotherapy is successful if a patient
improves at least 51% while others define success as the complete elimination of all
clinical signs. If the problems of terminology are coupled with the fact that the various investigators use different patients, allergens, concentrations, vehicles (aqueous
or alum-precipitated), and treatment protocols, it becomes obvious that it is difficult
to draw firm conclusions from the literature.

To simplify the discussion, it may be best to reduce the number of categories of
response to three: namely excellent, good, and poor. The authors define an excellent
response as 75% or greater reduction in symptoms or need for symptomatic therapy; a good response as 50–75% improvement; and a poor response as anything
below 50% improvement. These categories are very broad and are subject to interpretation by both the owner and the clinician. The definition of success varies
greatly, especially when owner expectations are considered. If the owner will accept
only complete resolution of all symptoms, the failure rate will be much higher.
Some owners rate immunotherapy successful if their pet's symptoms do not worsen
or only decrease moderately.

Since skin testing has been used much longer than serum testing to select both
patients and allergens for immunotherapy, most early published reports on the efficacy of immunotherapy are based on skin testing (see 'Immunotherapy results
based on skin testing versus serum testing' below). The average response rate based
on skin testing for each category and the range reported is as follows: excellent, 36%
(21–60%); good, 30% (21–42%); fair, 19% (14–24%); and poor, 22% (14–35%). The
ranges are clearly very wide and certain papers are more widely divergent.
Allowing for a failure rate of 22%, overall, one can say that there is a 78% response
rate to immunotherapy based on skin testing.

In a retrospective study of 146 dogs in Australia (Mueller, 1995), 77% of patients
reported an excellent to good response after eight months of immunotherapy. In a
survey of 144 dogs on immunotherapy for at least one year (Reedy and Miller,
1989), 64% of clients were satisfied with the program while 36% were not. In 42% of
the patients whose owners were satisfied with the program, immunotherapy was
the only medication necessary. Typically these dogs were symptom free as long as
the injections were continued. In another study (Garfield, 1992), 85% of clients rated
the improvement from immunotherapy as good to excellent within one year.

The clinician is reminded that most of these reports were uncontrolled studies. A
classic double-blind study with 51 dogs (Willemse, 1984) reported that 84% of
patients receiving allergen (not placebo) improved by more than 51%. In this same
study, owners reported that 23% of patients receiving placebo improved, while the
investigator rated the same group at 17%. This emphasizes the need for both the
clinician and the owner to rate improvement.

In the previous study, placebo injections included aluminum hydroxide as an
adjuvant. Since adjuvants stimulate the proliferation of reticuloendothelial cells, the
placebo injections may have modulated the animal's immune response. If true,

adjuvanted allergens may warrant further evaluation. In one uncontrolled study (Kunkle, 1980), 59% of patients on immunotherapy with aqueous extracts improved by 50% or more compared to 41% on alum-precipitated extracts. Since different immunotherapy schedules were used, it is difficult to compare results. The pyridine extraction is reported unsatisfactory for some allergenic extracts such as ragweed because it denatures some principal allergens (Lichtenstein, 1968). To date, efficacy with alum-precipitated pyridine extracts has been shown in humans for grass pollens (Starr and Weinstock, 1971).

Most clinicians have not observed that sex or breeding affects immunotherapy. In one study (Willemse, 1994), boxers and West highland white terriers were less responsive to immunotherapy. Some earlier reports (Scott, 1981) indicated that dogs treated with fewer allergens (i.e. 2–10) responded better than those treated with larger numbers of allergens (i.e. 12–20), but currently most investigators do not believe that the number of allergens in the immunotherapy injections affects the success rate. Seventy-eight percent of dogs on immunotherapy with 21 or more allergens compared to 72% with ten or less allergens (Angarano and MacDonald, 1991). In another study (Scott *et al.*, 1992), there was no significant difference in efficacy of immunotherapy for dogs receiving more than 15 allergens compared to that for those receiving 15 or less.

Pollen-allergic dogs responded better to immunotherapy than nonpollen-allergic dogs (81% versus 59%) and treatment with individual pollens was more successful than using mixed or grouped pollens (Reedy, 1979). In another study (Mueller, 1995), highly positive reactions to pollens indicated a 57.6% chance of a good to excellent improvement with immunotherapy, and this figure was 44% for highly positive reactions to house dust mites, 12.5% for highly positive reactions to molds, and 29.6% for strong insect reactions. Only 32% of patients with weak reactions responded.

Some investigators have reported that dogs over eight years of age are less likely to respond to injection immunotherapy than younger dogs (Austin, 1976; Willemse, 1994). Dogs allergy tested within three years of developing symptoms tended to have a greater chance of responding to immunotherapy compared to those tested after three years (Mueller, 1995). Of those tested within one year 71% improved with immunotherapy, while 60% of those tested between one and three years, and 57% of those allergic for more than five years improved with immunotherapy. In another study, 87% of atopic dogs with an onset before three years of age improved, while 73% with an onset between three and five years of age, and 25% with an onset after five years of age improved (Willemse, 1994). Others have not confirmed these results and report that the age of the patient does not appear to influence immunotherapy results (Scott, 1981).

Maintenance dosage may affect the immunotherapy results. In a clinical trial involving 133 dogs, Garfield (1992) reported that 85% of patients receiving high-dose specific allergens (i.e. 1 ml 40 000 PNU/ml) improved over 51% compared to 68% of those receiving low-dose specific allergen (i.e. 1 ml 10 000 PNU/ml). He also found no correlation between the number of positive intradermal skin tests and clinical improvement.

Immunotherapy results based on skin testing versus serum testing

Although there have been few controlled studies comparing immunotherapy results based on skin testing versus serum testing, some investigators have reported no significant difference in percentage of improvement between the two tests (Shirk, 1986; Sousa, 1990; Anderson and Sousa, 1992). The overall success rate reported for immunotherapy based on *in vitro* allergy testing is 59–66%, which approximates that reported for immunotherapy based on skin testing. There are also no reported differences in the success rates between commercial *in vitro* labs (Anderson and Sousa, 1992). When 112 dogs were serum tested using RAST and put on immunotherapy based on that test, 66% showed a moderate to excellent response (Shirk, 1986). In another study, dogs were both intradermal skin and serum tested, and then placed on immunotherapy based on the test results. Intradermal skin testing with individual allergens appeared to be the better method for confirming a diagnosis and selecting allergens for immunotherapy (Griffin and Rosenkrantz, 1991). However, in another study, combining both skin and serum (IgGd ELISA) tests produced superior immunotherapy results compared to those based on a skin or serum test alone (Willemse, 1994). Most investigators believe that *in vitro* testing alone should not be used to diagnose atopy, but rather as an aid for identifying important allergens (Anderson and Sousa, 1992).

As previously discussed, feline atopy is a newly reported allergic disorder, so there are very few published reports on the efficacy of immunotherapy in the cat. When 15 skin test-positive cats were treated with immunotherapy, 67% improved by at least 75% (Reedy, 1982). McDougal (1986) reported that 69% of atopic cats improved 75% or more with immunotherapy, three cats improved 50%–75%, and one cat responded poorly. These data indicate that atopic cats can respond to immunotherapy. However, one author (TW) does not believe that skin testing cats for atopy is valid and therefore immunotherapy based on these tests in cats is questionable.

Immunotherapy is an art and the response is best when the protocol followed for a specific patient is based on the individual patient's response. Most allergic patients experience some degree of benefit from immunotherapy. Whether the benefit from immunotherapy is worth the time, cost, inconvenience, and risk of adverse reactions, and whether equally satisfactory or even better relief of symptoms could be obtained by the appropriate use of medications are questions that cannot be answered at this time.

Long-Term Immunotherapy

There have been no reports of adverse effects from long-term immunotherapy (Reedy and Miller, 1989; Scott *et al.*, 1995). Extensive studies fail to reveal an increased incidence of collagenous, autoimmune, or lymphoproliferative disease in human patients treated with immunotherapy over many years (Malling and Weeke, 1993). The progress of the patient should be evaluated every 6–12 months and the duration of immunotherapy depends upon the response of the patient. The duration of treatment for the average human patient is 3–5 years (Patterson *et al.*, 1983). This will vary if the patient is being treated for pollens only versus non-pollens. For human grass pollen allergies, the effect of immunotherapy continues for at least six years after termination, while for perennial aeroallergens, such as the house dust mite, available data question the advisability of discontinuing immunotherapy (Malling and Weeke, 1993). Treatment periods of less than three years result in a high frequency of relapses. From experience with human venom allergy, immunotherapy should be continued for at least five years (VanMetre and Adkinson, 1993). In a study of 39 human patients with grass pollen allergy hyposensitized for approximately 2.5 years, the clinical effect was still present more than six years after termination of the treatment (Walker *et al.*, 1995). Some *in vitro* parameters tended to return to pretreatment level. Only 10% of dogs in one study (Willemse, 1994) were able to stop injection immunotherapy after an average treatment of 1.9 years.

Individuals differ in the duration of benefit they derive from immunotherapy if the injections are discontinued. In some patients, the improvement is long-lasting. In other patients minimal allergic symptoms may return that can be adequately managed by environmental control and occasional use of medication. For some patients, however, increasing symptoms develop after immunotherapy has been discontinued, and may require a reinstitution of injection treatment.

It has been reported (Baker, 1990) that some allergic pets will be permanently 'cured' after one or two years of immunotherapy. Some clinicians will maintain patients with injections every 2–4 weeks until they are symptom free for one year and then discontinue immunotherapy. However, most, if not all, patients will start to show allergic signs within one year after immunotherapy has been discontinued (Naclerio, 1995). For this reason, if a good improvement is seen with immunotherapy, most atopic dogs and cats should continue to receive booster injections every 2–4 weeks for life. On the other hand, continued administration of allergen extract year after year without clinical benefit to the patient is not considered proper medical practice.

Compliance

Immunotherapy is usually very slow, time consuming, and expensive. Compliance with an immunotherapy regimen obviously makes the difference between a successful or unsuccessful outcome. Noncompliance, which is defined as discontinuing immunotherapy before a reasonable trial (i.e. usually 9–12 months), is a significant problem in the treatment of chronic diseases. In a study on immunotherapy in a human pediatric practice (Lower *et al.*, 1993), after one year only 56% of patients were compliant. The better the educational approach to immunotherapy, the more likely it is to succeed. Close follow-up is needed and communication is essential. In another human study, there was a noncompliance rate of 10.77% for those who received their injections within the clinic (Tinkelman *et al.*, 1995b). This contrasted with a noncompliance rate in the remote population of 34.82%. Almost 50% of the noncompliant patients stopped injections before one year. One author (LMR) has a compliance rate of 84%, which stresses the importance of encouraging the clients to continue immunotherapy for at least the first year if not longer. Of 70 dogs no longer receiving immunotherapy in an Australian study (Mueller, 1995), 40% had discontinued the injections in less than six months, and 49% did so because of a lack of perceived improvement in allergic signs. Worsening of symptoms was the second most common reason (21%). Other reasons included difficulty in giving injections, expense, inconvenience, skepticism regarding the effectiveness of immunotherapy, concurrent illness, and even an improvement in symptoms.

When an owner has a pet who is improving with the immunotherapy, they will usually want to continue injections. If the owner does not appreciate any change, the temptation is to discontinue immunotherapy and return to symptomatic therapy. During the first year of immunotherapy, it is very important to stay in contact with the client at least every 3–6 months. If the owner does not report in on schedule, they should be called. Patients that are improving should continue injections. Patients showing slight or no response after six months of immunotherapy should make an appointment for re-evaluation. A schedule adjustment may improve a patient's response, but will not usually convert a nonresponder to one that is symptom free. Although the client and veterinarian would like a 100% success rate, that is not possible with the current state of the art. If immunotherapy does not completely 'cure' the patient, but significantly reduces the quantity of medications necessary to control the symptoms, immunotherapy should be considered somewhat of a success and be continued.

Immunotherapy Failures

Immunotherapy is considered a failure when a significant decrease in the patient's symptoms has not been achieved within one year, and 15–25% of the patients who undergo immunotherapy show little or no response. If client communication is not continued, the percentage will increase since owners often fail to recognize that a significant decrease in medication is beneficial for their pet. Some owners will call the immunotherapy a failure if their pet has to take any medication. Even in patients showing no response to immunotherapy, recheck appointments and phone calls are encouraged since clients may need this support.

As previously mentioned, the major cause of treatment failure is discontinuing immunotherapy before it has been given long enough to achieve a response (i.e. usually before 9–12 months of treatment). Another cause is failure to control environmental allergens, especially fleas. Most owners become lax about flea control, especially if an initial improvement is noted. Other causes of immunotherapy failure include skin infections, concurrent allergies (e.g. to food, contact), incorrect diagnosis, incorrect allergens, the pet's inability to respond, and other unknown factors. As previously stated, very few allergic patients need to be re-allergy tested. If there is no change with immunotherapy after 1–2 years, it should be discontinued. In all cases, the clinician should examine the patient before failure is declared. Unfortunately, some patients fail to respond to immunotherapy and can only be treated symptomatically.

References

Anderson RK, Sousa CA. *In vivo* vs *in vitro* testing for canine atopy. Workshop report. In Ihrke PJ, Mason IS, White SD (eds) *Advances in Veterinary Dermatology*, Volume 2. Pergamon Press, New York, pp. 425–427, 1992.

Angarano DW, MacDonald JM. Immunotherapy in canine atopy. In Kirk RW (ed.) *Current Veterinary Therapy* XI. W.B. Saunders Co, Philadelphia, 1991, pp. 505–508.

Austin VH. Atopic skin disease. *Mod. Vet. Pract.* **57:** 355–361, 1976.

Austin VH 1977 (unpublished data).

Baker E. *Small Animal Allergy.* Lea & Febiger, Philadelphia, pp.72–82, 1990.

Becker AB, Chung KF, Aizawa H, *et al.* Inhibition of the cutaneous response to antigen by a thromboxane-synthetase inhibitor (OKY-046) in allergic dogs. *J. Allergy Clin. Immunol.* **84(2):** 206–213, 1989.

Codner EC, Lessard P. Effect of hyposensitization with irrelevant antigens on subsequent allergy tests results in normal dogs. *Vet. Dermatol.* **3(6):** 209–214, 1992.

Connell JT, Klein DE. Protective effect of nasal sprays containing blocking antibody in hay fever. (Abstract) *J. Allergy* **45:** 115, 1970.

Cooke, RA. Active immunization in hayfever. *Laryngoscope* **25:** 108, 1915.

Creticos PS. Immunotherapy with allergens. *J. Am. Med. Assoc.* **268(20):** 2834–2839, 1992.

Creticos PS. Efficacy Parameters in Immunotherapy: A Practical Guide to Current Procedures. *Amer. Acad. Allerg. Immunol.* pp. 5–2, 1994.

Creticos PS. A review of oral immunotherapy. In Syllabus *Annu. Meet. Am. Coll. Allerg. Asthma & Immunol.* November 10–15, pp. 531–541, 1995.

DeBoer DJ. Survey of intradermal skin testing practices in North America. *J. Am. Vet. Med. Assoc.* **195:** 1357–1363, 1989.

Des Roches A. Specific immunotherapy prevents the onset of new sensitizations in monosensitized children. (Abstract) *J. Allergy Clin. Immunol.* **95(1):** 309, 1995.

deVries JE. Novel fundamental approaches to intervening in IgE-mediated allergic diseases. *J. Invest. Dermatol.* **102(2):** 141–144, 1994.

Durham SR. Grass pollen immunotherapy: inhibition of allergen induced late skin responses (LPR) is associated with an increase in IL-12 messenger RNA+ cells. (Abstract) *J. Allergy Clin. Immunol.* **95(1):** 304, 1995.

Esch RE. Role of proteases on the stability of allergen extracts. In Klein RG. *Regulatory Control and Standardization of Allergen Extracts.* Gustav Fischer Verlag, Stuttgart, pp. 171–177, 1990.

Evans R, Pence H, Kaplan H. *et al.* The effect of immunotherapy on humoral and cellular responses in ragweed hay fever. *J. Clin. Invest.* **57:** 1378–1380, 1976.

FDA Allergenic Products Advisory Committee. Recommendation to the FDA by FDA Allergenic Products Advisory Committee. *The AAAI News and Notes,* Winter, p. 13, 1986.

Garfield RA. Injection immunotherapy in the treatment of canine atopic dermatitis: comparison of 3 hyposensitization protocols. Presented at the Annual Members Meeting of the American Academy of the Veterinary Dermatologists & the American College of Veterinary Dermatology, **8:** 7–8, 1992.

Georgitis JW. Intranasal and inhalation therapies. In Syllabus *Annu. Meet. Amer. Coll. Allerg. Asthma & Immunol.* pp. 549–553, 1995.

Gergen PJ, Turkeltaub PC, Kovar MG. The prevalence of allergic skin test reactivity to eight common aeroallergens in the US population: results from the Second National Health and Nutrition Examination Survey. *J. Allergy Clin. Immunol.* **80:** 669–679, 1987.

Gleich GJ, Larison JB, Jones RT, *et al.* Measurement of the potency of allergy extracts by their inhibitory capacities in the radioallergosorbent tests. *J. Allergy Clin. Immunol.* **53:** 158, 1974.

Griffin CE. Insect and arachnid hypersensitivity. In Griffin CE, Kwochka KW, MacDonald JM (eds) *Current Veterinary Dermatology: The Science and Art of Therapy.* Mosby, St Louis, pp. 133–137, 1993a.

Griffin CE. Canine atopic disease. In Griffin CE, Kwochka KW, MacDonald JM (eds) *Current Veterinary Dermatology*. Mosby, St Louis, pp. 99–120, 1993b.

Griffin CE, Rosenkrantz WS. A comparison of hyposensitization results in dogs based on an intradermal protocol versus an *in vitro* protocol. *Proc. Acad. Vet. Allergy* **31**: 12–13, 1991.

Halliwell REW, Gorman NT. *Veterinary Clinical Immunology*. W.B. Saunders Co., Philadelphia, p. 247, 1989.

Halliwell, REW. Hyposensitization in the treatment of flea-bite hypersensitivity: results of a double-blind study. *J. Am. Anim. Hosp. Assoc.* **17**: 249, 1981.

Hsieh KH. Immunotherapy suppresses the production of MCAF and augments the production of IL-8 in asthmatic children. (Abstract) *J. Allergy Clin. Immunol.* **95(1)**: 308, 1995.

Iliopoulos O, Proud D, Adkinson F, *et al.* Effects of immunotherapy on the early, late, and rechallenge nasal reaction to provocation with allergen: changes in inflammatory mediators and cells. *J. Allergy Clin. Immunol.* **87**: 855–866, 1991.

Ishizaka K, Okaduira H, King TP. Immunogenic properties of modified antigen E. II. Ability of urea denatured antigen and polypeptide chain to prime T-cells specific for antigen E. *J. Immunol.* **114**: 110, 1975.

Ishizaka T, Ishizaka K. Biology of immunoglobulin E. Molecular basis of reaginic hypersensitivity. *Prog. Allergy*, **19**: 60–121, 1975.

Kuna P, Alam R, Kuzminska B, *et al.* The effect of preseasonal immunotherapy on the production of histamine releasing factor (HRF) by mononuclear cells from patients with seasonal asthma: results of a double-blind, placebo-controlled randomized study. *J. Allergy Clin. Immunol.* **83**: 816, 1989.

Kunkle GA. The treatment of canine atopic disease. In Kirk RW (ed.) *Current Veterinary Therapy* VII. W.B. Saunders Co., Philadelphia, pp. 453–458, 1980.

Lichtenstein LM, Norman PS, Winkenwerder WL. Antibody response following immunotherapy in ragweed hay fever. *J. Allergy* **41**: 49–57, 1968.

Lichtenstein LM. Histamine-releasing factors and IgE heterogeneity. *J. Allergy Clin. Immunol.* **81**: 814–820, 1988.

Lockey RF, Benedict LM, Turkeltaub PC, *et al.* Fatalities from immunotherapy and skin testing. *J. Allergy Clin. Immunol.* **79**: 660–677, 1987.

Lower T, Henry J, Mandik L, *et al.* Compliance with allergen immunotherapy. *Ann. Allergy* **70**: 480–482, 1993.

Maibach HI, Dannaker CJ, Lahti A, *et al.* Contact skin allergy. In Middleton E Jr, Reed CE, Ellis EF (eds) *Allergy: Principles and Practice*, 4th edition. Mosby, St Louis, p. 1632, 1993.

Malling HJ & Weeke B. Position paper: Immunotherapy. *Allergy* 48 **(14)**: 9–35, 1993.

Marsh DG, Lichtenstein LM, Norman PS. Induction of IgE-mediated immediate hypersensitivity to group I rye grass pollen allergens and allergoids in non-allergic man. *Immunology* **22**: 1013, 1972.

McDougal BJ. Allergy testing and hyposensitization for three common feline dermatoses. *Mod. Vet. Pract.* **81**: 629, 1986.

Mueller RS. Immunotherapy in 146 dogs with atopic dermatitis: A retrospective study. *Proc. Annu. Memb. Meet. Am. Acad. Vet. Dermatol. Am. Coll. Vet. Dermatol.* **11**: 38–40, 1995.

Naclerio R. A double-blind study of the discontinuation of ragweed immunotherapy. (Abstract) *J. Allergy Clin. Immunol.* **95(1)**: 305, 1995.

Nelson HS, Oppenheimer J, Vatsia GA, *et al.* A double-blind, placebo-controlled evaluation of sublingual immunotherapy with standardized cat extract *J. Allergy Clin. Immunol.* **92(2):** 229–236, 1993.

Nesbitt GH. Canine allergic inhalant dermatitis: A review of 230 cases. *J. Am. Vet. Med. Assoc.* **172(1):** 55–60, 1978.

Nesbitt GH. Canine atopy. *Compend. Cont. Ed.* **6:** 63–264, 1984.

Nielsen L. Antihistamine pretreatment reduces immunotherapy-induced side effects. (Abstract) *J. Allergy Clin. Immunol.* **95(1):** 307, 1995.

Nish WA, Charlesworth EN, Daris TL, *et al.* The effect of immunotherapy on the cutaneous late phase response to antigen. *J. Allergy Clin. Immunol.* **93(2):** 484–494, 1994.

Noon, L. Prophylactic inoculation against hayfever. Lancet **1:** 1572, 1911.

Norman PS, Lichtenstein LM, Ishizaka K. Diagnostic tests in ragweed hay fever: a comparison of direct skin tests, IgE antibody measurements, and basophil histamine release. *J. Allergy Clin. Immunol.* **52:** 210, 1973.

Patterson R, *et al.* Immunotherapy. In Middleton E Jr, Reed CE, Ellis EF (eds) Allergy: Principles and Practice, 2nd edition. CV Mosby Co, St Louis, 1983, p. 1120.

Platt-Mills TAE, Von Maur RK, Ishizaka PS, *et al.* IgA and IgG anti-ragweed antibodies in nasal secretions: quantitative measurements of antibodies and correlation with inhibition of histamine release. *J. Clin. Invest.* **57:** 1041, 1976.

Prinz JC, *et al.* Loss of Fc R2/CD23 expression on T and B lymphocytes during rush hyposensitization. In Ring J, Przybilia B. (eds) *New Trends in Allergy* III. Springer-Verlag, Berlin, pp. 105–108, 1991.

Reedy LM. Results of allergy testing and hyposensitization in selected feline skin diseases. *J. Am. Anim. Hosp. Assoc.* **18:** 618–623, 1982.

Reedy LM. Canine atopy. *Comp. Cont. Ed.* **1:** 550–556, 1979.

Reedy LM, Miller WH. (eds) *Allergic Skin Diseases of Dogs and Cats.* W.B. Saunders, Philadelphia, p. 130, 1989.

Rocklin RE. Clinical and immunologic aspects of allergen-specific immunotherapy in patients with seasonal allergic rhinitis and/or allergic asthma. *J. Allerg. Clin. Immunol.* **72(4):** 323–334, 1983.

Rosenbaum MR. The effects of mold proteases on the biological activity of pollen allergenic extracts in atopic dogs. *Proc. Annu. Memb. Meet. Am. Acad. Vet. Dermatol. Am. Coll. Vet. Dermatol.* **12:** 20, 1996.

Sampson HA. Adverse reactions to food. In Middleton E J Jr, Reed CE, Ellis EF (eds) *Allergy: Principles and Practice*, 4th edition. Mosby, St Louis, p. 1680, 1993.

Schick RO, Fadok VA. Responses of atopic dogs to regional allergens: 268 cases (1981–1984). *J. Am. Vet. Med. Assoc.* **189(11):** 1493–1496, 1986.

Schmeitzel LP. The effects of multiple intradermal skin tests on skin reactivity. *Vet. Allergist*, Summer, 1968.

Scott DW. Observations on canine atopy. *J. Am. Anim. Hosp. Assoc.* **17:** 91–100, 1981.

Scott DW, Miller WH, Griffin CE (eds) *Small Animal Dermatology*, 5th edition. W.B. Saunders, Philadelphia, pp. 514–517, 1995.

Scott KV, White SD, Rosychuk RAW. A retrospective study of hyposensitization in atopic dogs in a flea-scarce environment. In Ihrke PJ, Mason IS, White SD (eds) *Advances in Veterinary Dermatology* volume 2: Pergamon Press, New York, pp. 79–87, 1992.

Sharkey P. Rush immunotherapy: experience with a 1-day schedule. In Syllabus. *Annu. Meet. Amer. Coll. Allerg. Asthma & Immunol.* pp. 525–530, 1995.

Shirk ME. The canine RAST: A diagnostic procedure for allergic inhalant dermatitis. *Proc. Annu. Memb. Meet. Am. Acad. Vet. Dermatol. Am. Coll. Vet. Dermatol.* **26**: 32, 1986.

Sousa CA. Advances in diagnosis of allergic skin disease. In De Boer DJ (ed) *Advances in Clinical Dermatology.* W.B. Saunders, Philadelphia, pp. 1419–1427, 1990.

Starr MS, Weinstock M. Relationship between blocking antibody titres and symptomatic relief in hay-fever subjects treated with Allpyral. *Int. Arc. Allerg.* **41**: 157–159, 1971.

Sullivan TJ. Drug allergy. In Middleton E Jr, Reed CE, Ellis EF (eds). *Allergy, Principles and Practice*, 4th edition. CV Mosby Co, St Louis, pp. 1726–1746, 1993.

Tinkelman DG, Cole WQ, Tunno J. Immunotherapy: a 1-year prospective study to evaluate risk factors of systemic reactions *J. Allergy Clin. Immunol.* **95(1):** 8–14, 1995a.

Tinkelman DG, Smith F, Cole WQ, *et al.* Compliance with an allergen immunotherapy regime. *Ann. Allergy Asthma Immunol.* **74:** 241–246, 1995b.

VanMetre TE Jr, Adkinson NF Jr. Immunotherapy for aeroallergen disease. In Middleton E Jr, Reed CE, Ellis EF (eds) *Allergy: Principles and Practice*, 4th edition. Mosby, St Louis, pp. 1489–1509, 1993.

Walker SM, Varney VA, Jacobson MR, *et al.* Grass pollen immunotherapy: efficacy and safety during a 4-year follow-up study. *Allergy* **50:** 405–413, 1995.

Willemse A, Van den Brom WE, Rynberg A, *et al.* Effect of hyposensitization on atopic dermatitis in dogs. *J. Am. Vet. Med. Assoc.* **184:** 277, 1984.

Willemse T. Hyposensitization of dogs with atopic dermatitis based on the results of *in vitro* (IgGd ELISA) diagnostic tests. *Proc. Annu. Memb. Meet. Am. Acad. Vet. Dermatol. Am. Coll. Vet. Dermatol.* **10:** 61, 1994.

Wittich FW. Spontaneous allergy (atopy) in the lower animal: Seasonal hay fever (fall type) in the dog. *J. Allergy* **12:** 247–251, 1941.

Yunginger JW. What's new in allergy extract allergens? In Syllabus. *Annu. Meet. Amer. Coll. Allerg. Asthma. Immunol.* p. 332, 1995.

Appendix A: Fact Sheet for Allergen Extract Administration

Extract handling

1. The extract vials should be kept under refrigeration. Do not allow to freeze since this destroys the antigen.
2. Vials #1 and #2 should be discarded when the schedule indicates that they are finished even though there may still be extract in the vials. It is too dilute to be useful and the stability is short.
3. Vial #3 is the maintenance vial. When you are halfway through your last vial, please contact your veterinarian so that more extract can be ordered for your pet.

Immunotherapy schedule

1. The schedule for administration is attached. The injections are given weekly until maintenance (maximum dose). Once maintenance is reached, the interval between injections increases to once every two weeks. This dosage and interval will be continued until you have completed the injections in vial #3. At that point, if an improvement in symptoms has occurred, please order another vial and continue injections. If an improvement has not occurred, please contact this office to schedule a recheck examination.
2. Most owners feel that converting the schedule to actual calendar days and dates is helpful. If a big-blocked calendar is used, the dose can be indicated on the calendar.
3. This schedule is the standard schedule. Dose adjustments may need to be made for individual patients, but should only be done under the direction of your pet's veterinarian.

Allergen administration

1. The injections are given subcutaneously according to the schedule. It is optional who gives the injections. We recommend observing the first one in your veterinarian's office, and then if you choose, you give the second under supervision. After that, if you are comfortable administering injections, you can continue at home.
2. A new disposable needle and syringe should be used for each injection. Carefully save the used syringes and needles and return them to your veterinarian for safe disposal.
3. It is very important that each and every injection, especially during the initial phase of the protocol, is given when your pet can be observed for at least 30 minutes. The injections need not be given at the same time each day.
4. Your pet should not consume a large amount of food from one hour before to one hour after each injection. A snack or treat after the injection is allowed.
5. Heavy exercise should be avoided from one hour before to one hour after each injection. Walks are allowed.
6. If any adverse reactions (see below) are seen after an injection, no more injections

should be given until you have contacted your veterinarian. If your animal appears to be seriously ill, you should contact your local veterinarian or emergency clinic immediately.

Adverse reactions

1. Adverse reactions are very infrequent. Some pets will become more itchy during the initial phase of the schedule, but this should only be temporary and treated symptomatically. If it becomes severe, contact your veterinarian.
2. Aside from an increase in itchiness, adverse reactions are extremely rare and unlikely. If an adverse reaction is to occur, it will usually be within 30 minutes and there are usually early warning signs. If these early signs are ignored, a more severe adverse reaction may occur. If your pet is not its normal self after an injection, contact your veterinarian. Animals that sleep excessively, are hyperactive, or look uncomfortable after the injection may be showing the first signs of a vaccine reaction. Contact your veterinarian before any more injections are given.
3. Serious reactions are extremely rare, but can be life-threatening, and should never be ignored. Labored breathing, vomiting, diarrhea, collapse, or hives over most of the body require immediate veterinary attention. No further injections should be given until your veterinarian can review the case.

Points of information

1. Since immunotherapy does not reach 'full strength' immediately, most pets will not show any improvement during the loading phase.
2. Most pets who do respond usually do so within 6–9 months. A few will not respond until the end of the first year.
3. Since immunotherapy does not work immediately, medications can be used to lessen your animal's itchiness. Your veterinarian will make various suggestions, which you should follow. They should only be given on an 'as needed' basis. Excessive medication makes it impossible to determine whether immunotherapy is helping.
4. Routine immunizations should not be given on the same day as an allergy injection. If your pet develops an unrelated medical or surgical problem, contact your veterinarian to see how the immunotherapy schedule should be modified.
5. If an injection date is missed by up to one week, continue the schedule. If longer than one week has elapsed, contact your veterinarian before giving the next injection.

Appendix B: Schedule for Aqueous Immunotherapy (used at Cornell University, Ithaca, New York, USA)

Schedule A: Animals under 25 pounds

Day	Vial #1 (2000 PNU/ml)	Vial #2 (20 000 PNU/ml)
1	0.1	
3	0.2	
5	0.3	
7	0.4	
9	0.5	
11		0.1
13		0.2
15		0.3
17		0.4
19		0.5
26		0.5
40		0.5
61		0.5

After day 61, 0.5 ml of vial #2 is given every three weeks.

Schedule B: Animals over 25 pounds

Day	Vial #1 (2000 PNU/ml)	Vial #2 (20 000 PNU/ml)
1	0.1	
3	0.2	
5	0.4	
7	0.6	
9	0.8	
11	1.0	
13		0.1
15		0.2
17		0.4
19		0.6
21		0.8
23		1.0
30		1.0
44		1.0
65		1.0

After day 65, 1.0 ml of vial #2 is given every three weeks.

Appendix C: Hyposensitization Schedule (used at the Utrecht University, The Netherlands)

Week number	Volume (ml)	Concentration
0	0.1	10 000 PNU/ml
1	0.2	
2	0.4	
4	0.6	
6	0.8	
9	1.0	
12	1.0	
16	1.0	
20	1.0	

After week 20 the interval will become longer dependent upon the effect of the therapy; if possible the volume and concentration remain the same.

Appendix D: Immunotherapy Schedule (used by the Animal Dermatology Clinic, Dallas, Texas, USA)

Vial A (2000 PNU/ml)	Interval	Date given	Symptom score (itch) 0–10
1. 0.10 ml	7 days	_____	_____
2. 0.25 ml	7 days	_____	_____
3. 0.50 ml	7 days	_____	_____
4. 1.00 ml	7 days	_____	_____

Vial B (20 000 PNU/ml)	Interval	Date given	Symptom score (itch) 0–10
5. 0.10 ml	7 days	_____	_____
6. 0.25 ml	7 days	_____	_____
7. 0.50 ml	7 days	_____	_____
8. 1.00 ml	7 days	_____	_____
9. 1.00 ml	14 days	_____	_____
10. 1.00 ml	14 days	_____	_____
11. 1.00 ml	14 days	_____	_____
12. 1.00 ml	14 days	_____	_____
13. 1.00 ml	14 days	_____	_____
14. 1.00 ml	14 days	_____	_____
15. 1.00 ml	14 days	_____	_____

It is important to complete the injections on schedule. If improvement is noted, reorder a second vial and continue. If improvement does not occur, we suggest that you schedule a recheck.

-------------------6-------------------

Medical Management of Allergic Diseases

Introduction

With our current technology, allergic diseases are never cured (Griffin, 1993; Scott *et al.*, 1995). They are managed and this is best done by avoidance (e.g. for drug contact, or food hypersensitivity) or immunotherapy (e.g. for atopy). To use either of these methods of treatment, the animal's allergens must be defined by the appropriate allergy tests. Because of the expense and complexity of a thorough allergy evaluation, many owners initially decline such testing. Some allergic animals defy diagnosis and show no reactivity in any of the allergy tests performed. Lastly, there are some allergic animals who do not respond completely to immunotherapy or avoidance. For these animals, the symptoms must be controlled with various topical and systemic medications (Scott and Miller, 1993; Miller and Scott, 1994a). The specific protocol developed depends on the nature of the animal's disease and the desires and capabilities of the owner.

Allergic symptoms tend to worsen with advancing time. Early in the course of the disease, pruritus, the predominant sign of allergic skin disease in companion animals, is often easy to control. With time, pruritus often returns despite continuing previously effective treatments. The timing to treatment failure is variable. Some animals respond to the same treatments for years while others start itching again in a matter of months. Treatment failure can be explained by drug tachyphylaxis, a tolerance to the medications being used, or increasing severity of the underlying allergic condition. The latter appears to be most common. Accordingly, medical management is usually a dynamic process where treatments are adjusted according to the patient's needs.

Pruritus is a complex sensation (Shanley, 1988). Pruritic stimuli arising in the skin can be intensified or damped by emotional, biochemical, or other central factors. Since traditional cutaneous sensations (e.g. temperature, pain) reach the brain by the same nerve pathways that carry the pruritic stimuli, competing skin sensations can alter pruritus. Pruritus also tends to be cumulative. If a mildly itchy allergic dog is exposed to some additional pruritogenic stimulus (e.g. superficial bacterial folliculitis) its pruritus will increase significantly. Successful medical management of the allergic disease requires the correction or prevention of all additional pruritic stimuli.

Management Factors

The management of all allergic animals should be reviewed carefully. Animals housed outdoors can be at risk of increased itching because of boredom or excessive exposure to heat or cold. A well-designed kennel should prevent hot or cold exacerbations, but may not remove the stress of being kenneled. Very well insulated houses, especially those heated by wood stoves or non-humidified forced air, can be very drying. Since dry skin tends to be itchy, humidification should be suggested. The animal's diet and state of health should be reviewed. Poor diets or systemic illnesses that might cause skin disease or a feeling of ill health should be corrected. Lastly, and most difficultly, the pet's mental health should be reviewed. Conditions such as boredom and separation anxieties can intensify the pet's pruritus. Appropriate behavior modification will make it easier to treat the allergic pruritus.

Topical Treatments

Animals with allergic skin disease have inflamed pruritic skin. Environmental allergens may gain entrance to the body through the skin. Accordingly, routine and regular soaking or bathing of the animal can be beneficial and should be considered an important part of medical management. A 10–15 minute immersion in cool water or water treated with a colloidal oatmeal bath treatment can significantly lessen pruritus in some dogs for four or more hours.

A common complaint of allergic dog owners is that the dog licks its feet intensely when it returns from a walk outside, especially when it is wet or muddy outside. This increased pedal pruritus can be due to mechanical or thermal trauma sustained during the walk or by the accumulation of irritants or allergens between the dog's toes or pads. Some of these dogs derive great benefit from a foot bath. The feet are quickly rinsed in cool water when the dog reenters the house. Prolonged soaking is contraindicated and the feet must be dried thoroughly to prevent secondary colonization by bacteria or yeasts. Boots are sold for dogs and protect the feet from trauma and exposure to irritants or allergens. Some owners find them a great time saver since they do not then have to clean the dog's feet.

Since immersion has short-lived effects and does not clean the coat, most allergic dogs are bathed rather than soaked. Cats might also benefit from regular bathing, but it is impractical to impossible for most cats. The sensitivity of the animal's skin, the need for bathing, and the dog's response will dictate which shampoos are appropriate. In most cases, harsh antiseborrheic (e.g. coal tar), antiparasitic, or antibacterial (e.g. benzoyl peroxide) products are contraindicated. Mild products are most appropriate and include veterinary hypoallergenic grooming shampoos with or without moisturizers, colloidal oatmeal products, or mild antibacterial products (Kwochka, 1995). Any shampoo, especially if used too frequently, can dry an animal's skin and make its itching worse. To prevent this, it is best to avoid telling the owner how often to bathe the dog. Guidelines should be given about when bathing is appropriate and the owner should decide when to bathe based on the pet's response. With frequent bathing, especially during the winter, many dogs will develop a dry skin. This dryness can be minimized by the application of veterinary moisturizer as a spray or after-bath rinse.

Various veterinary shampoos and cream rinses containing an active antipruritic agent with the cleaning ingredients are available (Kwochka, 1995; Scott, 1995; Scott *et al.*, 1995). Currently, products containing diphenhydramine, 1% hydrocortisone, or pramoxine (a surface anesthetic agent) are available. These agents are absorbed through the skin during the bath and can interfere with the generation or transmission of the pruritic stimulus. If effective, the product must be used frequently to sustain the clinical response. No studies are available to indicate how effective each product is or whether one product is superior to another. The authors have used the various products and found, as expected, that some dogs respond to no product, some respond to all products, and some dogs respond better to one product than another. With a once or twice weekly application, no dog's pruritus was controlled completely with the product alone. With the expense and labor intensity of these treatments, many owners, especially of large dogs, will not make full use of them.

Allergic dogs are prone to develop secondary staphylococcal or *Malassezia* infections. When the infection is established, the dog's pruritus increases quickly and markedly. All allergic dogs whose 'allergies' suddenly worsen should be examined for fleas, other external parasites, or infection. If infection is found, it should be treated appropriately. Some allergic dogs have near constant infections. They respond to the appropriate antibiotic or antifungal treatments, but the infection recurs weeks later. These dogs may benefit from maintenance protocols discussed in Chapter 10.

Nonspecific modes of treatment tend to decrease, but not stop the animal's itching. If the animal is comfortably itchy both for itself and its owner, no further therapy is necessary. Usually additional therapy is necessary. The aim of medical therapy is to provide the desired results with the least side effects. Since many medications are available, it is often a matter of trial and error to find the best drug. Some owners are unwilling to experiment.

Anti-inflammatory Agents

Allergic diseases are inflammatory disorders and anti-inflammatory drugs can lessen or eliminate the signs of the disease. Many anti-inflammatory drugs exist and more are being developed. Today, corticosteroids, antihistamines, antidepressants, and special ω-6/ω-3 fatty acid supplements receive the widest use in animals.

There is little agreement among veterinarians, including the authors, on the place of corticosteroids in the management of allergic pruritus. Some individuals will avoid their use at all costs while others use them to the exclusion of all other treatments. Clearly, the latter should be avoided. Beyond that, the appropriateness of corticosteroid therapy depends on the case in question. Primary care veterinarians who see the young healthy allergic patient with a short allergy season find treatment with corticosteroids safe and effective. Dermatologists tend to be at the other end of the spectrum. They typically see animals with severe perennial allergies that need to be documented and treated with for example immunotherapy and strict dietary control. Both the primary care and referral veterinarian see cases that fall between the two extremes. The specific details of the case dictate the place of corticosteroids in its management.

Nonsteroidal agents

There are hundreds of potentially useful nonsteroidal agents, which may be of benefit to the allergic animal. Only a small number have been tested in dogs and cats and some are effective (Table 6.1) while others are of little or no benefit (Table

Table 6.1 *Oral agents useful in controlling allergic pruritus.*

Category	Drug name	Dosage for dogs	Dosage for cats
Corticosteroids	Dexamethasone	0.1 mg/kg q. 48–72 h	0.2 mg/kg q. 48–72 h
	Methylprednisolone	0.9 mg/kg q. 48 h	1.8 mg/kg q. 48 h
	Prednisolone	1.1 mg/kg q. 48 h	2.2 mg/kg q. 48 h
	Prednisone	1.1 mg/kg q. 48 h	2.2 mg/kg q. 48 h
	Triamcinolone	0.1 mg/kg q. 48–72 h	0.2 mg/kg q. 48–72 h
Antihistamines	Clemastine	0.05–0.1 mg/kg q. 12 h	0.15 mg/kg q. 12 h
	Chlorpheniramine	0.4 mg/kg q. 8 h	0.44 mg/kg q. 12 h
	Diphenhydramine	2.2 mg/kg q. 8 h	
	Hydroxyzine	2.2 mg/kg q. 8 h	
Antidepressants	Amitriptyline	1.0–2.0 mg/kg q. 12 h	
Fatty acids	DVM DermCaps™	1 cap/9.1 kg q. 24 h	1 ml/9.1 kg q. 24 h
	EfaVet™	1 cap/9.1 kg q. 24 h	1 cap/9.1 kg q. 24 h
	Gamma-linolenic acid	44 mg/kg q. 24 h	
	Eicosapentaenoic/ docosahexaenoic	60 mg/kg q. 24 h	
Mast cell stabilizer	Oxatomide		15–30 mg/cat q. 12 h

6.2). Very few are licensed for use in pets, and some which are extremely safe in humans (e.g. acetaminophen) can be toxic to animals. Before a clinical trial with a new drug is begun, the manufacturer of the drug should be contacted for any canine or feline pharmacologic or toxicologic data that might have been generated during the drug's development. These data should help define the safety of the drug and allow calculation of an appropriate dose. The efficacy will be determined by clinical trial. The doses given here have some proven efficacy with minimal–no

Table 6.2 *Oral agents of little benefit in controlling allergic pruritus in dogs.*

Category	Drug name	Dosage
Antihistamines	Astemizole	0.25 mg/kg q. 24 h
	Cimetidine	6 mg/kg q. 8 h
	Cyproheptadine	0.1 mg/kg q. 12 h
	Loratadine	0.4–1.0 mg/kg q. 24 h
	Terfenadine	5 mg/kg q. 12 h
	Trimeprazine	0.5 mg/kg q. 12 h
Antidepressants	Doxepin	1 mg/kg q. 8 h
Antioxidants	Vitamin C	30 mg/kg q. 12 h
	Vitamin E	400 IU q. 12 h
Miscellaneous	Acetylsalicylic acid	25 mg/kg q. 8 h
	Doxycycline	3 mg/kg q. 12 h
	Erythromycin	11 mg/kg q. 8 h
	Papaverine	150–300 mg/dog q. 12 h
	Zinc methionine	1 mg/kg q. 24 h

side effects. Various investigators talk of using higher doses with increased efficacy and no additional toxicity. Since their data are not published, it is impossible to determine the cost-effectiveness of their treatments. However, their comments highlight the variability of animals to tolerate and respond to any one particular drug. A drug that is of no benefit at a suggested dose may be effective at an increased dose. As long as the drug has a wide margin of safety and the owner is a careful observer of the patient, it is reasonable to consider dose increases, especially if a partial response is seen at a lower dose.

Most nonsteroidal agents act at one point in the inflammatory cascade rather than in the broad-based fashion of glucocorticoids (Griffin, 1993; Scott and Miller, 1993; Miller and Scott, 1994a; Scott *et al.*; 1995). Typically, they are not as effective as glucocorticoids in treating inflamed skin. If glucocorticoids will not stop the pruritus and inflammation, nonsteroidal agents are very unlikely to do so. However, nonsteroidal agents can prevent the skin from becoming inflamed if they are started just as the animal starts to itch or if they are preceded by a short course of glucocorticoids.

When all pruritic dogs or cats are considered together, it is clear that nonsteroidal agents are not as effective as glucocorticoids in the treatment of pruritus. However, in an individual case, one or more of the nonsteroidal agents may stop the animal's itching just as well as a glucocorticoid. The only way to determine the efficacy of the various agents is by a drug trial. If no response is seen in 14 days, the drug is ineffective and another should be used. Depending upon the number of drugs tested, the entire trial can be long, cumbersome, and unrewarding for about 50% of dogs and 25% of cats. Some owners will refuse to consider completion of the entire drug trial. Many clients will do some or all of the testing if given the option.

Where do nonsteroidal agents fit into the long-term management of allergic pruritus? Except with fatty acid supplements, an individual in the household must be available to administer the nonsteroidal agent to the dog every 8–12 hours on a regular basis. Cats are treated every 12–24 hours. Some agents, especially those that are not available in a generic formulation, are expensive. These and other limitations make the long-term management of allergic pruritus with nonsteroidal agents impractical in many households. Clients with pets that itch for 2–6 months usually find these treatments most acceptable. Other candidates for these treatments are pets awaiting specific allergy testing and those who have been allergy tested and are on immunotherapy and are waiting for its benefits to be seen.

Antihistamines

Antihistamines, or histamine blockers, can be beneficial in the treatment of allergic disorders (Scott and Buerger, 1988; Miller and Scott, 1990; Paradis *et al.*, 1991a, 1991b; Miller *et al.*, 1993; Miller and Scott, 1994b; Paradis, 1995; Scott *et al.*, 1994; Paterson, 1995). Antihistamines are compounds with varied chemical structures that can antagonize some of the actions of histamines. Some antihistamines may directly inhibit or stimulate mast cell secretion and alter the numbers or function of lymphocytes and other cell types influencing mast cell function (Miller and Scott, 1994a). Histamine blockers work by competitively antagonizing histamine at the receptor site on cell membranes. Two classes of histamine receptors, namely H_1 and H_2, are recognized. H_1 receptors mediate the classical allergic changes seen with histamine while the H_2 receptors mediate gastric acid secretion. H_2 receptors are also found on the membranes of mast cells, basophils, and lymphocytes. Endogenous histamine stimulates the receptors on these cells in a negative feedback fashion such that further histamine release is inhibited.

All H_1 blockers are antihistaminic, have some local anesthetic properties, and are anticholinergic (Scott and Miller, 1993; Miller and Scott, 1994a). Hydroxyzine, an anti-histamine that may stabilize mast cell membranes, is classified as a true ataractic drug with a psychotropic effect of producing calmness without depression or clouding of consciousness. Sedation is a common side effect of traditional H_1 blockers, but is mini-mal with the newer non-sedating products. Overdosage, either because of patient idiosyncrasies, gross overdosage, or decreased metabolism and excretion, can induce hyperexcitability, cardiac arrhythmias, and death (Scott and Miller, 1993; Miller and Scott, 1994a; Otto and Greentree, 1994). Since very few antihistamines are licensed for pets, specific contraindications for use are extrapolated from the human data. In gen-eral, antihistamines should be avoided or used with caution in animals with central nervous system disorders (e.g. seizure disorders, intracranial masses), glaucoma, car-diac arrhythmias, gastric and proximal duodenal spastic disorders, and urinary reten-tive disorders. Some antihistamines can be teratogenic so they should be avoided in pregnant animals. Antihistamines are metabolized by the liver and should be used with extreme caution in animals with decreased hepatic function. The simultaneous use of antihistamines and certain drugs is contraindicated in humans because hepatic clearance of these drugs alters the metabolism of the antihistamine and may cause antihistamine intoxication. To the authors' knowledge, these drug interactions have not been reported in animals, but it would seem prudent to avoid the various drug combinations. The drugs of most concern in veterinary dermatology are ketoconazole and itraconazole. They, and presumably all imidazole compounds, can increase the blood concentration of some antihistamines and corticosteroids.

Before 1988, most veterinarians dismissed H_1 blockers as ineffective in the treat-ment of allergic pruritus. Today, it is known that although any one particular antihistamine may not be effective in any more than 30% of treated dogs, antihista-mines as a group can be very useful (Scott and Buerger, 1988; Miller and Scott, 1990; Paradis *et al.*, 1991a, 1991b; Miller *et al.*, 1993; Miller and Scott, 1994b; Paradis, 1995; Scott *et al.*, 1994; Paterson, 1995). Dogs and cats are very individualistic in their response to a particular antihistamine. An animal may not respond to one antihista-mine, but may stop itching completely when another antihistamine is used. The only way to determine the efficacy of antihistamines in a particular animal is by sequential drug trials. If a drug is of minimal–no use after 14 days of administration, that drug should be discontinued and the next one started. If the animal's pruritus decreases by 50% or more during this initial treatment, the drug trial should be extended to see if the improvement increases and is sustainable. The maximal response may not be seen within 14 days (Paterson, 1995). Because allergic pruritus is modulated by numerous pruritogens, not just histamine, the number of dogs that experience a marked (but not complete) reduction in their pruritis with an anti-histamine is often greater than the number that stop itching entirely. The client should be asked to note these partially effective drugs. If no single drug is found to be satisfactory, the simultaneous use of several partially effective drugs may stop the pet's itching. This is discussed under combined treatments.

Most of the data on the efficacy of antihistamines and the other nonsteroidal agents were generated by non-blinded, typically non-placebo-controlled, clinical trials of 50 or fewer allergic animals ((Scott and Buerger, 1988; Miller and Scott, 1990; Paradis *et al.*, 1991a, 1991b; Miller *et al.*, 1993; Miller and Scott, 1994b; Paradis, 1995). With these scientific shortcomings, especially the small sample sizes, the specific figures given for efficacy (e.g. stops pruritus in 6.7% of dogs) must be viewed cautiously. Efficacy data have changed when a drug trial has been repeated in a different population of dogs (Paradis *et al.*, 1991a, 1991b; Miller *et al.*, 1993). However, no drug protocol proven to be of benefit in one study has been shown to be ineffective in another. The list of potentially useful antihistamines generated by these studies is shown in Table 6.1. The list of minimally effective products is shown in Table 6.2. As mentioned earlier, some investigators claim greater efficacy when increased doses are used. The doses listed in the various tables are those that produce minimal side effects and can be used as the baseline dosage in dose titration studies.

Some owners will not complete an entire antihistamine trial, but will try one or two. For them, it is appropriate to select a drug of high efficacy. For the dog, clemastine, chlorpheniramine, hydroxyzine, and diphenhydramine are most-to-least effective, respectively, in completely stopping pruritus (Scott and Buerger, 1988; Paradis *et al.*, 1991a, 1991b; Miller *et al.*, 1993). The rank order for decreasing pruritus by 50% or more is clemastine, hydroxyzine, diphenhydramine, and chlorpheniramine. For the cat, chlorpheniramine is superior to clemastine in stopping pruritus (Miller and Scott, 1990, 1994b). Neither drug has any real benefit in just reducing pruritus in the cat. Cats either respond completely or not at all. At the doses suggested in Table 6.1, side effects to H_1 blockers are uncommon. In decreasing order of frequency, side effects include drowsiness, anorexia, vomiting, diarrhea, and increased pruritus (Scott and Buerger, 1988; Miller and Scott, 1990; Paradis *et al.*, 1991a, 1991b; Miller *et al.*, 1993; Miller and Scott, 1994b; Scott *et al.*, 1994; Paradis, 1995). Drowsiness is usually transient and disappears in a week or less. Some mild sedation may be beneficial in hyperexcitable dogs who seem to itch out of proportion to the stimulus.

Cimetidine is a commonly used H_2 blocker. Alone, H_2 blockers have no dermatologic applications and could increase the severity of allergic reactions by inhibiting the negative feedback mechanism of histamines on mast cells. Some human data indicate that the combination of a H_1 blocker and cimetidine gives better results than those obtained with just the H_1 blocker. The expense of the drug has limited the number of studies in atopic dogs to one (Miller, 1989). When diphenhydramine (2.2 mg/kg q. 8 h) was given with cimetidine (6.6 mg/kg q. 8 h), no dog responded.

Antidepressants

Pruritus can originate centrally or peripherally (Shanley, 1988; Scott *et al.*, 1995). Animals with allergic skin diseases have peripheral pruritus but the intensity of the stimulus may be modulated centrally. Modulation is a commonly recognized phenomenon when the allergic dog stops itching while it is engaged in happy play. Itch is habit forming due to alteration of the cutaneous sensations, probable endorphin release, and other central affects. How much of an animal's pruritus is due to central affects is unknown. The recognition that antidepressant drugs can be beneficial in some nonpsychogenic dermatological disorders in humans has increased the interest in this avenue of treatment for allergic pets.

Tricyclic antidepressants have been most widely studied in dogs (Paradis *et al.*, 1991a; Miller *et al.*, 1995a; Griffin, 1993; Scott *et al.*, 1995). The exact mode of action of these drugs is unknown, but they bind with varying affinity to various receptors, including H_1, H_2, muscarinic, acetylcholine, noradrenergic, and serotonin receptors. The affinity of tricyclic antidepressants for H_1 and H_2 receptors is very marked, making them some of the most potent histamine blockers known. The list of contraindications for the use of antihistamines also apply for these drugs.

Two drugs, doxepin (1 mg/kg q. 8 h) (Paradis *et al.*, 1991a) and amitriptyline (1–2 mg/kg q. 12 h) (Miller *et al.*, 1992a), have been studied in the dog. In these studies, amitriptyline stopped or lessened pruritus in over 30% of treated dogs while doxepin was of no benefit in any dog. Amitriptyline was slightly less effective than clemastine in stopping allergic pruritus. Side effects seen with amitriptyline include sedation, vomiting, bizarre behavior, and clinically insignificant elevations of liver enzymes, especially alkaline phosphatase. Side effects seen with doxepin, given at 1 mg/kg q. 8 h include vomiting, somnolence, panting, and trembling. Griffin uses doxepin at 1–2 mg/kg q. 12 h and indicates that it can be tolerated and effective at this dosage (Griffin, 1993).

Although amitriptyline is suggested for the treatment of behavioral disorders in the cat, the authors have not been able to use it twice daily in allergic cats because all have developed significant side effects. Some investigators comment that it can be safe and effective when given once daily.

In 1994, one investigator gained national notoriety in the USA for his use of the antidepressant fluoxetine in dogs. Fluoxetine appears to selectively inhibit the reuptake of serotonin at the presynaptic neuronal membrane with no clinically important anticholinergic, antihistaminic, or anti-adrenergic activity. In the original interviews with the lay press the investigator suggested that fluoxetine (1 mg/kg q. 24 h) was safe and effective in the treatment of allergic or obsessive–compulsive disorders. In more recent reporting on his part, he acknowledges that fluoxetine has no place in the primary treatment of the average allergic dog (Melman, 1995). This supports the initial work with this drug done by Shoulberg who found minimal efficacy with some significant side effects (Shoulberg, 1990). Since pruritus is habit forming and can become an obsessive–compulsive behavior, treatment with fluoxetine or other antidepressants may have some place in the entire treatment protocol of selected cases. Until the safety and efficacy data on fluoxetine are published in a scientific fashion, the authors do not recommend its use.

Fatty acid supplements

In the late 1980s, the veterinary community was introduced to one of the most exciting methods of treatment of allergic pruritus, namely the use of Ω-6 and/or Ω-3 fatty acid supplements. Unlike the remainder of this text where trade names are avoided, specific product names are mentioned herein. Since it is difficult to obtain the specific formulation and stability data for a particular supplement, not all purportedly identical products can be expected to be identical in their clinical efficacy. Other products not mentioned may be equally or more effective, but data on their efficacy are not available.

In 1988, Scott reported that approximately 10% of the allergic dogs he treated with DVM DermCaps™ (DVM Pharmaceuticals, Inc., Miami, FL, USA) stopped itching with this treatment (Scott and Buerger, 1988). Miller corroborated these findings in 1989 when he reported that approximately 18% of his patients treated with DVM DermCaps™ stopped itching (Miller *et al.*, 1989). In the UK, Lloyd studied primrose oil (Ω-6 fatty acids), cold water marine fish oil (Ω-3 fatty acids), and an Ω-6/Ω-3 combination product (EfaVet™ Regular; Efamol Vet, London, UK) (Lloyd and Thomsett, 1989). He reported that all three supplements improved coat quality, but that the individual fatty acids did not reduce pruritus. The combination product was beneficial in reducing pruritus in 94% of his patients. Data generated by Harvey and Miller in the early 1990s have shown that over 50% of allergic cats can benefit from these treatments (Harvey, 1991; Miller *et al.*, 1993). Many of these early studies were not placebo controlled and therefore the specific figures on efficacy are subject to error. However, they have highlighted the probable benefit of fatty acid supplements and prompted many other investigations.

The essential nature of certain fatty acids and their metabolic pathways are well known (see Chapter 1) (Harvey, 1993; Horrobin, 1993). The Ω-6 and Ω-3 essential fatty acids are important for the structural integrity of membranes, for cholesterol transport, for the maintenance of the barrier layer of the skin, and for the generation of eicosanoids, especially the prostaglandins and leukotrienes. Interest in the role of the eicosanoids in health and disease has exploded in the last ten years. Eicosanoids have wide ranging affects including control of epidermal proliferation, modulation of the immune system at various points, and modulation of cutaneous inflammation (Harvey, 1993; Horrobin, 1993; Scott *et al.*, 1995). The two-series of eicosanoids are pro-inflammatory while the four- and five-series are less inflammatory or anti-inflammatory.

Why do some allergic dogs and cats respond to fatty acid supplementation? An obvious answer was dietary deficiency. Dietary deficiency has been discounted since all the studied animals were fed high-quality foods and their response was independent of the food they were eating. One of the theories on the pathogenesis of atopy in man suggests that affected individuals are deficient in the enzyme delta-6-desaturase (Horrobin, 1993; Scott *et al.*, 1995). Without sufficient quantities of this enzyme, fatty acid metabolism is abnormal, resulting in a relative or absolute excess of the pro-inflammatory eicosanoids. If such an enzymatic deficiency exists in atopic animals, supplementation with gamma-linolenic and/or eicosapentaenoic acids – fatty acids beyond the initial delta-6-desaturase blockade – would be expected to be beneficial. The responses seen in the initial studies using products with high levels of gamma-linolenic and eicosapentaenoic acids, support the theory of abnormal fatty acid metabolism in atopic dogs.

If irregularities in fatty acid metabolism are a central feature of atopy in animals, why are the response rates in the initial studies not greater? Since there are dozens of non-eicosanoid chemical mediators and modulators of pruritus, a complete response to treatments aimed at altering eicosanoid levels only would not be expected. However, since the DVM DermCaps™ and EfaVet™ Regular are very similar in formulation and dosage administered, various investigators revisited the issue of fatty acid supplements to try to determine whether response rates could be improved. Studies have focused on the efficacy of Ω-6 fatty acids alone, the Ω-3 fatty acids alone, the efficacy of Ω-6/Ω-3 combinations in various ratios, and the influence of the dose administered. The studies reported since the initial studies are difficult to compare and contrast because of their different subjects and study protocols. Basically, the early work can be summarized as follows: Ω-6 supplements at a dosage of 40 mg/kg/day, Ω-3 supplements at 16.5 mg/kg/day, or DVM DermCaps™ at double the manufacturer's recommended dose are no more effective than either DVM DermCaps™ or EfaVet™ Regular at the manufacturer's suggested dosage (Bond and Lloyd, 1992a, 1992b; Scarff and Lloyd, 1992; Scott *et al.*, 1992; Bond and Lloyd, 1994a). Studies then shifted to the effects of larger doses. Bond reported in several studies that the mean dosage of EfaVet™ Regular needed to control clinical signs in his dogs satisfactorily was approximately four times the manufacturer's suggested dose (Scarff and Lloyd, 1992). He and Lloyd switched some dogs, well controlled at four times the suggested dose to high dosages of pure Ω-6 or pure Ω-3 fatty acids (Bond and Lloyd, 1994a). The Ω-6 or Ω-3 content of the pure supplements was 1.25 or five times, respectively, greater then that taken in the combination product. When the dogs were switched from one product to another, there was no statistical difference in their response compared to that seen with the combination product. When Logas treated atopic dogs in a blinded fashion with either a marine lipid (Ω-3 dosage of 66 mg/kg/day) or corn oil (Ω-6 dosage of 130 mg/kg/day), the dogs did significantly better with the Ω-3 supplement (Logas and Kunkle, 1994). All these latest studies show that some animals may need very large doses of an appropriate supplement before a response is seen. What was not made clear was whether treatment should be begun with pure Ω-6 or pure Ω-3 or a combination product.

In 1994, Vaughn *et al.* published the results of a study where normal dogs were fed experimental diets containing Ω-6 and Ω-3 fatty acids in ratios of 5:1, 10:1, 25:1, 50:1, and 100:1. Leukotriene synthesis in the skin and neutrophils was measured. The dogs produced less pro-inflammatory and more anti-inflammatory eicosanoids when they ate the 5:1 or 10:1 diets. Vaughn's data indicates that both Ω-6 and Ω-3 fatty acids in the appropriate ratio are important in modulating inflammation. His work may help explain the sometimes conflicting results reported with supplementation. In those studies, no mention is made of the fatty acid content of the dogs' diet. Levels of the various fatty acids, especially the Ω-3 fatty acids, vary greatly from diet to diet. Depending on the type and amount of supplementation, the dog's total dietary Ω-6:Ω-3 ratio can be improved or worsened.

Scott and Miller performed an eight-week dietary trial in 18 atopic dogs with a commercial lamb and rice dog food (Ω-6:Ω-3 ratio of 5.5:1) and looked at the clinical response and the changes in blood and skin fatty acid profiles (Scott *et al.*, 1997). Their pruritus of eight of the 18 dogs was satisfactorily controlled with this diet. Seven of the eight responders had failed to improve when a fatty acid supplement was added to their original diet. With rare exception, the plasma fatty acid concentrations increased in all dogs during the dietary trial. All dogs had an abnormality in dihomo-gamma-linolenic acid metabolism, suggesting a delta-5-desaturase deficiency. Lloyd also recognized a delta-5-desaturase irregularity in one of his studies (Bond and Lloyd, 1992b). Scott and Miller also recognized a subset of dogs with an abnormality in linoleic acid metabolism, suggesting a delta-6-desaturase deficiency. The dogs whose pruritus did not decrease with the diet had this additional abnormality in fatty acid metabolism. If their data are substantiated in larger numbers of dogs, it would appear that all atopic dogs do have a defect in fatty acid metabolism. Some dogs are very abnormal. It would be very difficult to improve the pruritus in this latter subset with any fatty acid supplement.

To date, only three studies have been published on the efficacy of fatty acid supplements in the treatment of feline pruritus. Logas treated cats with a pure Ω-6 supplement and saw no response (Logas and Kunkle, 1993). Harvey and Miller, using EfaVet™ Regular (Harvey, 1991) or DVM DermCaps™ (Miller *et al.*, 1993), respectively, reported that over 50% of their patients improved with treatment.

All the studies performed to date indicate that fatty acid treatments can be very beneficial in atopic dogs and cats. These treatments are safe and are only contra-indicated in animals with a history of pancreatitis or fat intolerance. With the wide variation in the fatty acid content of commercial pet foods and the probability that not all atopic animals can metabolize fatty acids in an identical fashion, no one supplement at a specific dosage should be expected to be best for all animals. As with antihistamines, efficacy can only be determined by drug trial. In the veterinary literature, there are two schools of thought on the length of time necessary to prove or disprove efficacy of supplementation. One group indicates that a minimum of six weeks of treatment is necessary while the other indicates that 14–21 days is suffi-cient. If the purpose of the supplementation is to decrease pruritus, it will be seen in 21 days or less (Scott *et al.*, 1997). If improvement in coat quality, decrease in ery-thema, scale, or other cutaneous abnormalities is the focus, six or more weeks of treatment will be necessary to see the animal's maximal improvement.

What types of supplement should be tested? If the fatty acid profile of the animal's base diet is available, examination of the profile should suggest the type and amount of supplementation needed. Since it is very difficult to obtain these profiles, most cases will be treated on an empiric basis. Today, there are many different but seemingly identical fatty acid supplements. However, since their ingredients and processing are not identical it would be unreasonable to expect each product to perform in an identi-cal manner. Unless specific data on the efficacy of a particular product are available, it is probably best to avoid that product in the initial testing. A proven commercial supplement at the manufacturer's suggested dose should be used for the initial testing. If the proven product is ineffective, there is no clearcut answer as to what to do next. Options include megadosing the initial supplement, trial courses with each of the vari-ous other commercial supplements, dietary modification like the one tested by Scott and Miller, or supplementation with high dosages of Ω-3 fatty acids. Since megadosing the commercial combination products can be very expensive and commercial dog foods are generally low in Ω-3 fatty acid content, the authors suggest that the dog's diet is changed or a pure Ω-3 fatty acid supplement is tested next. The dosage should approach the 66 mg/kg/day suggested by Logas. If the second testing produces no results, subsequent testing would be on a hit-or-miss basis.

Corticosteroids

The cortex of the adrenal gland produces aldosterone, corticosteroids, and the sex steroids (Griffin, 1993; Scott, 1995; Scott *et al.*, 1995). In the dog and cat, cortisol is the primary corticosteroid produced. In the dog, the total corticosteroid secretion rate in prednisolone equivalents is 0.11–0.22 mg/kg/day. Corticosteroid production is under the control of the hypothalamic–pituitary–adrenal axis (HPAA). Adrenocorticotropic hormone (ACTH) is released from the pituitary under the influence of blood (plasma) cortisol concentration and higher influences. Plasma ACTH levels and con-sequently plasma cortisol levels are regulated by blood (plasma) cortisol levels, 'stress', and a diurnal rhythm.

Cortisol secretion is not constant throughout the day. In general, levels fluctuate according to a circadian (diurnal) rhythm, but marked changes can occur from hour to hour. Both ACTH and plasma cortisol levels are highest in the early morning and gradually decrease during the day. The cat, because of its nocturnal nature, appears to have a reversed rhythm with peak plasma levels occurring during the evening. Stress which can include fright, cold, exercise, or trauma can override the circadian rhythm and cause increased levels. Plasma cortisol levels, either endogenous or exogenous, act through a negative feedback loop to alter ACTH and cortisol secretion. Chronic steroid abuse will cause HPAA suppression. Severely suppressed animals are not able to respond to 'stress' and a shock-like condition can occur.

Adrenal corticosteroids have both glucocorticoid and mineralocorticoid activity. Glucocorticoids were introduced into clinical use in 1949. Modification of the basic steroid molecule has increased the glucocorticoid activity while decreasing the mineralocorticoid effects. The physiologic effects of pharmacologic plasma levels of glucocorticoids are caused by the alteration of glucose, protein, and lipid metabolism and a modulation of the immune response. Glucocorticoids modulate inflammation by altering macrophage function (decreased phagocytosis and decreased response to cytokines), altering lymphocyte function (decreased proliferation and decreased antigen processing), decreasing vascular permeability, decreasing the release of vasoactive amines, inhibiting prostaglandin and leukotriene synthesis, decreasing serum complement concentration, redistributing leukocytes, and stabilizing plasma membranes (Scott, 1995; Scott *et al.*, 1995). In general, glucocorticoids have a greater effect on leukocyte traffic than on function. The neutrophilia seen with glucocorticoid administration is caused by accelerated release from the bone marrow, an increase in the circulating half-life of the neutrophil, and a decrease in neutrophil egress from the blood. These changes decrease the number of neutrophils in the inflammatory site and lead to a decrease in inflammation. At therapeutic doses, glucocorticoids do not directly decrease antibody production. Steroid modulation of cellular interaction can result in a dampening of the humoral response.

The occurrence and severity of side effects seen with glucocorticoid administration depend upon the drug used, the route of administration, the frequency of administration, the duration of administration, the metabolic status of the animal, and idiosyncrasies of the animal (Scott and Miller, 1993; Miller and Scott, 1994a). Cats are resistant to but not immune from glucocorticoid side effects. Steroid side effects can be divided into those that are clinically obvious and those that are biochemical or immunologic.

Clinical side effects always include polydipsia, polyuria, and polyphagia. These signs are typically dose dependent. Some dogs will show profound signs even with very low doses. In many instances, the severity of these signs is associated with the use of prednisone or prednisolone. Switching the animal to an equipotent dose of another glucocorticoid with no mineralocorticoid activity usually decreases the polydipsia and polyuria to expected levels. Weight gain, personality changes, and excessive panting are other common findings.

With more chronic use or increased sensitivity on the animal's part, one sees muscle wasting, weakness, fat redistribution, and dermatologic changes. In dogs, the skin signs are a poor coat, which does not regrow well, thin skin, comedones, seborrhea, and an increased sensitivity to bacterial infection. Some dogs will develop calcinosis cutis. Cats, especially aged ones, will develop extremely fragile skin. Once the skin fragility is recognized, the damage is so advanced that managing these cats is extremely difficult. Internal changes include HPAA suppression, eosinopenia, neutrophilia, lymphopenia, hypercholesterolemia, hyperglycemia, elevation of the liver enzymes, and subnormal thyroid function.

Glucocorticoids are not innocuous and should be used carefully. Topical products have the widest margin of safety while injectable drugs are the most dangerous. Because of the widespread nature of allergic pruritus in animals, topical products have little application as the sole mode of treatment. In some cases, simultaneous use of topical and oral glucocorticoids will allow a lowering of the dose of oral glucocorticoid or the use of some nonsteroidal anti-inflammatory agents.

Topical glucocorticoids
Although the topical route of administration of glucocorticoids appears to be innocuous to owners, all or most of the drug will be absorbed into the animal's body where it acts like an oral or injectable product. Since far fewer mg of drug are given by the topical route, clinical side effects are not usually seen. However, even short courses of a potent topical glucocorticoid can induce HPAA suppression, will interfere with allergy tests, and can alter the animal's metabolism (Griffin, 1993; Scott, 1995; Scott et al., 1995). Abuse of a potent topical product in a small area will cause localized cutaneous Cushing's disease (e.g. epidermal atrophy, hair loss, comedones). Use over wide areas will cause full-blown iatrogenic hyperadrenocorticism. Since topical glucocorticoid preparations are expensive and most allergic animals itch in wide areas, have haired skin, and tend to lick off topical medications, they have limited use in allergic pets as the sole mode of treatment. They are most useful in animals with allergic otitis externa or with focal areas of intense pruritus.

With topical products, not only does one have to select the drug, but also the vehicle. Topical glucocorticoids are available in a cream, ointment, gel, lotion, or spray form. For acute eruptions, lotions or gels should be used, while creams and ointments are reserved for chronic lesions (Scott et al., 1995). A potent glucocorticoid will be needed to gain control of a pre-existing inflammation. For the skin, the drug will have to be applied three or four times daily, while once or twice daily will suffice in the ears. For maintenance treatment, the frequency of administration is decreased and a less potent agent is used. No studies are available in animals suggesting that one topical steroid is more effective than another. Betamethasone valerate is a commonly used potent product and 1% hydrocortisone receives widest use for maintenance therapy.

Many allergic dogs and cats have both itchy skin and ears. The animal's body and otic pruritus can be stopped with oral glucocorticoids but the dosage required to stop both is usually higher than that needed to stop the body itching. Appropriate use of an otic glucocorticoid will allow a significant reduction in the systemic dosage. Allergic otitis externa is an inflammatory ceruminous otitis with or without secondary colonization or infection by bacteria, *Malassezia* yeast, or both. Infection is determined by cytologic examination of any exudate. Successful ear treatment requires the removal of the excess cerumen, elimination of any infecting organisms, and a reduction in the inflammation. Ear cleaners will be needed in all cases to remove the wax, pus, and old medication. The choice of the otic medication depends on whether the ears are infected or just inflamed. With infection, one of the many glucocorticoid–antibiotic–antifungal products is typically used. Once the infection has resolved, the medication should be changed since these products usually contain potent glucocorticoids and the anti-infectives are no longer needed. Two authors (WHM, LMR) find that a solution of 1% hydrocortisone and 2% Burow's solution in propylene glycol is very effective for the treatment of non-infected allergic otitis externa. A once-daily application controls the symptoms in many allergic animals. The product is inexpensive and because of its propylene glycol base is an effective ear cleaner. Thus the owner can both clean and medicate with only one application.

Oral glucocorticoids

The oral route of glucocorticoid administration is usually preferred since the dosage can be carefully controlled and the drug can be discontinued quickly if necessary (Griffin, 1993; Scott and Miller, 1993; Miller and Scott, 1994a; Scott, 1995; Scott *et al.*, 1995). Many veterinarians administer an injection of a glucocorticoid, usually of a repositol nature, and follow it with oral medication. This practice should be discouraged since it increases the cost and potential risk of steroid therapy and is usually no more effective than appropriate oral therapy.

If oral glucocorticoids are to be used at anti-inflammatory doses for two weeks or less, any drug can be used and gradual tapering before withdrawal is unnecessary. Although the rare dog will show signs of glucocorticoid insufficiency when the medication is stopped abruptly, most dogs will not since significant adrenal suppression will not occur with this short course of treatment. In most clinics, prednisone or prednisolone is the oral glucocorticoid of choice. Although there are pharmacologic differences between them, they seem to be interchangeable in most animals. For dogs, the initial dose of prednisolone used to treat very pruritic animals is 1.1 mg/kg q. 24 h. Obviously, the initial dose can be reduced if the patient's condition warrants it. Cats receive 2.2 mg/kg q. 24 h. Some cats with a glucocorticoid-responsive dermatitis will show no response to this dose of prednisolone, but will stop scratching completely when an equipotent dose of dexamethasone is used.

Traditionally, the daily dose of prednisolone is divided and 50% is given twice daily. Most dogs and cats respond just as well when the full dose is given once daily. Once-daily therapy is less labor intense for the owner, especially of cats, and tends to minimize the clinical side effects. Most dogs who take their prednisolone only in the morning will not wake the owner up in the middle of the night to urinate (Scott *et al.*, 1995). If another oral glucocorticoid is the drug of choice in a clinic or is needed for an individual case, it should be administered at an equivalent dose. For instance, dexamethasone and triamcinolone are considered by some to be ten times more potent then prednisolone (Griffin, 1993; Scott *et al.*, 1995). Accordingly, the anti-inflammatory dose of dexamethasone or triamcinolone for dogs and cats is 0.1 mg/kg q. 24 h and 0.2 mg/kg q. 24 h, respectively.

Oral glucocorticoids are far from innocuous and prolonged usage, especially at high dosage, puts the animal at risk of developing side effects. This is especially true in old animals or when the animal has an intercurrent medical problem. Clearly, a week or two of treatment in the young healthy animal will have no longlasting affects. Treatment for six months or more will induce some longlasting metabolic and pathologic changes. Intermediate courses of treatment may or may not be problematic. There are no clearly defined standards that help the practitioner decide when alternatives to glucocorticoids should be sought for the pet who itches for 1–6 months. One author (WHM) believes that alternatives to glucocorticoids should be investigated when the pruritus persists for two months or longer while the other authors use glucocorticoids only for a short period of time or when all else fails.

If long-term glucocorticoid therapy is necessary, daily therapy is contraindicated. For maintenance therapy, alternate-day therapy should be used as this minimizes HPAA suppression and the catabolic side effects of glucocorticoids (Scott and Miller, 1993; Miller and Scott, 1994a; Scott, 1995). Minimization is the key word! Alternate-day therapy does not eliminate the deleterious side effects, but only keeps them, hopefully, to an acceptable level. Because of their short half-lives, prednisone, prednisolone, or methylprednisolone are the only drugs to be used.

Alternate-day glucocorticoids are minimally effective in eliminating pre-existing inflammation. Daily treatments are needed to return the skin to normal. If daily treatments are stopped too soon, alternate-day therapy may be ineffective. The common practice of dispensing glucocorticoids with very specific and inflexible instructions (e.g. give the dosage twice daily for three days, then once daily for three days, and then on alternate days) can cause some treatment failures if the dosage is reduced before the inflammation has resolved. The best treatment protocol is one individualized to the patient's needs. The client should be given guidelines on what is expected from the steroid for his or her pet and be told to administer the drug daily until the goals are met. The client should also be told to return for an examination if the desired results are not seen within a certain number of days. After the acute symptoms have resolved, the therapy is switched to the alternate-day regimen and then the dose is decreased to the lowest possible acceptable level. There are two commonly used protocols to achieve alternate-day administration. In the first, the loading dose of prednisolone is given daily until healing is satisfactory, typically 5–7 days. At that point, the same dose is administered every other day for 7–14 days. If the animal's pruritus is well controlled, the alternate-day dose is gradually reduced to the lowest acceptable level. In the other protocol, the glucocorticoid is given daily until healing has occurred and then the daily dosage is gradually reduced to the lowest acceptable level. This dosage is then increased by 50–75% and is given every other day. If the animal remains symptom free, the dosage is gradually reduced. The holding dosage is given every other morning and can be adjusted up or down as needed. Nocturnal cats may do better with evening administration. The rare pet will only need treatment once or twice weekly.

When glucocorticoids are used for chronic maintenance therapy, the final dose should be one where the animal is comfortably itchy. If the allergic dog or cat is itch free, the glucocorticoid dosage is too high and should be reduced further. By maintaining the animal at a low level of pruritus, the natural progression or regression of the disease can be followed. In many patients, the maintenance dose of the glucocorticoid will have to be increased to compensate for the increasing severity of the allergic symptoms. Because trivial levels of pruritus can predispose some dogs to secondary bacterial or *Malassezia* infections and some cats are either completely itch free or are mutilating themselves, some animals have to be maintained in the itch-free state. For these animals, the dosage is titrated to the point where symptoms first appear and is then increased slightly. Periodic attempts to lower the dosage should be made to determine the animal's current glucocorticoid requirement.

Not all animals can be successfully maintained with alternate-day prednisolone treatment. Common complaints include excessive polyuria and polydipsia, even at low drug dosages, and unacceptable levels of pruritus on the off day, especially during the evening. As mentioned before, some animals are disproportionately polyuric and polydipsic when they take prednisone or prednisolone. Switching to methylprednisolone, a glucocorticoid with no mineralocorticoid activity, usually solves the problem. However, the expense of this drug can preclude its use in large dogs. There are many ways to deal with the animal whose pruritus is intolerable on the off day. The animal can be treated with a lower dosage of prednisolone on a daily basis, the animal can receive most of its prednisolone on an alternate-day basis with a small dosage administered on the off day, or a more longlasting drug like dexa-methasone or triamcinolone can be substituted for the prednisolone. Obviously, the lowest possible drug dosages are used in all three scenarios. All these protocols can be effective, but are more hazardous then alternate-day prednisolone treatment. The animal is exposed to a more constant source of exogenous glucocorticoid, which will suppress the HPAA and, more importantly, does not give the tissues time to repair themselves. With any of these protocols, the question is not if glucocorticoid side effects will be seen, but rather when and to what extent will they be seen.

Animals receiving chronic glucocorticoid therapy, especially with a non-alternate-day prednisolone regimen, should have a complete physical examination at least twice yearly. Since dogs taking chronic corticosteroids are prone to urinary tract infections, a urinalysis should be evaluated at each visit. Blood work is run as needed. If clinical or laboratory abnormalities are detected or reach an unacceptable level, the therapy can be modified or, if glucocorticoids are the only effective form of therapy, the owner can be informed that changes are occurring and must be followed carefully.

Injectable glucocorticoids

Parenteral glucocorticoids vary in potency, the route of administration, and the rate of absorption from the injection site. The basic steroid molecule is conjugated to an ester base. Modification of the ester base changes its water solubility, which alters its rate of absorption. The hemisuccinate and phosphate bases have a very high water solubility with complete absorption in 30–60 minutes. The acetate, diacetate, tebutate, acetonide, and hexacetonide bases give poor water solubility with absorption in 2–14 days.

Parenteral glucocorticoids, even those with the hemisuccinate or phosphate bases, do not have an immediate onset of action. The mechanism of action of glucocorticoids is via the generation of cell specific proteins and because of the time necessary to generate these proteins, the earliest change that can be seen after an intravenous injection is one hour, with the maximum effect seen in eight hours. Because of this delayed onset, glucocorticoids should not be considered as the first line of defense in life-threatening allergic reactions. Since oral drugs are typically absorbed in 30 minutes or less, injections are not needed for immediate relief.

Parenteral glucocorticoids are administered subcutaneously, intramuscularly, or intralesionally. The intralesional route is really subcutaneous (sublesional) administration as it is very difficult to administer intralesional glucocorticoids with a needle and syringe. Intralesional steroids can cause as many side effects as subcutaneous or intramuscular glucocorticoids.

The place of parenteral steroids in the management of chronic pruritus in dogs is debated. The authors do not use repositol glucocorticoids in dogs and believe that their frequent use is inappropriate for the management of allergic pruritus in most cases. Use of extremely longlasting products is contraindicated in all cases. Regardless of the product used, the precise daily dose released and the duration of action is extremely variable. With repositol forms, the duration of HPAA suppression and molecular tissue damage far outlasts the clinical anti-inflammatory effects. If repositol drugs are to be used, they should be reserved for cases where anti-inflammatory therapy is required for two weeks or less, once or twice a year (Miller and Scott, 1994a; Scott *et al.*, 1995).

Many dermatologists, including the authors, use repeated injections of repositol glucocorticoids in cats. Young healthy cats are more resistant to steroid side effects and can be safely treated with multiple injections of methylprednisolone acetate (5 mg/kg) (Scott and Miller, 1993; Scott *et al.*, 1995). Most young cats show no permanent deleterious side effects when they are given injections every third month. If the cats is aged or requires more frequent injections, oral glucocorticoids should be considered.

Some owners report that oral medications do not work as well as injections. This is typically due to an insufficient oral dose of medication and can be corrected by increasing the dose or changing the drug. If parenteral drugs are the only effective glucocorticoid for an animal, the long-term prognosis is very guarded.

Combination Treatments

Since cutaneous inflammation is a very complex process and the various non-steroidal agents discussed previously have a very focused area of activity, many individual agents may not be potent enough to provide partial or complete relief from pruritus. Partial efficacy is recognized when the nonsteroidal agent reduces the animal's pruritus by 50% or more, but not enough to consider treatment successful (Scott and Buerger, 1988; Paradis *et al.*, 1991a). Simultaneous treatment with two or more agents with different modes of action can be beneficial in both dogs and cats.

A variety of studies on the efficacy of the combination of a fatty acid supplement and an H_1 blocker have been published (Paradis *et al.*, 1991b; Bond and Lloyd, 1992a; Paterson, 1995; Scott and Miller, 1995). In one group of experiments, the animals showed no improvement with the administration of the standard dosage of either the antihistamine or fatty acid supplement (Paradis *et al.*, 1991b; Bond and Lloyd, 1992a; Scott and Miller, 1995). In another study, the treated dogs had responded partially to the antihistamine, but the response was not sufficient for long term control (Paterson, 1995). The results of the experiments showed that the combination of two ineffective drugs could stop pruritus in some animals and would increase the performance of a partially effective drug. The authors are also aware of many cases in dogs where a partially effective antihistamine or antidepressant became effective when a fatty acid supplement was added to the treatment regimen.

The potential for synergism between fatty acid supplements and antihistamines has prompted many investigators, including the authors, to start their antihistamine and antidepressant trials in combination with a fatty acid supplement. The fatty acid supplement is started first. If an incomplete or no response is seen after 21 days of administration, an antihistamine or an antidepressant is added, one at a time, to the treatment regimen. If a combination is of minimal benefit after 7–14 days of simultaneous use, the ineffective drug is replaced with another until a satisfactory combination is found or until all combinations are proven ineffective. When an effective combination is found, the question arises as to whether the response is due to the antihistamine or antidepressant alone or the combination of drugs. The question is answered by dropping the antihistamine or antidepressant. If the animal's pruritus returns to its pre-trial level, the antihistamine or antidepressant is important and the fatty acid supplement can be discontinued.

The steroid-sparing effects of antihistamines or fatty acid supplements have also been demonstrated (Miller, 1989; Paradis *et al.*, 1991a, 1991b; Bond and Lloyd, 1994b). In one study, the combination of the antihistamine trimeprazine and prednisone was effective in a greater percentage of dogs then either drug alone (Paradis *et al.*, 1991a). In the same study, the authors reported that the addition of trimeprazine to a well-established alternate-day glucocorticoid regimen allowed a 30–50% reduction in the prednisone dosage for 75% of the dogs. The steroid-sparing effects of fatty acid supplements have also been demonstrated. When atopic dogs with an established alternate-day glucocorticoid protocol were given either DVM DermCaps™ or EfaVet™, most dogs were able to have their maintenance level of glucocorticoids reduced by 25–50% (Miller, 1989; Bond and Lloyd, 1994b). To the authors' knowledge, no studies have been performed to determine whether the combination of a fatty acid supplement and an antihistamine or antidepressant would have maximal steroid-sparing effects.

Beyond trials with the combination of an antihistamine or antidepressant and a fatty acid supplement, complex treatment protocols should be approached carefully in most allergic animals. The use of three or more drugs increases the confusion, expense, and labor intensity of the treatment. Some clients can become so disenchanted with complex treatments that they elect to return to glucocorticoids. The prime candidate for simultaneous treatment with three or more drugs is the dog or cat whose pruritus can only be controlled with a high-dose glucocorticoid protocol. Many owners of these animals will try anything to help their pet. Drugs should be selected carefully so that drug similarities or interactions do not intoxicate the animal.

Nonsteroidal Anti-inflammatory Drugs

By convention, the term nonsteroidal anti-inflammatory drug (NSAID) is reserved for those compounds that inhibit prostaglandin synthesis (Scott and Buerger, 1988). Individual compounds can have additional actions. Aspirin and phenylbutazone are the classic NSAIDs. Many newer NSAIDs (e.g. acetaminophen, ibuprofen) are marketed for humans and more are being developed. Most NSAIDS are highly protein bound resulting in prolonged effects, but this can also cause pharmacokinetic interactions by displacing other agents from their protein binding sites. Gastrointestinal ulceration and bleeding can occur as a result of the irritation of these drugs and/or because these drugs decrease the protective prostaglandin production. Bleeding disorders, nephrotoxicity, and drug eruptions can also occur with many of these agents.

Aspirin is the most widely used NSAID in veterinary medicine. In addition to interrupting prostaglandin synthesis, it also dampens the actions of prostaglandins and inhibits the formation of kinins. When Scott tested the antipruritic activity of aspirin at very high doses (25 mg/kg q. 8 h) in atopic dogs, the results were very disappointing (Scott and Buerger, 1988). His data suggest that prostaglandins are not a major mediator of pruritus in the dog. If true, other NSAIDs would be expected to be equally as ineffective as aspirin.

Antioxidants

All normal individuals form small amounts of free radicals (superoxide, hydroxyl, and peroxide) during normal metabolic processes. Large quantities are generated with cellular injury. Free radicals perpetuate the initial insult by further damaging tissues. The hydroxyl radical is most reactive and can initiate lipid peroxidation and cause cell membrane damage. Free radicals can be neutralized by enzymatic and nonenzymatic antioxidants. Nonenzymatic agents include vitamin C, vitamin E, and reduced glutathione. Glutathione peroxidase, catalase, and superoxide dismutase are the major enzymatic systems. DMSO (dimethyl sulfoxide) is a well known chemical free radical scavenger.

When vitamin E (400 IU q. 12 h) or vitamin C (30 mg/kg q. 12 h) was given to atopic dogs, no dog's pruritus improved (Miller, 1989; Miller *et al.*, 1992b). These data suggest that either free radicals play no significant role in allergic pruritus or that nonenzymatic antioxidants are not potent enough to neutralize the free radicals. Orgotein, a copper–zinc superoxide dismutase, was licensed for use in the dog. Although some initial work showed encouraging anti-inflammatory results, the product was withdrawn from the market before it was evaluated in allergic diseases. It is unknown whether other individual antioxidants or combinations would have any effect on allergic pruritus.

Mast Cell Stabilizers

Mast cell stabilizers have no direct anti-inflammatory effects. They stabilize membranes and inhibit the degranulation of sensitized mast cells. As mentioned previously, hydroxyzine may have some cell stabilizing effects. The authors have used experimental mast cell stabilizers in dogs and found them to be very effective after a 2–3 week lag phase. None of these drugs has reached the market. One report indicates that the mast cell stabilizer oxatomide can be beneficial in about 50% of atopic cats when used at 15–30 mg/cat q. 12 h (Prost, 1993).

Unproven Agents

A variety of other potentially useful antipruritic agents have been tested and have been shown to be of minimal benefit (see Table 6.2) (Scott and Buerger, 1988; Miller, 1989; Scott and Cayatte, 1993; DeBoer *et al.*, 1994; Paradis, 1995). We are presently in the era of gene manipulation, cytokine isolation and purification, and immunologic modulation to help human patients with acquired immunodeficiency syndrome (AIDS). All these efforts may well produce some agents of benefit to allergic pets.

Autoimmune and immune-mediated skin disorders are well known in veterinary dermatology and are treated with immunosuppressive agents, which have wide-ranging immunological effects (Scott *et al.*, 1995). Treatment protocols are well established. Since allergy can be considered a state of immunologic hyperreactivity, it stands to reason that immunosuppressive agents might be of some benefit. Treatment with the agents discussed below is radical, expensive, potentially life-threatening, and of unproven benefit. These treatments should be considered only as a last resort when the animal has failed to respond to all conventional treatments. Prolonged discussions with the client are necessary to ensure that he or she understands the experimental nature of these treatments.

Cytotoxic agents

The antimetabolite azathioprine and the alkylating agent chlorambucil are the two most commonly used immunosuppressive agents in veterinary dermatology (Griffin, 1993; Scott *et al.*, 1995). Among their other effects these agents decrease antibody production and decrease the number of leukocytes. Because of cats' sensitivity to it, azathioprine is used primarily in dogs at a dose of 1.5–2.5 mg/kg q. 24 h. When cats with dermatological disorders are treated with a cytotoxic agent, chlorambucil at a dose of 0.1–0.2 mg/kg q. 24 h is typically used. As would be expected, either agent can cause myelosuppression and a variety of other side effects. The reader should thoroughly familiarize him or herself with either product before using it. To the authors' knowledge, this method of treatment has only been used in the dog (Miller and Scott, 1994). Typical of the protocols used to treat autoimmune skin diseases, the drug is given daily until maximal benefit is seen, typically after 2–3 weeks. At this point, the drug is administered on an alternate-day basis for maintenance therapy. In the reported cases, the dogs' pruritus was reduced, but not eliminated with treatment. The authors are also aware of cases where no response was seen.

Gold salt therapy (chrysotherapy)

Chrysotherapy is used in the treatment of rheumatoid arthritis and certain autoimmune skin diseases (Scott *et al.*, 1995). Among their effects, gold compounds can stabilize lysosomal membranes, decrease migration and phagocytic activity of macrophages and neutrophils, inhibit prostaglandin synthesis, and suppress immunoglobulin synthesis. Aurothioglucose is the most widely used gold compound in veterinary medicine and is administered at a dose of 1 mg/kg intramuscularly once weekly after two test doses. A lag phase of 6–12 weeks is common. Reported side effects are few, but nephrotoxicity and bone marrow suppression can be seen. During the induction phase of therapy, urinalysis should be run weekly and a hemogram should be run bimonthly.

Tetracycline and niacinamide

Tetracyclines possess a variety of anti-inflammatory and immunomodulatory properties including decreased antibody production, inhibition of lipases and collagenases, and inhibition of prostaglandin synthesis (White *et al.*, 1992). Niacinamide can block antigen–IgE-induced histamine release, prevent degranulation of mast cells, inhibit phosphodiesterases, and decrease protease release.

Tetracyclines have been used successfully in man to treat a variety of noninfectious skin diseases including acne, rosacea, panniculitis, bullous pemphigoid, and sterile eosinophilic pustulosis (Scott *et al.*, 1995). Aside from one study on the effects of doxycycline on atopic pruritus in dogs (Scott and Cayatte, 1993), the anti-inflammatory effects of tetracyclines in inflammatory dermatoses of the dog and cat remain untested. In the atopic study, no dog experienced any relief with treatment. As a sole agent, niacinamide also remains untested in animals.

When the combination of tetracycline and niacinamide was given to dogs with either discoid lupus erythematosus or pemphigus erythematosus, 25–65% of the dogs responded (White *et al.*, 1992). Anecdotally, this combination has also been used to treat successfully some dogs with dermatomyositis, sterile granulomatous disorders, sterile panniculitis, metatarsal fistulas in German shepherds, hereditary lupoid dermatosis of the German shorthaired pointer, and lupoid onychodystrophy (Rosychuk, 1995). At the onset of treatment each drug is given three times daily. Dogs over 10 kg of body weight receive 500 mg of tetracycline and 500 mg of niacinamide. Dogs weighing less than 10 kg receive 250 mg of each drug. Once a response is seen, the frequency of administration is decreased to twice daily and then once daily if possible. Side effects are reported to be uncommon and include anorexia, vomiting, diarrhea, hyperexcitability, depression, and lameness.

To the best of the authors' knowledge, tetracycline and niacinamide remain untested in the treatment of allergic pruritus. The actions of niacinamide suggest that it could be very effective.

References

Bond R, Lloyd DH. Randomized single-blind comparison of an evening primrose oil and fish oil combination and concentrates of these oils in the management of canine atopy. *Vet. Dermatol.* **3:** 215, 1992a.

Bond R, Lloyd DH. A double-blind comparison of olive oil and a combination of evening primrose oil and fish oil in the management of canine atopy. *Vet. Rec.* **131:** 558, 1992b.

Bond R, Lloyd DH. Double-blind comparison of three concentrated essential fatty acid supplements in the management of canine atopy. *Vet. Dermatol.* **4:** 185, 1994a.

Bond R, Lloyd DH. Combined treatment with concentrated essential fatty acids and prednisolone in the management of canine atopy. *Vet. Rec.* **134:** 30, 1994b.

DeBoer DJ, Moriello KA, Pollet RA. Inability of short-duration treatment with a 5-lipoxygenase inhibitor to reduce clinical signs of canine atopy. *Vet. Dermatol.* **5:** 13, 1994.

Griffin CE. Canine atopic disease. In Griffin CE, Kwochka KW, MacDonald JM (eds) *Current Veterinary Dermatology.* Mosby Year Book, St Louis, 1993, p. 133.

Harvey RG. Management of feline miliary dermatitis by supplementing the diet with essential fatty acids. *Vet. Rec.* **128:** 326, 1991.

Harvey RG. Essential fatty acids and the cat. *Vet. Dermatol.* **4:** 175, 1993.

Horrobin DF. Medical uses of essential fatty acids (EFAs). *Vet. Dermatol.* **4:** 161, 1993.

Kwochka KW. Shampoos and moisturizing rinses in veterinary dermatology. In Bonagura JD (ed.) *Kirk's Current Veterinary Therapy XII*. W.B. Saunders, Philadelphia, 1995, p. 590.

Lloyd DH, Thomsett, LR. Essential fatty acid supplementation in the treatment of canine atopy. A preliminary study. *Vet. Dermatol.* **1:** 41, 1989.

Logas DB, Kunkle GA. Double-blinded study examining the effects of evening primrose oil on feline pruritic dermatitis. *Vet. Dermatol.* **4:** 181, 1993.

Logas D, Kunkle GA. Double-blinded crossover study with marine oil supplement containing high-dose eicosapentaenoic acid for the treatment of canine pruritic skin disease. *Vet. Dermatol.* **5:** 99, 1994.

Melman SΛ. Use of Prozac in animals for selected dermatological and behavioral conditions. *Vet. Forum* August: 19, 1995.

Miller WH Jr. Non-steroidal anti-inflammatory agents in the management of canine and feline pruritus. In. Kirk RW (ed). *Current Veterinary Therapy X*. Philadelphia. W.B. Saunders, 1989, p. 566.

Miller WH Jr. Fatty acid supplements as anti-inflammatory agents. In Kirk, RW (ed.) *Current Veterinary Therapy X*. Philadelphia. W.B. Saunders, p. 563, 1989.

Miller WH Jr, Scott DW. Efficacy of chlorpheniramine maleate for the management of allergic pruritus in cats. *J. Am. Vet. Med. Assoc.* **197:** 67, 1990.

Miller WH Jr, Scott DW, Wellington JR. A clinical trial on the efficacy of clemastine in the management of allergic pruritus in dogs. *Can. Vet. J.* **34:** 25, 1993.

Miller WH Jr, Scott DW. Medical management of chronic pruritus. *Compend. Cont. Ed.* **16:** 449, 1994a.

Miller WH Jr, Scott DW. Clemastine fumarate as an antipruritic agent in pruritic cats. Results of an open clinical trial. *Can. Vet. J.* **35:** 502, 1994b.

Miller WH Jr, Griffin CE, Scott DW. Clinical trial of DVM Derm Caps in the treatment of allergic diseases in dogs. A nonblinded study. *J. Am. Anim. Hosp. Assoc.* **25:** 163, 1989.

Miller WH Jr, Scott DW, Wellington JR. Nonsteroidal management of canine pruritus with amitriptyline. *Cornell Vet.* **82:** 53, 1992a.

Miller WH Jr, Scott DW, Wellington JR. Investigation of the antipruritic effects of ascorbic acid given alone and in combination with a fatty acid supplement to dogs with allergic skin disease. *Canine Pract.* **17:** 11, 1992b.

Miller WH, Jr, Scott DW, Wellington JR, *et al.* Efficacy of DVM Derm Caps liquid in the management of allergic and inflammatory dermatoses of the cat. *J. Am. Anim. Hosp. Assoc.* **29:** 37, 1993.

Otto CM, Greentree WF. Terfenadine toxicosis in dogs. *J. Am. Vet. Med. Assoc.* **205:** 1004, 1994.

Paradis M, Scott DW, Giroux D. Further investigations on the use of nonsteroidal and steroidal antiinflammatory agents in the management of canine pruritus. *J. Am. Anim. Hosp. Assoc.* **27:** 44, 1991a.

Paradis M, Lemay S, Scott DW. The efficacy of clemastine (Tavist), a fatty acid-containing product (DVM Derm Caps), and the combination of both products in the management of canine pruritus. *Vet. Dermatol.* **2:** 17, 1991b.

Paradis M. Nonsteroidal antipruritic drugs. *Proc. Eur. Soc. Vet. Derm.* **12:** 203, 1995.

Paterson S. Additive benefits of EFAs in dogs with atopic dermatitis after partial response to antihistamine therapy. *J. Sm. Anim. Pract.* **36:** 389, 1995.

Prost C. Les dermatoses allergiques du chat. *Pract. Med. Chirurg. Anim. Comp.* **28:** 151, 1993.

Rosychuk RAW. Newer diseases and therapies in veterinary dermatology. *Proceedings of the Fall Skin Seminar.* DVM Pharmaceuticals, Inc., Key West, p. 18, 1995.

Scarff DH, Lloyd DH. Double blind, placebo-controlled crossover study of evening primrose oil in the treatment of canine atopy. *Vet. Rec.* **131:** 97, 1992.

Scott DW. Rational use of glucocorticoids in dermatology. In Bonagura, JD (ed). *Kirk's Current Veterinary Therapy XII.* Philadelphia, W.B. Saunders, 1995, p. 573.

Scott DW, Buerger RG. Nonsteroidal anti-inflammatory agents in the management of canine pruritus. *J. Am. Anim. Hosp. Assoc.* **24:** 425, 1988.

Scott DW, Cayatte SM. Failure of papaverine hydrochloride and doxycycline hyclate as antipruritic agents in pruritic dogs. Results of an open clinical trial. *Can. Vet. J.* **34:** 164, 1993.

Scott DW, Miller WH Jr. The combination of an antihistamine (chlorpheniramine) and an omega-3/omega-6 fatty acid-containing product (DVM Derm Caps) in combination, and the fatty acid supplement at twice the manufacturer's recommended dosage. *Cornell Vet.* **80:** 381, 1990.

Scott DW, Miller WH Jr, Decker GA, *et al.* Failure of terfenadine as an antipruritic agent in atopic dogs: Results of a double-blinded, placebo-controlled study. *Can. Vet. J.* **35:** 286, 1994.

Scott DW, Miller WH Jr, Decker GA, *et al.* Comparison of the clinical efficacy of two commercial fatty acid supplements (EfaVet and DVM Derm Caps), evening primrose oil, and cold water marine fish oil in the management of allergic pruritus in dogs. A double-blinded study. *Cornell Vet.* **82:** 319, 1992.

Scott DW, Miller WH Jr, Griffin, CE. *Muller and Kirk's Small Animal Dermatology,* 5th edition. W.B. Saunders, Philadelphia, 1995.

Scott DW, Miller WH Jr, Reinhart GA, *et al.* Effect of an omega-3/omega-6 fatty acid-containing commercial lamb and rice diet on pruritus in atopic dogs: Results of a single-blinded study. *Can. J. Vet. Res.* **61:** 145, 1997.

Scott DW, Miller WH Jr. The combination of an antihistamine (chlorpheniramine) and an omega-3/omega-6 fatty acid-containing product (DVM Derm Caps Liquid) for the management of pruritic cats. Results of an open clinical trial. *N. Z. Vet. J.* **43:** 29, 1995.

Scott DW, Miller WH Jr. Medical management of allergic pruritus in the cat, with emphasis on feline atopy. *J. S. Afr. Vet. Assoc.* **64:** 103, 1993.

Shanley KJ. Pathophysiology of pruritus. *Vet. Clin. North Am.* **18:** 971, 1988.

Shoulberg N. The efficacy of fluoxetine (Prozac) in the treatment of acral lick and allergic-inhalant dermatitis in canines. *Proc. Am. Acad. Vet. Derm. and Am. Coll. Vet. Derm.* **7:** 31, 1990.

Vaughn DM, Reinhart GA, Swaim SF, *et al.* Evaluation of effects of dietary n-6 to n-3 fatty acids ratios on leukotriene B synthesis in dog skin and neutrophils. *Vet. Dermatol.* **5:** 163, 1994.

White SD, Rosychuck RA, Reinke ST, *et al.* Use of tetracycline and niacinamide for treatment of autoimmune skin disease in 31 dogs. *J. Am. Vet. Med. Assoc.* **200:** 1497, 1992.

7
Food Hypersensitivity

Introduction

Simplistically, an adverse reaction to a food is any abnormal or exaggerated clinical response to the ingestion of a food or a food additive. Reactions may be due to a food allergy (hypersensitivity) or food intolerance with an immunologic or a non-immunologic basis, respectively. The terminology used to describe adverse reactions to foods is confusing because of variations in the interpretation of the terms. In an attempt to standardize nomenclature, the American Academy of Allergy and Immunology (AAAI) and the National Institute of Allergy and Infectious Disease (NIAID) has proposed (AAAI, 1984) the following definitions: 'The terms food allergy and food hypersensitivity are used synonymously and describe a group of diseases that are characterized by an abnormal or exaggerated immunologic response to the ingestion of specific food allergens. Food allergy can be subdivided into two broad categories: IgE-mediated (Type I) hypersensitivities and those that occur by non-IgE-mediated immune mechanisms. Food intolerance is a term used to describe an abnormal physiological response to an ingested food or food additive that is not immunologic in nature and may include idiosyncratic, metabolic, pharmacological, or toxic responses. Food intolerances are believed to make up the majority of human adverse reactions to foods, but it is unknown if this is also true in dogs and cats.

On a clinical basis, it is very difficult to distinguish between a food hypersensitivity and a food intolerance. Dietary elimination and challenge incriminates the food, but does not define the mechanism. To make a firm diagnosis of food allergy, evidence of immunologic reactivity must be demonstrated, but this is often impractical in small animals. The terms food allergy and food hypersensitivity have been traditionally used to describe all adverse reactions to foods, including reactions that may truly be food intolerance.

The majority of well-characterized human food allergic reactions are IgE-mediated (Type I) hypersensitivities, although non-IgE-mediated immune mechanisms may be responsible for a variety of hypersensitivity disorders. Adverse reactions to food can be manifested by cutaneous, respiratory, gastrointestinal, neurologic, or hematologic signs. Symptoms may be restricted to one organ system or involve multiple organ systems. Even within one organ system, the signs of an adverse food reaction are not specific.

Pathogenesis

Ingested food represents the greatest foreign antigenic load confronting the immune system. During the digestive process the gastrointestinal barrier, by both immunologic and nonimmunologic mechanisms, blocks foreign antigens from entering the body proper. Although the 'gut-associated lymphoid tissue' (GALT) must mount a rapid and potent response against potentially harmful foreign substances and pathogenic organisms, it must also remain unresponsive to enormous quantities of nutrient proteins. In the vast majority of individuals, tolerance develops to food allergens that are constantly gaining access to the body proper, but the means by which it develops is not completely understood.

Although antibodies of all immunoglobulin classes can be produced after oral administration of antigen, laboratory studies in mice (Mowat *et al.*, 1982) show that a single feeding of a protein antigen results in suppression of systemic IgM, IgG, and IgE antibody responses as well as cell-mediated immune responses. This is believed to be due to activation of CD8$^+$ suppressor cells residing in the GALT. In the susceptible host, a failure to develop or a breakdown in oral tolerance may result in a variety of hypersensitivity responses to an ingested food antigen.

Food-allergic disorders may involve more than one hypersensitivity mechanism. Type I and Type IV hypersensitivity reactions have been documented in food hypersensitivity. The IgE produced in response to a food antigen can sensitize bowel mast cells or mast cells anywhere in the body. There is also evidence for Type III hypersensitivity reactions to foods, but these findings are inconsistent and unclear. Until proven otherwise, it is best to consider the signs of a food hypersensitivity as due to a Type I, III, or IV hypersensitivity reaction. The significance of the circulating serum concentration levels of IgA and IgG directed against foods is uncertain since they can be found not only in patients with food hypersensitivities but also in normal non-food allergic individuals and patients with other disorders.

Complete digestion of food protein results in the production of free amino acids and small peptides, which are probably poor antigens. Thus an incompletely digested food protein has a greater potential to incite an allergic response (Roudebush *et al.*, 1994). Hypersensitivity reactions to dietary allergens may induce dysfunction in the intestine's mucosal barrier, disturb the physiological protein transfer, and consequently lead to excessive permeation of intact proteins. The manner in which antigen is transported across the small intestinal mucosa has a profound effect on the initiation of the immune response. Aberrant antigen absorption can lead to an exaggerated immune response, thereby broadening the sensitivity. Increased intestinal permeability to macromolecules may be hypothesized as part of the primary defect in permeability (Roudebush *et al.*, 1994).

One human study has indicated that patients with atopic dermatitis and food hypersensitivity have subclinical malabsorption, which is reversed when food allergens are removed from the diet (Sampson, 1993). The increased susceptibility of young infants to allergic food reactions is believed to be the result of immunologic immaturity and to some extent immaturity of the gut. In atopic children, the enteric mucosa may be the first tissue to become sensitized to inhalant allergens (Scala, 1995). It is not known why foods provoke different constellations of symptoms in different individuals. Our understanding of the basic immunopathologic mechanisms in food allergy remains incomplete.

Prevalence

The true incidence of food hypersensitivity in small animals is unknown. Based on the great numbers and sales of commercial 'hypoallergenic' diets for dogs and cats, the public perception of the importance of allergic reactions to foods is obviously quite high. While early studies indicated that the overall incidence of food hypersensitivity in small animals was less than 1% of the total population (Walton, 1967), more recent investigators have found that food hypersensitivities may be more prevalent than previously thought (Baker, 1974).

In dogs, the reported incidence of food hypersensitivity varies from 1–5% of all skin conditions and up to 23% of cases of nonseasonal allergic dermatitis (Baker, 1974; Reedy and Miller, 1989; Scott *et al.*, 1995; Walton, 1967). From 1–6% of all feline dermatoses are reported to be due to food hypersensitivity (Carlotti *et al.*, 1990). Food hypersensitivity is the third most common canine allergic skin disease and the second most common in the cat (Scott *et al.*, 1995). Cats appear to have a higher incidence of food allergies than dogs (MacDonald, 1993). The incidence of non-dermatologic food allergies in small animals, such as gastrointestinal and neurologic conditions, is unknown. Obviously, food hypersensitivity can occur in conjunction with other allergic conditions. In one study (White and Sequoia, 1989), 43% of dogs with food allergy dogs also had another concurrent allergic condition such as atopy. Food hypersensitivity can be difficult to diagnose and document in a patient with multiple forms of allergy.

The U.S. Department of Agriculture has estimated that 'some 15% of the (human) population may be allergic to some food ingredients or ingredient', as recorded in the Federal Register (U.S. Department of Agriculture, 1983). In clinical surveys, 8% of children younger than six years of age have evidence of food intolerance, and 2–4% experience reproducible allergic reactions to foods. Studies suggest that 70–80% of human infants 'outgrow' their food hypersensitivity (Sampson, 1993). Similar studies are not available in adults, although some surveys suggest that 1–2% of the general adult population are sensitive to foods or food additives. Only 8% of human patients with suspected food allergy had symptoms confirmed by oral food challenge (Bock, 1987).

Food Allergens

Foods are composed of proteins, carbohydrates, and lipids. In general, the major food allergens that have been identified are water-soluble glycoproteins, which have molecular weights ranging from 10 000–60 000 daltons. Most are stable to treatment with heat, acid, and proteases, but cooking and the process of digestion can create novel antigens. Although virtually any food or food additive can cause an allergic reaction, a few food allergens are believed to be responsible for the majority of food-allergic reactions. Egg, peanuts, and cows' milk account for 80% of allergic reactions in American children, and peanuts, nuts, and seafood account for most reactions in American adults (Sampson, 1993). Fish is a major allergen in Scandinavian children. Food hypersensitivity to peanuts appears to be increasing in the USA and does not tend to be 'outgrown'.

Walton (1967) reported that milk was the cause of food hypersensitivity in 23% of dogs in Great Britain, while wheat accounted for 10%, beef 13%, and eggs 3%. Harvey (1993), also reporting on dogs from Great Britain, found that cereals (28%), dairy products (28%), and beef (8%) were the most common allergens. Results of dietary provocation in 21 dogs with proven food hypersensitivity in the USA revealed that beef, cows' milk, wheat, soybean, chicken, chicken eggs, and corn were the principal allergens (Jeffers *et al.*, 1991). In cats in the USA the most common food allergens, based on dietary challenge, are fish (42%) and dairy products (14%) (White and Sequoia, 1989). Walton reported that milk (7%) and beef (5%) were the most common food allergens in cats in Great Britain. Other reported food allergens in small animals include lamb or mutton, pork, rabbit, horsemeat, turkey, clam juice, whale meat, rice, potatoes, oat meal, maize, kidney beans, and chocolate, as well as food preservatives and food additives (Scott *et al.*, 1995). One investigator (Harvey, 1993) reported that 52% of food-allergic dogs were allergic to only one allergen and 48% were allergic to more than one.

Cows' milk is a complex food containing at least 20 protein components (Sampson, 1993). The milk-protein fractions are subdivided into casein proteins (76–86%) and whey proteins (14–24%). β-lactoglobulin is the most allergenic component, followed by casein, lactalbumin, and bovine serum albumin (Reedy and Miller, 1989). The antigenicity of some of the milk proteins is altered by heat. Bovine serum albumin is the most heat-labile component, whereas α-casein is the most heat-stable. β-lactoglobulin also is relatively heat-resistant. Whole milk, skimmed milk, and powdered milk are equally antigenic. Harvey (1993), reported that dogs that were allergic to cows' milk could not eat cheese and vice versa. Cross-reactivity has been demonstrated in humans between milk proteins in cows, goats, and sheep (Sampson, 1993). However, Jeffers *et al.* (1996) found no significant cross-reaction in dogs between beef and cows' milk. Milk and milk products are easily recognized on food labels, but milk components such as casein, casinate, lactose, and whey, which are common food ingredients, may go unrecognized as milk. Milk proteins are also found in a variety of food that might not be suspected of containing milk, such as canned tuna, hot dogs, and other nondairy products (Yunginger, 1995).

Lamb or mutton is commonly fed to dogs and cats in many parts of the world and is subsequently a frequent cause of food allergy in those countries (Walton, 1967). Since lamb was rarely used in commercial pet foods in the USA, American veterinarians commonly recommended it as the principal protein source for home-cooked food allergy elimination test diets (see 'Elimination diets' on page 182). However, in the last few years, some commercial pet food manufacturers have been using lamb or mutton in 'hypoallergenic' diets. This has led the public and some veterinarians to erroneously conclude that lamb is somehow 'hypoallergenic' and not only incapable of causing food allergy, but may even prevent the development of food allergy. The authors wish to repeat that *any food substance* is capable of causing a food allergy.

Fish, unlike other food allergens, appears to be more susceptible to manipulation, such as heating and lyophilization, than other foods (Sampson, 1993). Some human patients who were allergic to fresh cooked salmon or tuna could ingest canned salmon or tuna without difficulty. It is presently unclear whether fish proteins cross-react. The most well-characterized fish allergen is parvalbumin of cod fish, allergen M (*Gad c 1*). Scombroid fish (tuna and mackerel) can contain large amounts of histamine if they are spoiled or subjected to high storage temperatures (Reedy and Miller, 1989).

Soybeans, which are legumes and an inexpensive source of high-quality protein, are commonly added to many commercial pet foods. Four major protein fractions have been identified and they appear to be equally allergenic. Soy-allergic individuals have been reported as having no symptoms after ingesting soy oil, but

European investigators (Porras *et al.*, 1985) have detected some soy protein in soy oil products.

Wheat and other cereal grains are common causes of food allergy, especially in dogs. The globulin and glutenin fractions are believed to be major allergenic fractions in IgE-mediated reactions. Extensive cross-reactivity has been noted between the cereal grains, especially between buckwheat and rice (Yamada *et al.*, 1995), and between wheat, rye, and barley. The extent of cross-reaction between grains and grasses is unclear, but it has been reported that human patients with grass pollen allergies have an increased incidence of food allergies (Boccafogli *et al.*, 1994). The authors would like to remind readers that rice, which is commonly used in elimination or hypoallergenic diets, has been reported to cause adverse food reactions in dogs.

Closely related food groups may contain allergens that cross-react clinically, such as legumes, seafoods, and animal products (Guilford, 1992), but within a species, animal products do not consistently cross-react. An individual allergic to cows' milk may be able to eat beef and inhale cow dander (Reedy and Miller, 1989). Patients allergic to beef should obviously avoid veal as well as other bovine products such as liver, sweetbreads, and gelatin. The extent of cross-reaction between chicken protein and chicken eggs is currently unclear. IgE antibodies from egg-allergic children have been shown to cross-react with egg proteins of other birds (Sampson, 1993). Chicken egg yolk is considered less allergenic than egg white, which contains 23 different glycoproteins.

Hidden allergens can also be a problem in food allergies. Mixed vegetable oils can contain any variety or number of oils such as corn and soy. Animal fats, meat by-products, and meat-and-bone meal may contain beef, pork, or chicken. Many canned meats, including human baby food meats, such as lamb, beef, and turkey usually contain 'gravy', which indicates wheat flour. Sodium caseinate, a milk protein, is often added to canned tuna to improve the packing qualities (Yunginger, 1995). Natural vitamin A may contain fish. The term parve designates food that contains neither meat, fowl, nor milk. Food starch or modified food starch can be made from wheat, corn, sorghum, arrowroot, tapioca, or potato. Certain medications often include a binder such as calcium or magnesium stearate made from the stearic acid of pork, beef, or lamb fat. Flavoring agents in medications or treats are commonly not specified, but often consist of pork, beef, or fish. Some popular dog treats contain wheat, soybean, meat (unspecified), milk, fish, corn, and barley as ingredients.

Clinical Presentation

Clinical signs of food allergy are very variable and can involve the skin, gastro-intestinal tract, respiratory tract, central nervous system, or combinations of these systems. The skin is a frequent target organ for IgE-mediated food hypersensitivity reactions. Ingestion of food allergens may lead to the rapid onset of cutaneous symptoms or aggravate more chronic conditions. The cutaneous signs of a food hypersensitivity are varied, nonspecific, and can mimic many other dermatologic conditions.

In the dog, the most common clinical presentation of food hypersensitivity is nonseasonal generalized pruritus with or without lesions. The pruritus is of varying severity and the distribution is often indistinguishable from that seen with atopy.

Rosser (1993a) reported that 80% of 51 food hypersensitive dogs had pruritus of the ears and pinnae, while 61% chewed the feet, and in 53%, the inguinal area. Other signs included localized pruritus, flea allergy-patterned pruritus (Figure 7.1), erythema, papules, recurrent episodes of acute moist dermatitis, recurrent pyodermas, epidermal collarettes, bilateral or unilateral otitis externa, seborrhea (Figure 7.2), edema of the eyelids, urticaria, hives, and angioedema. One author (TW) reports that ventral papular dermatitis is a common feature of food hypersensitivity in dogs. Although systemic anaphylaxis from foods has been reported in humans, it has not been reported in small animals. Any sign may occur alone or in combination with others. Nondermatologic symptoms such as gastrointestinal and neurologic symptoms may occur with or without skin lesions. Concurrent allergies are common and include flea bite hypersensitivity, atopy, and allergic contact dermatitis. Rosser (1993a) reported on two dogs with idiopathic epilepsy that responded to an elimination diet and relapsed when challenged.

It is estimated that 10–15% of animals with dermatologic signs of food hypersensitivity may have concurrent gastrointestinal signs (Carlotti *et al.*, 1990), such as vomiting, diarrhea, bloating, and cramping. Stools may contain occult blood, polymorphonuclear neutrophils, and eosinophils. The incidence of concurrent gastrointestinal signs would be much higher if the occurrence of flatus, borborygmus, or subtle bowel changes were included. Griffin (Scott *et al.*, 1995) observed that pruritic dogs who had more than three bowel movements day (normal 1.5/day) were more likely to have food allergies.

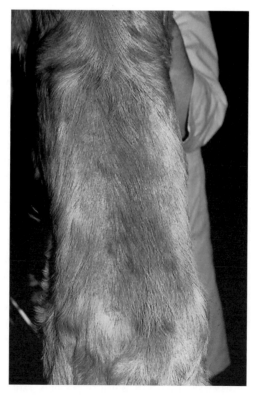

Figure 7.1   *Traumatic hair loss over the lower back.*

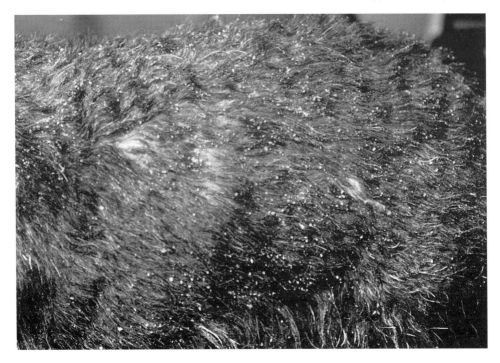

Figure 7.2   *Seborrhea sicca due to a food hypersensitivity.*

There appears to be no age, sex, or breed predisposition. Symptoms can begin at any age. In one study (Rosser, 1993a), the initial age of onset of symptoms was less than one year old in 33%, 1–3 years of age in 51%, and 4–11 years of age in 16%. The youngest was two months old and the oldest was 11 years of age. Any breed may be affected, including mixed breeds, but Rosser (1993a) also reported soft-coated wheaten terrier, dalmatian, west Highland white terrier, collie, Chinese shar pei, Lhasa apso, cocker spaniel, springer spaniel, miniature schnauzer, and Laborador retriever at risk of developing food hypersensitivity. MacDonald (1993) reported that food hypersensitivities, in the southeastern part of the USA, were more common in Chinese shar peis and poodles.

Clinical signs of food allergy in cats are also varied with the most common being pruritus, traumatic alopecia, and miliary dermatitis (Figure 7.3). The pruritus may be generalized, but is often localized to the face, neck, or ear region (Plate 3). In one study of 13 cats with food hypersensitivity (Rosser, 1993b), the ears were involved in 69% and the face in 62%. There was a generalized distribution in 8%. Other reported signs include eosinophilic plaques and lymphocytic–plasmacytic colitis (Nelson *et al.*, 1984). One cat with chronic diarrhea was diagnosed as having duodenal lymphosarcoma on two separate endoscopic biopsies. After medical treatment failed to help, the cat was placed on an elimination diet, and the clinical signs resolved, but returned with each food challenge (Wasmer *et al.*, 1995). As with dogs, there is no age, sex, or breed predisposition. Concurrent allergies such as flea bite hypersensitivity and atopy are not uncommon in cats with food hypersensitivity.

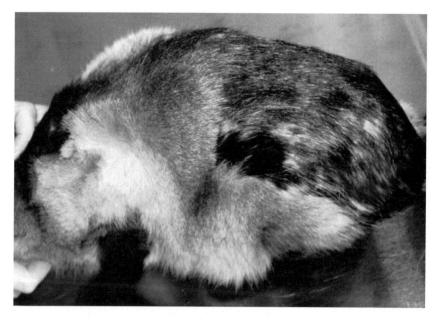

Figure 7.3   *Traumatic hair loss over the lower back of a cat with a food hypersensitivity to fish.*

A history of dietary change or absence of dietary change is not usually helpful in food hypersensitivity. This may be due to common allergens in most pet foods. Walton (1967) reported a two-year sensitization in his food hypersensitive cases. Although food hypersensitivities in small animals typically cause perennial symptoms, the authors have seen dogs and cats with seasonal or episodic food reactions. Seasonal symptoms due solely to the ingestion of seasonal allergens are rare in pets. A more likely cause would be a perennial borderline food hypersensitivity that becomes symptomatic with an increase in pollens. This could be due to cross-reactions between food allergens and pollen allergens or the threshold phenomenon. Cross-reactions between inhaled and ingested allergens such as between grass pollens and cereal grains are common in humans, but have been poorly documented in small animals. If both the pollen allergy and food allergy are borderline, symptoms would only occur when both were present. Episodic food reactions that occur when the patient only eats the offending allergen periodically are rare, and are more likely to be due to food intolerance (non-immunologic) than food hypersensitivity. The authors have seen episodic adverse food reactions when pizza was fed to a dog, a dog ate garbage, and a cat ate a mouse.

Although variable, the response to glucocorticoids can often be useful in the clinical history of a patient with food allergy. As a general rule, dogs and cats with food hypersensitivities do not respond as well to glucocorticoid therapy as patients with other types of allergies, such as atopy. For example, for a cat with severe facial pruritus that does not respond to adequate glucocorticoid therapy, one of the first rule-outs would be food allergy. The reason for this poor response in some patients is unknown. However, a good response to glucocorticoids does not exclude food hypersensitivity from the differential diagnosis. A complete response to systemic glucocorticoids has been reported in 39% (Rosser, 1993a) to 50% (Scott *et al.*, 1995) of food hypersensitive dogs and 64% of food hypersensitive cats (Rosser, 1993b).

Diagnostic Approach

In many diseases, the clinical manifestations, history, and available laboratory tests are often characteristic or even pathognomonic of the causative agent(s). This is not the case with food hypersensitivity, which can mimic many other conditions, both allergic and nonallergic. Depending on the signs and history, food hypersensitivity should always be considered in the differential diagnosis. Important rule-outs include atopy, flea bite hypersensitivity, scabies, infections (bacterial, yeast, and fungal), drug reactions, and idiopathic seborrhea.

There is a great need for simple and reliable diagnostic tests in food hypersensitivity. The ideal test should have high reliability, be able to document that the patient's symptoms are caused by certain allergen(s), and demonstrate that the offending allergen is causing the symptoms through an immunologic mechanism. Since the immunologic mechanisms of food hypersensitivity may be multiple and more than one mechanism may be involved in the same patient, it is highly unlikely that a single laboratory test will determine the immunologic nature of all food hypersensitivity reactions. Currently, in veterinary medicine, the diagnosis of food hypersensitivity is based predominantly on clinical grounds and the demonstration of an immunologic response to a food allergen is difficult and impractical. Four methods that are employed in the diagnosis of food hypersensitivity (Table 7.1) include:

- elimination diet;
- intradermal skin or *in vivo* tests;
- serum or *in vitro* tests – for example the radioallergosorbent test (RAST) and enzyme-linked immunosorbent assay (ELISA)
- gastroscopic food sensitivity testing.

Elimination diets

The standard method of diagnosis of any adverse food reaction involves dietary elimination, challenge, and provocation. Before an elimination diet is started, concurrent problems such as fleas or infections should be resolved first. Improvement following antimicrobial therapy does not rule-out food hypersensitivity as the underlying cause. The restrictive diet must be individualized based on the list of ingredients in the pet's typical diet, including snack foods and flavored medications. It is important that the pet owner understands that every ingredient the pet has been eating is suspect and must be avoided during the test period. Since most commercial pet foods share similar ingredients, switching from one brand or type to another is not adequate. A short period of fasting coupled with the use of cathartics may hasten the pet's response, but are usually not necessary or readily accepted by most owners. One indiscretion by any family member, friend, or neighbor can invalidate the test and mean restarting from the beginning. Pets that roam freely, hunt, or eat garbage cannot be adequately tested unless they are confined. In multiple pet households, the suspected food hypersensitive pet must not eat the other pets' food. Cat litter boxes must be removed from the dog's access since ingestion of cat feces can be a point source of a 'food' allergen.

Home-cooked elimination diets

A strict home-cooked elimination test diet is recommended for the diagnosis of food hypersensitivities in small animals. For the dog, a protein and a carbohydrate source must be selected while only a protein source is selected for the cat. If the pet has not eaten a diet containing lamb, it can be used for the protein source. If lamb has been fed over several months, it cannot be used. Other potential protein sources include rabbit, venison, goat, fish, turkey, and horsemeat depending upon the pet's previous eating habits. The protein source can be boiled, broiled, or baked. If ground lamb is used, boiling is preferred to remove excess fat. If whole fish is used, it can be cooked in a pressure cooker to dissolve the bones. Boiled rice or potatoes are commonly used as carbohydrate sources. A large supply of meat and carbohydrates can be cooked separately in advance, stored in plastic bags, frozen, and then thawed and heated as needed. For feeding, the rice or potatoes are mixed with the protein source at a ratio of 5:1 to 2:1. Water may be added to the ration if this diet is constipating.

Since sudden dietary changes can cause gastrointestinal disturbances, the new ingredients should be introduced slowly over 3–4 days. Most cats will take longer to adjust to the dietary change. Approximately the same volume as the normal ration is fed. For some pets, the amount may need to be increased, but do not overfeed. While the test diet is being fed, the pet should not receive anything else – no table foods, rawhide chew sticks, dog bones, or flavored medications should be given. Dogs who need to chew can have overcooked meat or unflavored nylon bones. If a

Table 7.1   *Diagnostic tests for food allergy.*

Type of test	Example
SCREENING	
Diagnostic elimination diets	Home-cooked elimination diets Commercial 'hypoallergenic' diets
Skin testing	Intracutaneous Patch testing
Serum testing	RAST ELISA
Less commonly used tests	Serum specific IgG, IgM, or IgA antibodies Leukocyte histamine release Circulating immune complexes Lymphokine production Lymphoblast transformation Intestinal mucosal biopsy Organ culture (jejunal biopsy) challenge Sublingual provocation Subcutaneous provocation Leukocyte cytotoxic test Serum specific IgG4 antibodies Neutrophil chemotactic assay
VERIFICATION	
Elimination–challenge test	

medication is necessary, such as a heartworm preventative, the unflavored form should be used.

Commercial 'hypoallergenic' diets

In theory, a hypoallergenic diet is one that is less likely to produce or aggravate a food hypersensitivity by containing only a limited number of allergens (e.g. only one protein and one carbohydrate source). The hope is that the aggravating allergen is avoided. Unfortunately, many commercial 'hypoallergenic' diets, even those advertised as containing only rice and lamb, also include other ingredients that may perpetuate the allergic symptoms, such as milk, soy, wheat, corn, and poultry products (Brown *et al.*, 1995). For this reason, commercial 'hypoallergenic' diets are not recommended as the initial test elimination diet. There are many commercial 'hypoallergenic' diets currently on the market and new ones frequently introduced. The authors prefer to use these diets for maintenance after the diagnosis of food hypersensitivity has been established and the food allergen is known (see 'Treatment' on page 185).

Response time

Most food hypersensitive patients will show some improvement with the elimination diet within 3–4 weeks, but some may take as long as 6–10 weeks. In one report (Harvey, 1993), all of 25 food hypersensitive dogs responded within three weeks. However, Rosser (1993a), reported that 30% of his 51 cases responded within 1–3 weeks, 53% within 4–6 weeks, and the remainder within 7–10 weeks.

Challenge

If an improvement is noted with the elimination diet, the patient should be challenged with the old diet. If no relapse is seen, treats are introduced. The time required to provoke an adverse response varies. As a general rule, the longer it takes for clinical signs to resolve on the elimination diet, the longer it can take for the offending dietary component to reinitiate those signs. The duration of time between challenge and the onset of clinical signs is significantly different between dogs with intolerance to cereal (8.3 days) and those intolerant to dairy products (4.1 days) (Harvey, 1993), but none required longer than 14 days to relapse. When food hypersensitive cats were challenged (Rosser, 1993b), symptoms returned within 15–30 minutes in two of them, 24 hours in two cats, 2–3 days in four cats, 6–8 days in four cats, and 10 days in one cat.

If symptoms do not recur with challenge, the improvement was coincidental. If symptoms do recur, the diet should be switched back to the elimination diet. If the patient improves a second time on the elimination diet, a food hypersensitivity or intolerance has been documented. If the symptoms decrease significantly, but not completely, the pet may have a food hypersensitivity concurrent with some other disease. The authors have had clients who reported that the elimination diet reduced but did not eliminate their pet's symptoms, indicating concurrent problems (e.g. food plus atopy or food plus flea).

Provocative challenge testing is necessary to identify the allergen and is done by adding one pure food ingredient to the restrictive diet every 7–14 days. Only one food ingredient (e.g. beef, milk, wheat) is added at a time. In humans, the double-blind, placebo-controlled oral food challenges (DBPCFC) to diagnose food allergy are labeled the 'gold standard' for the diagnosis of food allergies (Sampson, 1993). If the signs recur or intensify during the challenge period, the pet cannot tolerate this ingredient and it should be discontinued. Once the symptoms return to the prechallenge state, the next food ingredient is added until the entire list of test foods (Table 7.2) is completed. When the elimination–challenge test gives an equivocal result, it should be repeated. The diagnosis of food allergy is considered established when withdrawal of the suspected allergen from the diet leads to a complete resolution of symptoms and three successive challenges with the causative allergen duplicates presenting symptoms (Goldman *et al.*, 1963). Unfortunately, these stringent conditions are rarely met in veterinary practice. Although hypersensitivities undoubtedly exist, there is no way that a clinician can distinguish hypersensitivity from the other putative mechanisms of dietary intolerance.

In vivo and *in vitro* testing

Skin testing and serologic testing are used in humans to identify specific IgE antibodies to a food allergen. Test results may or may not be clinically significant. Probable reasons for this lack of accuracy include alterations in the antigenic composition of food antigens as a result of cooking, processing, digestion, and metabolism. Some investigators (Goldman *et al.*, 1963) have noted that certain milk-sensitive patients have negative skin and serum test results to the native protein, but are positive for the enzymatic digest of β-lactoglobulin. The reliability of skin and serum testing also varies widely from one food to another. The clinical significance of positive skin and serum tests must be proven by provocative challenge.

Skin testing not only detects the presence of antibody, but also the releasability of mediators from mast cells. In man, skin testing is an acceptable means of excluding immediate food allergy, but only 'suggestive' of indicating clinical hypersensitivity (Sampson, 1993). Intradermal testing for food antigens has a high incidence of false-positive results (60–65%) whereas negative skin tests confirm the absence of IgE-mediated reactions (negative predictive accuracy greater than 95%). Commercial food extracts are apparently not as accurate as pure fresh foods for skin testing. Approximately 41% of human allergists routinely skin test for food allergies. In veterinary medicine, skin testing for food allergy remains unproven. The sensitivity of skin testing for food allergy in dogs (i.e. proportion of subjects with disease that will have a positive test for the disease) has been found to be 33% and the specificity (i.e. proportion of subjects without the disease who have a negative reaction), 50.5% (Kunkle and Horner, 1992). Serum testing for food allergies in dogs is even less

Table 7.2   *Foods for challenge testing.*

Beef	Fish
Chicken	Corn
Pork	Soy
Chicken	Wheat
Lamb	Brewer's yeast
Egg	Milk

accurate than skin testing. ELISA testing was found to have a positive predictive value of only 40% and RAST testing was judged unreliable (Jeffers *et al.*, 1996). Based on these studies, skin and serum tests are not recommended for the diagnosis of food allergies in dogs. The reliability of skin and serum testing for food allergies in cats is currently unknown.

Other diagnostic techniques

Other *in vivo* and *in vitro* tests are available in human medicine to aid in the diagnosis of a food hypersensitivity. Cytotoxic types of tests have not been shown to be reliable or reproducible and should not be used (Sampson, 1993). However, basophil or leukocyte histamine release assays are specific and reproducible tests. These tests are unproven in veterinary medicine and their technical difficulties limit their usefulness.

Gastroscopic food sensitivity testing (GFST) involves endoscopic observation of gastric mucosal reactions following exposure to pure food extracts. This technique has only been performed on a small number of dogs (Guilford *et al.*, 1994) and needs to be studied further before the usefulness of the test is known. An interesting observation has been that the sensitivity of the procedure appears to be enhanced by preceding testing with a hypoallergenic diet ('unmasking').

Skin biopsies are of little value in the diagnosis of food hypersensitivities. The changes – a superficial perivascular dermatitis with some hyperplastic epidermal changes – are common to most hypersensitivity disorders. Strict food trials remain the preferred method of diagnosis of food hypersensitivity in small animals.

Treatment

The best therapy for food hypersensitivity is strict avoidance. In order to do this completely the offending allergen(s) must first be known. Unless the veterinary clinician provides an unequivocal diagnosis of food hypersensitivity, a large percentage of the pet population will continue to have their diets altered based on misconceptions of food hypersensitivity. Most pets with food hypersensitivities can usually eat a specially selected commercial 'hypoallergenic' diet. The list of ingredients is compared with the results of the provocative challenge testing and a suitable diet is selected. If the pet cannot tolerate the 'hypoallergenic' diet, the diet either has some hidden allergen(s) or the patient is also allergic or intolerant to additives, artificial flavors, dyes, or preservatives. Another similar commercial 'hypoallergenic' diet should be tried. Canned diets require fewer preservatives than dry foods and may therefore be better tolerated (Guilford, 1992). White (1986) reported that 54% of his patients with food hypersensitivity who responded to home-cooked lamb and rice experienced a flare when fed canned rice and lamb. The reasons for this are unknown.

Approximately 20% of food hypersensitive dogs cannot consume any commercial diet and must be maintained on a home-cooked diet (Scott *et al.*, 1995). Prolonged feeding of a strict unbalanced diet will lead to malnutrition, metabolic abnormalities, and eating disorders. Supplementation with fats, vitamins, and minerals is essential to ensure nutritional adequacy (Table 7.3). Prolonged feeding of a single protein source

Table 7.3   *Maintenance hypoallergenic diet for dogs and cats. (From Lewis and Morris, 1984.)*

Dietary constituent	Amount
Lamb	4 oz
Cooked rice	1 cup
Vegetable oil	1 teaspoon
Dicalcium phosphate	1½ teaspoons
Balanced unflavored vitamin and mineral supplement	
	Yield: ²/₃ pound (530 kcal)

may increase the likelihood of developing a hypersensitive reaction to that protein. Reedy (1994) reported that a cat hypersensitive to fish developed a hypersensitivity to lamb after being strictly fed lamb for two years.

In man, especially in children, spontaneous remission of food hypersensitivity has been recognized (Sampson, 1993). This phenomenon may result from the development of immunologic tolerance due to maturation of the immune system and/or the digestive system. These findings have not been reported in animals. Challenge with the offending food every six months or so would be necessary to prove or disprove a spontaneous remission. Very few owners are willing to do this.

There have been no appropriately designed clinical trials that have demonstrated efficacy for the use of injection immunotherapy, oral desensitization, or subcutaneous provocation and neutralization for food hypersensitivity (Sampson, 1993). Other investigators have challenged the accepted perception (misperception) that immunotherapy is not effective for the treatment of food allergy. Further controlled studies with adequate numbers of patients must be performed to prove efficacy, to establish criteria for therapy, and to assess the most efficacious treatment regimen, the length of treatment, the extent of protection afforded, and the potential long-term risks. Safer vaccines should be developed. With the recent explosion in our knowledge about IgE regulation, a more direct form of immunomodulation may become available.

References

American Academy of Allergy and Immunology/National Institute of Allergy and Infectious Disease (NIH). *Adverse Reactions to Foods.* Anderson JA, Sogn DD (eds), NIH Publication 84–2442, pp. 1–6, 1984.

Baker E. Food allergy. In Chamberlain KW (ed.) *Vet. Clin. North Am., Symposium on Allergy in Small Animal Practice*, volume 4. WB Saunders, Philadelphia, 79–89, 1974.

Boccafogli A, Vicentini L, Camerani A, *et al*. Adverse food reactions in patients with grass pollen allergic respiratory disease. *Ann. Allergy* **73**: 301–308, 1994.

Bock SA. Prospective appraisal of complaints of adverse reaction to food in children during the first 3 years of life. *Pediatrics* **79**: 683–688, 1987.

Brown CM, Armstrong PJ, Globus H. Nutritional management of food allergy in dogs and cats. *Compend.* **17**: 637–659, 1995.

Carlotti DN, Remy I, Prost C. Food allergy in dogs and cats: a review and report of 43 cases. *Vet. Dermatol.* **1:** 55–62, 1990.

Goldman AS, Anderson DW, Sellers WA, *et al*. Milk allergy: oral challenge with milk and isolated milk proteins in allergic children. *Pediatrics* **32:** 425–443, 1963.

Guilford WG. What constitutes a hypoallergenic diet? *Proc. ACVIM Forum* **10:** 674, 1992.

Guilford WG, Strombeck DR, Rogers Q, *et al*. Development of gastroscopic food sensitivity testing in dogs. *J. Vet. Internal. Med.* **8:** 414–422, 1994.

Harvey RG. Food allergy and dietary intolerance in dogs: a report of 25 cases. *J. Small Animal Pract.* **34:** 175–179, 1993.

Jeffers JG, Shanley KJ, Meyer EK. Diagnostic testing of dogs for food hypersensitivity. *J. Am. Vet. Med. Assoc.* **198:** 245–250, 1991.

Jeffers JG, Meyer EK, Sosis EJ. Responses of dogs with food allergies to single ingredient dietary provocation. *J. Am. Vet. Med. Assoc.* **209:** 608–611, 1996.

Kunkle G, Horner S. Validity of skin testing for diagnosis of food allergy in dogs. *J. Am. Vet. Med. Assoc.* **200:** 677–680, 1992.

Lewis LD, Morris M Jr. (eds) *Small Animal Clinical Nutrition*, 2nd edition Topeka, KS, USA: Mark Morris Associates, 1984.

MacDonald JM. Food allergy. In Griffin CE, Kwochka KW, MacDonald JM (eds) *Current Veterinary Dermatology*. Griffin Mosby, St. Louis, p. 121, 1993.

Mowat AM, Strobel S, Drummond HE, *et al*. Immunological responses to fed protein antigens in mice. I. Reversal of oral tolerance to ovalbumin by cyclophosphamide. *Immunology* **45:** 105–113, 1982.

Nelson RW, Dimperio ME, Long GG. Lymphocytic-plasmacytic colitis in the cat. *J. Am. Vet. Med. Assoc.* **184:** 1133–1135, 1984.

Porras O, Carsson B, Fallstrom SP, *et al*. Detection of soy protein in soy lecithin, margarine, and occasionally soy oil. *Int. Arch. Allergy Appl. Immunol.* **78:** 30–32, 1985.

Reedy LM. Food hypersensitivity to lamb in a cat. *J. Am. Vet. Med. Assoc.* **204:** 1039, 1994.

Reedy LM, Miller WH Jr. *Allergic Skin Diseases of Dogs and Cats.* WB Saunders, Philadelphia, pp. 147–158, 1989.

Rosser EJ. Diagnosis of food allergy in dogs. *J. Am. Vet. Med. Assoc.* **203:** 259–262, 1993a.

Rosser EJ. Food allergy in the cat: a prospective study of 13 cats. In Ihrke PJ, *et al* (eds) *Advances in Vet. Dermatol. II.* Pergamon Press, New York, p. 33, 1993b.

Roudebush P, Gross KL, Lowry SR. Protein characteristics of commercial canine and feline hypoallergenic diets. *Vet. Dermatol.* **5:** 69–74, 1994.

Sampson HA. Adverse reactions to food. In Middleton E Jr, Reed CE, Ellis EF (eds) *Allergy: Principles and Practice*, 4th edition, Mosby, St. Louis, pp. 1661–1686, 1993.

Scala G. House dust mite ingestion can induce allergic intestinal syndrome. *Allergy* **50:** 517–519, 1995.

Scott DW, Miller WH Jr, Griffin CE. *Small Animal Dermatol.* 5th Edition. WB Saunders, Philadelphia, pp. 528–535, 1995.

U.S. Department of Agriculture. Rules and Regulations. *Fed. Regist.* 1983, **48:** 32749.

Walton GS. Skin responses in the dog and cat to ingested allergens: observations on 100 confirmed cases. *Vet. Record.* **81:** 709–713, 1967.

Wasmer ML, Willard MD, Helman RG, *et al*. Food intolerance mimicking alimentary lymphosarcoma. *J. Am. Anim. Hosp. Assoc.* **31:** 463–466, 1995.

White SD. Food hypersensitivity in 30 dogs. *J. Am. Vet. Med. Assoc.* **188:** 695–698, 1986.

White SD, Sequoia D. Food hypersensitivity in cats: 14 cases. *J. Am. Vet. Med. Assoc.* **194:** 692–695, 1989.

Yamada K, Urisu A, Morita Y, *et al.* Immediate hypersensitive reactions to buckwheat ingestion and cross allergenicity between buckwheat and rice antigens in subjects with high levels of IgE antibodies to buckwheat. *Ann. Allergy Asthma Immunol.* **75:** 56–61, 1995.

Yunginger JW. Current views. In *Allergy and Immunology: Food Allergies and Hidden Substances.* Current Views, Inc., November 1995.

——8——
Allergic Contact Dermatitis

Introduction

The term contact dermatitis can be used in two ways, either to describe any rash resulting from substances touching the skin or as a synonym for allergic contact dermatitis. Substances coming in contact with the skin can cause dermatitis by allergic and/or nonallergic mechanisms. When an allergic mechanism is involved, the resulting rash is called allergic contact dermatitis. Irritant dermatitis, which is non-immunologic and more common than allergic contact dermatitis, results from contact with a substance that chemically damages the skin, such as acids, alkalis, solvents, surfactants, detergents, dessicants, enzymes, and oxidants. The irritant effect differs from one agent to another and may occur after a single contact with a strong irritant such as battery acid or require repeated contact with milder irritants (i.e. a cumulative irritant), such as with detergents and solvents. Some substances, such as cement, can be both an irritant and an allergen.

Irritant dermatitis is the result of direct damage to keratinocytes by the offending compound. The concentration of the chemical is critical in determining the severity of skin lesions. At the most severe end of the spectrum of irritant dermatitis is a chemical burn. The mildest lesions can be transient epidermal edema. A sensitization phase is not required. There are no diagnostic tests for determining whether a dermatitis is caused by an irritant, but by definition, an irritant would probably affect most normal individuals.

Allergic contact dermatitis results when a substance comes into contact with skin that has undergone an acquired specific alteration in its reactivity. This altered reactivity is the result of previous skin exposure and the development of specific T cells against the contactant (i.e a type IV hypersensitivity reaction; cell-mediated immunity). Because of the immunologic basis of allergic contact dermatitis, only a few individuals in an exposed population will develop signs of the disease. Allergic contact dermatitis is more common in animals with an inflammatory skin disease such as atopy, irritant dermatitis, or seborrhea, because of the compromised epidermal barrier and easier penetration of the skin (Olivry *et al.*, 1990). Moisture also facilitates contact between the patient and the allergen. Poison ivy and poison oak dermatitis is the best known example of human allergic contact dermatitis and illustrates that the sensitivity is acquired; individuals not exposed (e.g. Europeans) do not show this type of allergy.

In photocontact dermatitis, photoallergens, which tend to be simple chemicals, must first be activated by the absorption of light. With subsequent exposure to long-wave ultraviolet light (UVA, wavelength 320–400 nm of sunlight), dermatitis occurs only in the sites exposed to light (Maibach *et al.*, 1993). Some photoallergens induce a longlasting sun sensitivity and patients so affected are called persistent light reactors. Phototoxic skin reactions are not immunologically based. In man, allergic photocontact dermatitis is caused mainly by fragrances, Compositae plants, sunscreens, and certain systemically administered drugs such as phenothiazines and certain antibacterial chemicals (Maibach *et al.*, 1993). A photosensitivity confined to unpigmented skin, which produced vascular thrombosis and subsequent infarction similar to lesions seen in bovine and ovine photosensitivity (Araya and Ford, 1981) was reported in a kennel of harrier hounds (Fairley, 1994). The responsible photodynamic agent was not identified. Contact urticaria is characterized by a transient wheal and flare response rather than a persistent dermatitis and may be immunologic or nonimmunologic (Maibach *et al.*, 1993). The immunologic form is believed to be a type of immediate hypersensitivity.

Pathogenesis

The contactant may be a complete allergen, a low molecular weight substance, or a photoallergen. Most contactants are simple chemicals or haptens, which after penetrating the skin must be conjugated to carrier skin proteins before they become allergenic. The haptens involved in allergic contact dermatitis may be electrophilic, lipophilic, or prohaptens. Some contact allergens such as certain plants, preservatives, and drugs share chemical properties and cross-react. The hapten–protein complex is phagocytized by Langerhans' cells, which have a macrophage lineage, reside in the epidermis, and cover most skin surfaces as a regularly distributed network. After hapten pinocytosis, the Langerhans' cell migrates via the afferent lymphatics to the parafollicular cortex of a regional lymph node, where it presents the allergen to naive T lymphocytes through accessory signals such as interleukin (IL)-1 secretion. These sensitized T cells proliferate and then migrate back to the entire skin.

Once the sensitization process has started, it requires a minimal span of 5–10 days up to a year or longer for clinical allergy to be demonstrable. Following a later contact with the same allergen, sensitized T lymphoyctes release lymphokines such as IL-2R at the contact site. IL-1 concentrations are reported to be increased in human suction blister fluid of allergic patch test when compared to irritant reactions (Maibach *et al.*, 1993). Interferon (IFN) α has also been reported (Scott *et al.*, 1995) to be a critical mediator in classic contact hypersensitivity. These lymphokines induce polyclonal lymphocyte proliferation, attract polymorphonuclear cells, retain inflammatory cells at the site, activate phagocytosis, and cause increased vascular permeability with extravasation of blood cells and plasma proteins. The resultant induration, erythema, and pruritus observed clinically are probably directed at the elimination of the allergen. Lesions do not appear immediately following subsequent contact, but typically occur within 24–48 hours, though this latent period can vary from a few hours up to five days (Reedy and Miller, 1989). Clinical lesions can occur anywhere on the body where the allergen is applied and not just at the initial site. This type of delayed or contact-type allergy can be transmitted by lymphocytes, but not by serum. Once sensitized, allergic contact dermatitis persists for decades, but reactivity will decrease if exposure is limited. Allergic contact dermatitis in the dog may have a different pathogenesis from that in other species, and can vary from one dog to another, depending on the allergen(s) involved (Scott *et al.*, 1995). Species variation in allergic contact dermatitis has also been reported in laboratory animals. For example, guinea pigs can be induced to develop allergic contact dermatitis more easily than rabbits or rats, and some strains of guinea pigs are more susceptible than others (Polak, 1980). In man, mononuclear cells are the predominant infiltrating cell (Maibach *et al.*, 1993). In some dog studies (Thomsen and Thomsen, 1989), the neutrophil has been the predominant inflammatory cell. Other studies (Fadok and Gross, 1993; Merchant *et al.*, 1993; Walder and Conrol, 1994; Frank and McEntee, 1995) have implicated eosinophils as a cellular component of allergic contact dermatitis in the dog.

Prevalence

Problems in the accurate differentiation between allergic contact and irritant dermatitis mean that the true incidence of allergic contact dermatitis in dogs and cats is unknown, but it is probably uncommon to rare. The reasons for this low incidence are unknown, but may be related to the protective nature of the pelage, the poor ability of dogs and cats to develop Type IV hypersensitivity reactions, or other mechanisms. Dogs and cats can be sensitized, but most are exposed to many potential contact allergens throughout their lives and never develop clinical sensitivity (Reedy and Miller, 1989). Of canine dermatology cases 1% (Walton, 1977) to 10% (Nesbitt, 1977; Grant, 1980) were reported to be caused by allergic contact dermatitis. Cats can become sensitized to chemical contactants experimentally (Schultz and Maguire, 1982). The incidence of allergic contact dermatitis in cats is unknown, but is probably rare. Allergic contact dermatitis has been reported in a horse (Reddin and Steven, 1946).

It has been estimated that 20–30% of human dermatology patients have allergic contact dermatitis and that 25–60% of North American people are sensitive to poison ivy and poison oak (Maibach *et al.*, 1993). There is marked variation in the susceptibility to develop allergic contact dermatitis. Some patients are easily sensitized while a small segment of the normal, nonallergic population, perhaps 5%, cannot be sensitized, even to potent agents such as dinitrochlorobenzene (DNCB). Certain individuals are genetically more prone than others to develop contact sensitivity. Experimental studies in humans (Walker *et al.*, 1967) show a trend toward genetic clustering. Patients capable of becoming sensitized are more likely to have children susceptible to sensitization than patients who are not easily sensitized, and patients sensitized to one chemical are more likely to become sensitized to another. There is also evidence that certain strains of laboratory animals (Walker *et al.*, 1967) possess a genetic predisposition to develop contact sensitivity, but to date there are no data to suggest that genetic factors are operative in companion animals.

The relationship between human allergic contact dermatitis and atopic dermatitis is complex and controversial. Patients with atopic dermatitis have a relatively high incidence of allergic contact hypersensitivity to topical drugs, but as a group these patients are more difficult to sensitize than normal, nonallergic control subjects (Maibach *et al.*, 1993). Human atopics are known to have decreased responsiveness to classic contact sensitizers such as DNCB. The relatively high incidence of contact sensitivity in these patients results from the frequent application of a wide variety of topical agents to inflamed skin. Interestingly, approximately 20% of dogs with allergic contact dermatitis are also atopic (Nesbitt, 1977; Thomsen and Kristensen, 1986). Aeroallergen contact sensitivity has also been reported in atopic humans (De Groot and Young, 1989) and dogs (Joshua, 1956; Frank and McEntee, 1995). This only indicates that the transcutaneous route is involved in atopy (Olivry *et al.*, 1995) and does not imply a delayed hypersensitivity mechanism.

Certain individuals are more prone than others to develop contact sensitivity. In humans, the young or the elderly are more difficult to sensitize than young adults or those of middle age (Maibach *et al.*, 1993). Age of onset of allergic contact dermatitis in dogs and cats is controversial. Repeated exposure to or application of a potent allergen over large areas of the body to damaged or inflamed skin in high concentrations or under occlusion increases penetration and favors sensitization.

Etiologic Agents

The causes of contact allergy are many, varied, and constantly changing. Virtually any drug, chemical, or plant can cause sensitization, depending upon its sensitizing potential, the degree of exposure, and the extent of percutaneous penetration. As previously stated, in North America, poison ivy and poison oak are the most common causes of plant allergic contact dermatitis in humans but, to date, poison ivy and poison oak contact allergies have not been reported to occur naturally in small animals. Patients allergic to poison ivy and poison oak may cross-react to chemically related materials such as mangoes or lacquer made from certain trees. *Primula obconica* and chrysanthemums have frequently been incriminated as etiologic agents in Europe (Maibach *et al.*, 1993). In the dog, naturally occurring contact allergy has been reported to certain plants such as wandering Jew (*Tradescantia fluminensis*) (Kunkle and Gross, 1983), *Hippeastrum* (Willemse and Vroom, 1988), Asian jasmine (Merchant *et al.*, 1993), oleander (Werner, 1993), and dandelion leaves (Dunstan *et al.*, 1993).

Topical medications are a common cause of contact allergy in man. Reactions are seen in animals, but at a low incidence, probably because topical drugs are used less frequently. In man, neomycin, ethylenediamine, certain topical anesthetics, formaldehyde, and lanolin are very common sensitizers. In animals, neomycin is the most common sensitizer (Reedy and Miller, 1989). Topical products such as those containing coal tars or insecticides are suspected of causing sensitization, but since these agents are irritants, the reaction may not be a true allergic phenomenon. With topical medications, the sensitization can be due not only to the drug or active ingredient, but also the vehicle, fragrances, stabilizers, or preservatives (e.g. parabens, parachlorometaxylenol, dichlorophene). Studies have suggested that human allergy to topical corticosteroids themselves occurs at a frequency of 3–5% (English *et al.*, 1990). Patch test reactions to a topical steroid are often subtle, but clinically relevant and a frequently missed diagnosis. Human patients presensitized to corticosteroids may also react to systemic corticosteroids (Lauerma *et al.*, 1991). Lanolin and its derivatives occasionally cause persisting and unsuspected allergic contact dermatitis because of their incorporation in many ointment bases. Detergents, shampoos, soaps, cosmetics, fragrances, dyes, glues, nickel, chromium, cobalt, rubber products, and topical antimicrobial agents have been reported as causes of allergic contact dermatitis in humans.

Aside from plants and medications, other reported contact allergens in the dog include plastics (e.g. bowls, toys, flea collars), carpet deodorizer (Comer, 1988), cedar wood (Clark and Taylor, 1993), leather, motor oil, dishwashing detergents (Fadok and Gross, 1993), floor waxes, wool, synthetic rugs, fertilizers, cement (dichromates and nickel) (Olivry, 1993), insecticides, and mop sprays (Schwartzman, 1974). In a Danish study (Thomsen and Kristensen, 1986), 63% of dogs studied were mono-sensitive and 23% were sensitive to two allergens. The sensitizer(s) in plastics for animals is unknown, but flea collar dermatitis in dogs was reported to be caused by dichlorvos (Muller, 1970). When studied in humans, flea collar dermatitis was found to be an irritant dermatitis (Cronce and Alden, 1968).

Reports of contact dermatitis in cats are few (Walton, 1977; Willemse, 1980; Halliwell and Gorman, 1989: Calderwood Mays and Messinger, 1993) and involve for example flea collars, neomycin, and carpet deodorant. Allergic contact dermatitis has been reported in a horse (Reddin and Steven, 1946), which was patch test positive to a combination of saddle soap and leather conditioner, but neither of these separately. According to the author, the condition did not recur following a switch to a noncolored saddle soap, which suggested a dye as the allergen.

Clinical Presentation

Obviously, the distribution of lesions in contact dermatitis will be confined to areas of contact, but also depends upon the nature of the contactant. Because of the natural protection provided by the pelage, lesions resulting from environmental contact allergens are mostly confined to sparsely haired or hairless areas of the body such as the abdomen, scrotum, perineum, chin, ventral tail, ventral neck, ventral chest, pressure points, and feet. Scott (1989) reported that scrotal lesions in the dog are commonly irritant reactions rather than allergic contact dermatitis. Lesions are rarely dorsal. Pododermatitis, which is common, usually affects the ventral inter-digital areas and not the thick pads themselves. However, if the contactant is a sub-stance on a flat smooth surface such as a floor wax, the skin between the pads may not be affected. Contactants on an irregular surface, such as carpet fibers or plants, may affect the entire palmar and plantar surfaces of the paw and distal extremity. Although not absolute, atopics tend to have lesions on the dorsum of the paw while animals with contact dermatitis have disease on the palmar and plantar surfaces. As a general rule, the more chronic the allergy, the more widespread the eruption since pruritus damages the skin and removes hair, which exposes new areas.

Topical medication reactions would be expected to occur at the site of application, but since animals can spread the medication by scratching or licking, lesions can also occur around the area of application as well as on the foot or in the mouth used to scratch or lick the area, respectively. Medications applied to the whole body such as shampoos, dips, rinses, sprays, and powders produce generalized lesions. Intertriginous areas such as the axillary or inguinal regions or the skin between the pads are usually most severely involved since they tend to accumulate material, which is held in intimate contact with the skin.

The early clinical features of allergic contact dermatitis include erythema, swelling, papules, and plaques (Figure 8.1 and Plate 4). Bullae or vesicles are rare. Pruritus can vary from mild to severe. As the disease progresses, crusting, alopecia, lichenification,

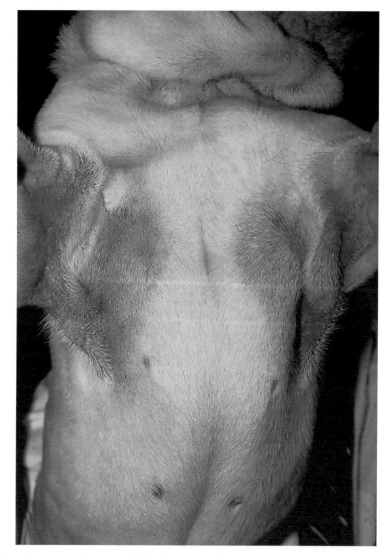

Figure 8.1   *Alopecia, erythema, and lichenification of the ventral abdomen of a dog sensitive to a floor wax.*

and hyperpigmentation appear. Secondary pyodermas are common and have been reported in 40% of cases (Nesbitt, 1977). The clinical features of allergic contact dermatitis are not distinctive and the differential diagnosis includes irritant contact dermatitis, atopy, food allergy, scabies, skin infections (bacterial, *Malassezia*, or fungal), seborrheic dermatitis, hookworm dermatitis, and *Pelodera* dermatitis.

Although there is apparently no sex predisposition for allergic contact dermatitis in dogs, in one study (Thomsen and Kristensen, 1986), 73% were males. There may be a genetic predisposition; in the previous reference, of 22 confirmed cases of allergic contact dermatitis in Denmark, 50% were in German shepherds, which comprised only 16% of the dog population. Over 20% of canine cases of allergic contact dermatitis in England have been found to occur in yellow Laborador retrievers (Walton, 1977). Other breeds reported at increased risk include poodles (Muller, 1967), golden retrievers, wire-haired fox terriers, Scottish terriers, and West Highland white terriers (Olivry *et al.*, 1990).

Diagnostic Approach

The diagnosis of allergic contact dermatitis is not a neat orderly process involving first the history, next the physical, and then diagnostic test results, but rather a continuing interaction using information obtained at each of these steps and rule-outs. The history can be of a seasonal or nonseasonal nature depending upon the type of contactant. As a general rule, seasonal allergies suggest an outdoor source. If multiple animals are involved or if the pruritus truly precedes the lesions, allergic contact dermatitis is very unlikely. If the history indicates that the problem started simultaneously with an environmental change, irritant dermatitis is more likely. Although allergic contact dermatitis can be produced in dogs after a 3–5 week sensitization, most naturally occurring cases follow a longer period of exposure, usually more than two years and rarely less than six months (Walton, 1977; Thomsen and Kristensen, 1986). However, in one study (Nesbitt, 1977), 50% were 2–12 months old and one case occurred in a twelve-week-old dalmatian (Werner, 1993). After the physical examination and routine diagnostic tests are completed, a tentative diagnosis of allergic contact dermatitis may be made.

Skin biopsies in allergic contact dermatitis are often similar to those of other types of dermatitis and are therefore not specific or diagnostic. However, skin biopsies can be helpful, especially if obtained from an early lesion, preferably one less than 48 hours old, and they should be performed to rule out other diseases. Since microscopic changes are present before macroscopic alterations are visible, the variations in histologic features are largely a result of lesion duration and range from mild to severe. Also, microscopic changes can vary from field to field in the histologic sections. Cardinal features of allergic contact dermatitis include epidermal intercellular edema (spongiosis) and infiltration with mononuclear cells, neutrophils, and eosinophils. Other changes include acanthosis, parakeratosis, and secondary bacterial or *Malassezia* infections. If there is epidermal necrosis, an irritant dermatitis is a more likely diagnosis (Walder and Conroy, 1994).

The most commonly used tests for the diagnosis of allergic contact dermatitis include an isolation (avoidance) technique or patch testing (open or closed). Before performing any test for allergic contact dermatitis, the patient should first be bathed in a hypoallergenic shampoo to remove any residual contactants from the hair and skin. Also corticosteroids must be discontinued for at least 3–6 weeks before testing.

Isolation techniques

Isolation techniques can be used to support the diagnosis of a contact dermatitis, but do not distinguish between irritant and allergic contact dermatitis. If the owners are very dedicated, the offending substance can be identified. Ideally, the pet should be removed from the suspect agent or environment for 10–30 days. Boarding in a veterinary hospital is preferred. Isolation in the home is very difficult and requires confining to a kennel, play pen, or basement. Care must be taken to avoid any contact with suspected allergen(s) such as grass, and cement. If an improvement is noted while not exposed, the diagnosis of contact dermatitis is supported but not proved. Provocative exposure testing is then necessary. If the signs recur upon re-exposure, usually after 48–72 hours up to ten days, the diagnosis is supported.

If the suspect contactant is something simple like a food bowl or a toy, the isolation procedure is straightforward. If an environmental agent is involved, the procedure is much more complicated. If the pet is normal with no allergies when hospitalized and the signs recur when the pet returns to its natural environment, a great deal of detective work will be necessary. Suspect agents like carpets and floor cleaners are placed in the 'clean' room one at a time in sufficient quantity so that the pet will touch them. Allergic reactions should not occur for several days. If a reaction occurs, the substance is removed and the pet is immediately bathed. If the history suggests multiple sensitivities, the testing should be continued once the skin has returned to normal. Obviously this type of testing requires a very dedicated owner and a cooperative pet.

Patch testing

Patch tests are used to determine whether a patient has a Type IV hypersensitivity to specific substances. Suspect agents at a nonirritating concentration are placed in pure form on bare normal skin and the test site is examined 48–72 hours later for signs of reaction (erythema and edema). Patch testing is the only practical test for demonstrating contact allergy; it not only confirms a diagnosis, but also gives some idea of the allergen involved. Patch testing is indicated in any unusual dermatitis that does not respond to treatment as expected.

Patch testing can be carried out in an open or a closed fashion. The back or lateral thorax are common test sites. The test area should be clipped at least 24 hours before the test since clipper irritation can cause false positive reactions. Trauma to the test site will invalidate the test, so an Elizabethan collar and foot bandages should be used. Hospitalization is advised. As a general rule, liquids (e.g. shampoos, dips, disinfectants) should be tested at the same concentrations that they are used.

Walton has suggested some concentrations and vehicles for patch testing dogs. Petrolatum is the standard diluent. Some chemicals such as chlorhexidine and formalin produce false-negative patch tests when diluted with petrolatum. Topical medicaments are usually applied to inflamed skin, whereas patch testing must be done on normal skin. Inflamed skin may be more permeable than normal skin, and consequently poorly penetrating medicaments, notably neomycin, frequently give false-negative patch test results. If the topical medicament is relatively nonirritating under patch test conditions, penetration can be safely enhanced by increasing the patch test concentration and thus overcoming false-negative tests with that particular medicament. For example, patch testing for neomycin sensitivity is performed with 20% neomycin, even though the usual concentration of neomycin in topical applications is 0.5%.

Open patch testing
The test materials suspended in the appropriate vehicle or diluted as indicated are

rubbed on the skin and the test sites are examined daily for five days. To prevent bleeding of one test antigen into another, the test sites should be widely separated. Thus, the number of tests should be kept small. The test site must be protected from water, dirt, and self-trauma.

False negatives may be caused by lack of penetration and false positives by inflammation from self trauma. Because of these problems, open patch testing is often unsatisfactory in veterinary medicine.

Closed patch testing

The closed or occlusive patch test is currently the best diagnostic test for allergic contact dermatitis. A nonstandard form of this test consists of placing a suspension of the suspect material on the skin under a piece of gauze, taping the gauze in place, and leaving the material under occlusion for 48–72 hours. Some knowledge of the suspect material is needed and a large area of normal skin is required. False negatives and slippage of the bandage are common problems. Positive results should always be checked on normal, nonallergic pets to rule out irritant reactions. Different vehicles (water, alcohol, petrolatum) and concentrations of the suspected allergen should be tested. This nonstandard test is reserved for uncommon allergens not provided in a standardized patch test kit, such as plants. Detergents, shampoos, and soaps should be diluted before patch testing (0.1–2% in water) but even these concentrations may be irritating under patch test occlusion.

In human medicine, standardized commercial patch test kits are available and these include common sensitizers at nonirritating concentrations. Currently there are no commercial kits available in veterinary medicine. The human European Standard Battery test, which is recommended by the International Contact Dermatitis Research Group, has been tested and reported effective in diagnosing canine allergic contact dermatitis (Thomsen and Kristensen, 1986; Willemse, 1986; Olivry and Heripret, 1989). The test allergens consist of 22 extracts of metals, rubbers, chemicals, animal derivatives, and vegetal products in a petrolatum base (Table 8.1, Plate 5). Some allergens included in the battery are mixtures. If a mixture produces a positive reaction, additional tests can be performed with individual extracts. If kept in the dark below 4°C, the test kit has a shelf-life of approximately two years. The allergens in this test have proved to be nonirritating to both humans and dogs (Olivry *et al.*, 1990). In one study (Olivry and Heripret, 1989), this test confirmed over 50% of suspected cases of allergic contact dermatitis with no false positives in normal, nonallergic dogs. Avoidance and elimination of causative substances was successful in 32 of 54 dogs. Advantages of this test include the use of standardized allergens, the small surface area required, and ease of application and interpretation.

Interpretation of patch test results

The patch test is read at 48 and 72 hours. Willemse (1986) reported that positive test reactions which become stronger with additional time were more likely to be due to allergic contact dermatitis (Plate 6). From a practical point of view, it is usually not possible to distinguish between true-positive and false-positive reactions, but the difference between allergic and irritant reactions may be determined from the configuration of the test site reaction and by dilution. Irritant patch test reactions are usually limited to the test patch, while allergic reactions usually extend beyond

Table 8.1   *The European Standard Battery of Allergens.*

Allergen	Conc. (%)	Environmental sources and uses
Potassium dichromate	0.5	Cement, dyes, leathers, alloys, oils, paints
Neomycin sulfate	20.0	Antibiotic in topical medications
Thiuram mix	1.0	Rubbers, preservatives, insecticides, fungicides
Paraphenylene diamine	1.0	Dyes, antioxidants, inks
Cobalt chloride	1.0	Cement, alloys, dyes, paints, furs, oils
Benzocaine	5.0	Topical medications
Formaldehyde (in water)	1.0	Disinfectants, detergents, preservatives, plastics, leathers
Colophony	20.0	Adhesives, waxes, glues, inks, linoleums, leathers
Quinoline mix	6.0	Topical medications
Balsam of Peru	25.0	Topical medications, aromatics, deodorants
PPD mix, black rubber mix	0.6	Black rubbers, oils
Wool alcohols/lanolin	30.0	Topical medications, leathers, furs, polishes
Mercapto mix	2.0	Rubbers, oils, anti-infectives, fungicides
Epoxy resin	1.0	Plastics, glues, adhesives, paints, varnishes, inks
Paraben mix	15.0	Preservatives, glues, polishes
Butyl phenol	1.0	Shoe repairing, glues
Carba mix	3.0	Rubbers, insecticides, fungicides
Fragrance mix	8.0	Perfumes, topical medications, detergents, oils
Ethylene diamine	1.0	Stabilizers, insecticides, fungicides, rubbers
Quaternium 15	1.0	Anti-infective, fungicide, preservative
Nickel sulfate	5.0	Alloys, stainless steel, detergents, paints, cements
Primin	0.01	Primula (cross-reactions with other quinones)

the test patch. Also, in allergic pets, a ten-fold dilution of the allergen will still result in a positive reaction while negative results will usually be obtained in dogs with an irritant reaction.

   All true-positive reactions are significant, but they may not be clinically relevant. The reaction could indicate an old sensitivity or portend a future problem. The history must be examined to determine if the allergen is in the environment. More troublesome problems are false-positive and false-negative reactions. False-negative results can be due to failure to include all the appropriate test antigens or because of poor antigen penetration. Poor site occlusion or protection can affect penetration as can the concentration of the antigens.

Treatment

Avoidance is curative; however, this requires identification of the causative agent. If this is possible, a mild dermatitis will resolve spontaneously in 7–14 days. More severe reactions heal more slowly. Bathing to remove any residual contactant will hasten the response and corticosteroids can be used to lessen the pruritus and inflammation. A common failing is to use an inadequate quantity of systemic steroid in the initial stages. Oral prednisone (1 mg/kg for dogs and 2 mg/kg for cats) for 7–14 days is preferred (Scott and Miller, 1995). Antihistamines do not suppress the acute inflammation in allergic contact dermatitis, but may provide patient comfort because of their sedating side effects. Topical medicaments should be avoided as they can irritate or become 'new' sensitizers. Although hyposensitization (topical, oral, injection) to certain contactants has been shown to be possible in humans (Kligman, 1958), the process is tedious, not always successful, and temporary. Once hyposensitization is stopped, sensitivity usually returns to its previous level within 6–10 months. In mice and humans, ultraviolet light (UVB) (Troost *et al.*, 1995) induces specific hyporesponsiveness when administered simultaneously with allergen. This may be through depletion of Langerhans' cells and downmodulatory effects on T cell-mediated responses to contact allergens. If the offending allergen cannot be identified or removed, symptomatic therapy with corticosteroids will be necessary (see Chapter 6). Frequent bathing can decrease the allergen load and thus lower the necessary dose of corticosteroid.

References

Araya OS, Ford EJH. An investigation of the type of photosensitization caused by the ingestion of St John's Wort (*Hypericum perforatum*) by calves. *N. Z. Vet. J.* **35:** 27–30, 1981.

Calderwood Mays MB, Messinger LM. Carpet deodorant contact dermatitis in a cat. *Proc. Annu. Memb. Meet. Am. Acad. Vet. Dermatol./Am. Coll. Vet. Dermatol.* **9:** 67, 1993.

Clark EJ, Taylor JBH. Cedar wood-induced allergic contact dermatitis in a dog. *Proc. Annu. Memb. Meet. Am. Acad. Vet. Dermatol./Am. Coll. Vet. Dermatol.* **9:** 68, 1993.

Comer KM. Carpet deodorized as a contact allergen in a dog. *J. Am. Vet. Med. Assoc.* **193(2):** 1553–1554, 1988.

Cronce PC, Alden HS. Flea collar dermatitis. *J. Am. Med. Assoc.* **206:** 1563, 1968.

De Groot AC, Young E. The role of contact allergy to aeroallergens in atopic dermatitis. Contact *Dermatitis* **21:** 209–214, 1989.

Dunstan RW, Rosser EJ, Kennis R. Histologic features of allergic contact dermatitis in four dogs. *Proc. Annu. Memb. Meet. Am. Acad. Vet. Dermatol./Am. Coll. Vet. Dermatol.* **9:** 69, 1993.

English JS, Ford G, Beck MH, *et al.* Allergic contact dermatitis from topical systemic steroids. Contact *Dermatitis* **23:** 196, 1990.

Fadok VA, Gross TL. Generalized allergic contact dermatitis induced by topical dishwashing detergent in a dog. *Proc. Annu. Memb. Meet. Am. Acad. Vet. Dermatol./Am. Coll. Vet. Dermatol.* **9:** 66, 1993.

Fairley RA, Mackenzie IS. Photosensitivity in a kennel of harrier hounds. *Vet. Dermatol.* **5(1):** 1–7, 1994.

Frank LA, McEntee MF. Demonstration of aeroallergen contact sensitivity in dogs. *Vet. Allerg. Clin. Immunol.* **3(3):** 75–80, 1995.

Grant DI, Thoday KL. Canine allergic contact dermatitis: A clinical review. *J. Sm. Anim. Pract.* **21:** 17–27, 1980.

Halliwell REW. Gorman NT. *Veterinary Clinical Immunology.* W.B. Saunders, Philadelphia, 1989, pp. 253–258.

Joshua JO. Some allergic conditions in the dog and cat. *Vet. Rec.* **68:** 682, 1956.

Kligman AM. Hyposensitization against *Rhus* dermatitis. *Arch. Dermatol.* **78:** 47, 1958.

Kunkle GA, Gross TL. Allergic contact dermatitis to *Tradescantia fluminensis* (wandering Jew) in a dog. *Comp. Cont. Educ.* **5:** 925, 1983.

Lauerma A, Reitamo S, Maibach HI. Systemic hydrocortisone/cortisol induces allergic skin reactions in presensitized subjects. *J. Am. Acad. Dermatol.* **24**: 182, 1991.

Maibach HI, Dannaker CJ, Lahti A. Contact skin allergy. In Middleton E Jr, Reed CE, Ellis EF (eds), *Allergy: Principles and Practice*, 4th edition. Mosby, St Louis, pp. 1605–1641, 1993.

Merchant SR, Hodgin EC, Lemare SL. Eosinophilic pustules and eosinophilic dermatitis secondary to patch testing a dog with Asian jasmine. *Proc. Annu. Memb. Meet. Am. Acad. Vet. Dermatol./Am. Coll. Vet. Dermatol.* **9**: 64, 1993.

Muller GH. Contact dermatitis in animals. *Arch. Dermatol.* **96**: 423–426, 1967.

Muller GH. Flea collar dermatitis in animals. *J. Am. Vet. Med. Assoc.* **157**: 1616, 1970.

Nesbitt GH. Contact dermatitis in the dog: A review of 35 cases. *J. Am. Anim. Hosp. Assoc.* **13**: 155–163, 1977.

Olivry T. Allergic contact dermatitis to cement: A delayed hypersensitivity to dichromates and nickel. *Proc. Annu. Memb. Meet. Am. Acad. Vet. Dermatol./Am. Coll. Vet. Dermatol.* **9**: 63, 1993.

Olivry H, Heripret D. Use of a closed patch test technique in the diagnosis of allergic contact dermatitis in the dog. *Proc. Acad. Vet. Allergy Annual Meeting*, pp. 11–12, 1989.

Olivry T, Preland P, Heripret D, *et al.* Allergic contact dermatitis in the dog. *Vet. Clin. North Am. (Small Anim. Pract.)* **20**: 1443–1456, 1990.

Olivry T, Moore PF, Nayden DK. Characterization of the inflammatory infiltrate in canine atopic dermatitis. *Proc. Annu. Memb. Meet. Am. Acad. Vet. Dermatol./Am. Coll. Vet. Dermatol.* **11**: 98–100, 1995.

Polak L. Immunologic aspects of contact sensitivity. *Monogr. Allergy* **15**, 1980.

Reddin L, Steven DW. Allergic contact dermatitis in the horse. *North. Am. Vet.* **27**: 561, 1946.

Reedy LM, Miller WH Jr. *Allergic Skin Diseases of Dogs and Cats.* W.B. Saunders, Philadelphia, pp. 159–169, 1989.

Schultz KT, Maguire HC. Chemically induced delayed hypersensitivity in the cat. *Vet. Immunol. Immunopathol.* **3**: 585, 1982.

Schwartzman RM. Contact dermatitis. In Kirk RW (ed.) *Current Veterinary Therapy*, V. W.B. Saunders, Philadelphia, p. 405, 1974.

Scott DW. Recent advances in the diagnosis and management of contact dermatitis. *World Small Anim. Vet. Med. Assoc. Annual Meeting*, Harrogate, UK, 1989.

Scott DW, Miller WH Jr, Griffin CE. *Small Animal Dermatology*, 5th edition. W.B. Saunders, Philadelphia, pp. 523–528, 1995.

Thomsen MK, Kristensen F. Contact dermatitis in the dog: A review and clinical study. *Nord. Vet. Med.* **38**: 129, 1986.

Thomsen MK, Thomsen HK. Histopathological changes in canine allergic contact dermatitis patch test reactions: A study on spontaneously hypersensitive dogs. *Acta Vet. Scand.* **30**: 379, 1989.

Troost RJJ, *et al.* Hyposensitization in nickel allergic contact dermatitis: Clinical and immunologic monitoring. *J. Am. Acad. Dermatol.* **32**: 576–583, 1995.

Walder EJ, Conrol JD. Contact dermatitis in dogs and cats: Pathogenesis, histopathology, experimental induction and case reports. *Vet. Dermatol.* **5(4)**: 149–162, 1994.

Walker FB, Smith PD, Maibach HI. Genetic factors in human allergic contact dermatitis. *Int. Arch. Allerg. Appl. Immunol.* **32**: 453, 1967.

Walton GS. Allergic contact dermatitis. In Kirk RW (ed.) *Current Veterinary Therapy* VI. W.B. Saunders, Philadelphia, pp. 571–575, 1977.

Werner A. Contact allergic dermatitis in a young Dalmatian dog. *Proc. Annu. Memb. Meet. Am. Acad. Vet. Dermatol./Am. Coll. Vet. Dermatol.* **9:** 65, 1993.

Willemse T. Crusting dermatoses in cats. In Kirk RW (ed.) *Current Veterinary Therapy* VII. W.B. Saunders, Philadelphia, pp. 469–472, 1980.

Willemse TW. Contact dermatitis. *Eur. Soc. Vet. Dermatol.* Annual Meeting, Paris, 1986.

Willemse TW, Vroom MA. Allergic dermatitis in a Great Dane due to contact with *Hippeastrum*. *Vet. Rec.* **122:** 490–491, 1988.

9

Arthropod Hypersensitivity Disorders

Introduction

The phylum Arthropoda includes four classes which are of veterinary importance (Soulsby, 1982; Bowman, 1995). Of these, the Insecta (insects) and Arachnida (arachnids) can cause dermatologic disease. Worldwide, there are thousands of species of insects and arachnids. Some species are well-known causes of traumatic dermatitis, e.g., pinnal fly dermatitis caused by *Stomoxys calcitrans* (Bowman, 1995; Scott *et al.*, 1995), while most others are or were thought to be of no dermatologic significance. For years, the only insects thought to be of allergic significance to pets were fleas, bees, wasps, and hornets. Important allergenic arachnids included ticks, parasitic mites, and environmental mites. Today, it is well known that other insects and arachnids will induce an IgE antibody response in dogs and cats. In some cases (e.g. mosquito bite hypersensitivity) the significance of the allergic antibody response has been proven (Mason and Evans, 1991; Ihrke and Gross, 1994). In other cases, clinical allergy is suspected, but not proven (Holtz, 1990; Griffin, 1993; Gross, 1993; Buerger, 1995; Willis and Kunkle, 1996). With the increased use of insect and arachnid antigens in intradermal and serologic allergy testing, the role of these parasites in canine and feline allergy should be defined.

Insect Hypersensitivity Disorders

Over 70% of the known arthropods are insects (Soulsby, 1982; Bowman, 1995). These insects can be problematic for animals because they:

- feed on the animal;
- inject some allergenic saliva or venom while feeding on or stinging the animal;
- leave potentially allergenic body parts or excreta where the animal can inhale, ingest, or transdermally absorb them.

The injection route of sensitization is well know since flea bite hypersensitivity is the most common allergic skin disease of the dog and cat. The role of inhaled, ingested, or transdermally absorbed allergens is uncertain.

Flea bite hypersensitivity

Fleas are insect parasites of dogs, cats, pigs, people, rodents, rabbits, and birds. In addition to being annoying, fleas can be vectors for various diseases and can produce allergic reactions in certain individuals. Fleas are the most common external parasite of companion animals and are an important cause of skin disease. In flea infested areas, fleas are believed to be a major factor in more than 50% of small animal dermatology cases (Scott *et al.*, 1995).

Anatomy and life cycle

Fleas (order Siphonaptera) are small wingless insects with laterally compressed bodies and a thick, brown chitinous cuticle (Soulsby, 1982; Dryden, 1993a; Bowman, 1995). The cuticle is covered with a thin lipid layer, the epicuticle. The epicuticle is impermeable to water but freely permeable to lipids and lipid-soluble substances (Bowman, 1995). Powerful legs adapted for jumping enable fleas to readily transfer from host to host. There are over 2000 species and subspecies. Worldwide, *Ctenocephalides* spp., especially *C. felis felis*, are most problematic for dogs and cats but *Pulex irritans*, *Echidnophaga gallinacea*, *Spilopsyllus cuniculi*, and *Tunga penetrans*, as well as others are important in certain instances (Dryden, 1993a, 1993b; MacDonald, 1995; Scott *et al.*, 1995).

All adult fleas are host-dependent blood-sucking ectoparasites of warm-blooded animals. Although adult fleas can leave their host and survive in a standard household environment, they will die relatively quickly unless a new host is found. Accordingly, fleas should be considered permanent rather then transient parasites. Most species, especially when hungry, show limited host specificity. During feeding, specialized mouthparts pierce the host's skin to siphon blood. Saliva is injected into the wound to prevent the blood from clotting. Hosted adult fleas can live for long periods without feeding but a blood meal is necessary for reproduction.

Fleas develop by complete metamorphosis (Figure 9.1) (Dryden, 1993a, 1993b; MacDonald, 1995). The life cycle of *C. felis felis* has been extensively studied and is used throughout this discussion. Data developed for the cat flea may not apply to other species. Copulation occurs after a blood meal and the female can lay up to 20

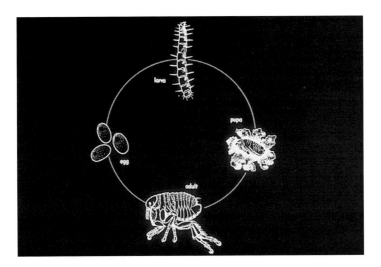

Figure 9.1 *Life cycle of the flea showing percentages of each stage at any given time. (Courtesy of L. Veith, Vet-Kem Corp., Des Plaines, IL.)*

eggs at one time. Most egg laying appears to occur at night while the animal is sleeping. With multiple feedings, the female can lay up to 50 eggs/day. Flea eggs are small, ovoid, white, and nonsticky (Figure 9.2). Typically, the eggs are laid on the host and fall into the environment for development. Since egg laying is heaviest on the sleeping animal, napping and sleeping areas will be most heavily infested. The female poultry flea, *E. gallinacea*, burrows into the host's skin and lays her eggs there. The eggs hatch on the host and the larvae fall into the environment to complete their development. The female cat flea can lay over 1000 eggs in the first 50 days of her life and over 2000 during her entire lifetime.

There are three larval stages called instars. The eggs hatch to first-instar larvae, which when newly hatched are creamy yellow in color, legless, and maggot-like with masticating mouth parts and two posterior hooked processes called anal struts (Figure 9.3). The struts are used for locomotion, grasping, and holding. The larvae are very active, negatively phototactic, and positively geotactic. From the hatch site, they quickly crawl into cracks in the flooring, deep into upholstery and carpets, or under organic debris to avoid sunlight (Dryden, 1993a; Robinson, 1995). Very little food is necessary for development, but the larvae do ingest organic matter, especially blood-containing fecal pellets, which fall from the host. The first-instar larvae do not travel far from the site of hatching. Second-instars will migrate more widely and can infest areas 1 m or more from the hatch site (Robinson, 1995). Shortly after molting, the third instar spins an oval sticky cocoon in which it pupates (Figure 9.4) to form the adult. Depending on the presence or absence of appropriate stimuli for emergence (e.g. pressure, carbon dioxide tension, and heat) adult fleas can emerge from the cocoon in a matter of days or stay in a state of suspended animation for long periods (Dryden, 1993a). Pre-emerged adults can lay dormant for as long as 140 days under appropriate environmental conditions.

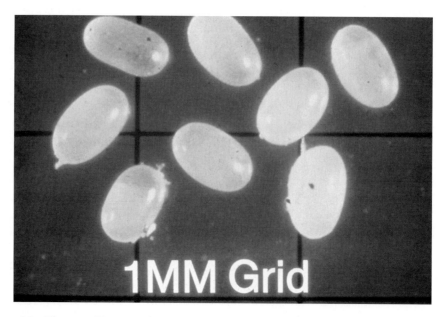

Figure 9.2   *Flea eggs. (Courtesy of Vet-Kem Corp., Des Plaines, IL.)*

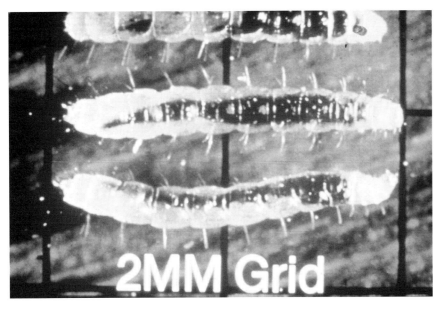

Figure 9.3   *Flea larvae. (Courtesy of Vet-Kem Corp., Des Plaines, IL.)*

The rate of development of the flea through its various life phases depends greatly on the local temperature and humidity (Dryden, 1993a, 1993b). Moderate temperatures (18–27°C) and high humidity (70–80%) favor rapid development while low temperatures and humidity slow development. Although the general weather conditions in an area may be not be conducive (e.g. hot and dry) for flea development, the

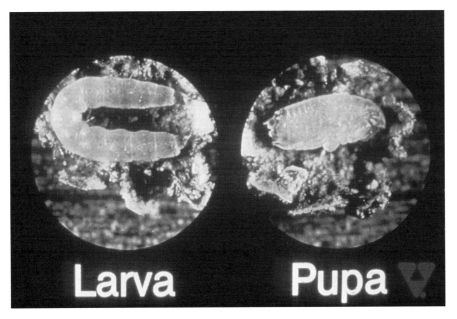

Figure 9.4   *Flea larva and pupa exposed in a cocoon. (Courtesy of Vet-Kem Corp., Des Plaines, IL.)*

climatic conditions deep within carpets or in organic debris can be very different. Under good conditions, cat flea eggs hatch in 1–10 days, the larval phase lasts 5–11 days, and adults begin to emerge from the cocoon five days after pupation. With environmental modifications, the typical 21–28-day life cycle can be accelerated to 12–14 days or slowed to as long as 174 days. Temperatures above 35°C (90°F) and relative humidities below 50% favor dehydration and death of larvae. Hard rains outside can drown larvae and pupae. Very cold temperatures, for example, less than 1°C (33.8°F) are lethal to all phases of the cat flea. Pre-emerged adults may be able to survive these cold temperatures, provided the cocoon is well protected.

In the controlled laboratory environment, newly emerged cat fleas are very hardy and can survive for long periods (Dryden 1993a, 1993b). Under household conditions with for example room temperatures of 22.5–24°C (72.5–75.2°F) and relative humidities of 60–78%, most nonhosted, nonfed adult fleas are dead in 12–14 days. With higher temperatures or lower humidity, nonhosted, nonfed fleas die more quickly. Once the cat flea has fed, its metabolism requires a near constant source of blood. Permanent separation from the host after feeding results in rapid death in a matter of days. Adult feeding fleas can survive on their host for over 100 days.

Host distribution
Although the common names for fleas (e.g. dog flea, cat flea) might imply some host specificity, no such specificity exists (Scott *et al.*, 1995). Hungry fleas will feed from almost any warm-blooded animal. Most species of fleas appear to be able to complete their life cycle while feeding on an 'unnatural' host. For example, *C. felis felis* thrives on dogs, raccoons, opossums, squirrels, and a variety of other wild and domestic animals. However, *C. canis* does not develop past the first larval phase when it is hosted on cats.

Most species of fleas move freely over an animal's body and can be found almost anywhere. *E. gallinacea* has a predilection for the facial region and *S. cuniculi* has a preference for the pinna and preauricular area (Scott *et al.*, 1995).

Clinical disorders
During feeding, the flea injects its saliva into the wound to prevent blood clotting. Flea saliva is a complex substance and is both irritating and allergenic. The saliva of *C. felis felis*, *P. irritans*, and *P. simulans* share common antigens (Scott *et al.*, 1995). Accordingly, an animal bothered by the bite of one species of flea is likely to be sensitive to the bites of any other species of flea. Since the flea bite is both mechanically and chemically irritating, all normal animals will develop an inflammatory papule at the site of the bite. The poultry flea (*E. gallinacea*) and the chigoe or sand flea (*T. penetrans*) burrow into the host's skin and cause severe local damage. The animal's response to the bites of the flea dictates what type of dermatitis it will develop.

Flea bite dermatitis.   Flea bite dermatitis is a nonallergic condition caused by the irritation of the flea bite. The severity of the dermatitis should be proportional to the number of fleas the animal harbors. Normally, one or two fleas should not produce any clinical dermatitis. As a clinical entity in most veterinary practices, flea bite dermatitis is very uncommon. Most pet owners living in flea regions know that flea bites will bother their pet. When their dog or cat starts to nibble at the arrival of the first few fleas, the owner either ignores the chewing or examines the pet for fleas. If the initial nibbling is ignored, the scratching and chewing will escalate as the flea load increases. At this point, fleas will be obvious. Most concerned owners will treat the fleas without seeking veterinary advice.

The clinical signs of flea bite dermatitis are a variably pruritic papular eruption. In the dog, common areas of involvement include the lower back, tail, posterior and medial thighs, and the inguinal region. In the cat, crusted papules are found between the shoulder blades and along the lower back. Some cats have no primary lesions and just groom excessively, especially over the lower back and in the inguinal region. In true flea bite dermatitis, the severity of the clinical signs is related to the number of fleas present. Some nervous pets or those with very sensitive skin will itch out of proportion to the number of fleas present and will appear to be flea allergic.

The diagnosis of flea bite dermatitis is made by physical examination and demonstration of the flea or flea excreta. A skin test with flea antigen should show no immediate or delayed reaction.

Flea bite hypersensitivity. This is a pruritic, papulocrustous dermatitis in animals that have become sensitized to antigenic material in flea saliva. Flea bite hypersensitivity, also called flea allergy dermatitis, is the most common allergic skin disease of the dog and cat worldwide. The incidence varies with the climate, flea population, and allergic susceptibility of the pet population. Atopic patients are very prone to develop flea bite hypersensitivity (Scott *et al.*, 1995; Willis and Kunkle, 1996).

The distinction between nonallergic flea bite dermatitis and flea bite hypersensitivity can sometimes be difficult. In nonallergic flea bite dermatitis, there is usually a direct relationship between the number of flea bites and the degree of reaction. In pets suffering from another allergic disorder (e.g. atopy, food hypersensitivity) or who are allergic to flea bites, this relationship does not always exist. In the very allergic patient, a few flea bites can produce a severe allergic reaction.

Pathogenesis
The pathogenesis of flea bite hypersensitivity has been extensively studied in the dog (Halliwell, 1984; Halliwell and Longino, 1985; Halliwell and Schemmer, 1987; Scott *et al.*, 1995). Flea saliva contains histamine-like compounds, enzymes, polypeptides, amino acids, aromatic compounds, and fluorescent materials (Halliwell, 1984; Greene *et al.*, 1993a, 1993b; Trudeau *et al.*, 1993; McKeon and Opdebeech, 1994; Scott *et al.*, 1995). Gel filtration studies have shown many polypeptide bands, approximately 15 of which appear very important (Greene *et al.*, 1993a). Some of these antigens have been synthesized from flea messenger RNA (Greene *et al.*, 1993b). Studies to identify the important antigens have shown that there is no one antigen important in all flea allergic dogs or cats. Beyond that, controversy exists. Some groups report that the most reactive fractions are in the 40–58 kD range (Greene *et al.*, 1993a, 1993b; Trudeau *et al.*, 1993) while others find most reactivity above 66 kD (McKeon and Opdebeech, 1994). One group finds a clear difference in reactivity between flea allergic and flea nonallergic animals (Greene *et al.*, 1993a) while another finds no such difference (McKeon and Opdebeech, 1994). The reasons for these differences are unknown, but may relate to study design. Future studies should clarify these issues. The antigens are known to induce a

Type I hypersensitivity, Type IV hypersensitivity, and basophil hypersensitivity reactions. Late-phase IgE-mediated reactions may also be important.

The orderly process of sensitization and desensitization demonstrated in the guinea pig does not occur in dogs and cats. In many instances, delayed reactions precede the development of immediate reactions, but delayed reactions have been documented as occurring at the same time or even after the onset of immediate reactions. In general, most flea allergic dogs have both immediate and delayed skin test reactivity while only 5–10% show either an immediate or a delayed reaction but not both. Delayed reactions can occur at 4–8 hours, 24 hours, or 48 hours.

In studies on the pathogenesis of flea allergy in the dog, Halliwell showed that dogs who were exposed to fleas periodically developed positive skin tests within 2–12 weeks while animals who were exposed to fleas constantly developed their reactions much later and to a lesser extent (Halliwell, 1984). The episodically exposed animals typically had detectable serum concentrations of IgE and high serum levels of IgG against flea antigen while the continuously exposed dogs had little detectable antibody of either class (Halliwell and Longino, 1985). This data suggest that continuous exposure can lead to a state of partial or complete immunologic tolerance. If the constantly exposed dogs were switched to an intermittent exposure, they developed skin test reactivity and an IgE and IgG antibody response, which suggests that their tolerance was lost. Once a dog developed reactivity, it persisted for the length of the study (44 weeks) rather than being lost early as in the guinea pig.

Type I and Type IV hypersensitivity reactions have been documented in the dog, but the variable histologic picture and the fact that delayed reactions can occur from 4–48 hours suggests that another immunologic mechanism may be present. A late-onset IgE reaction and cutaneous basophil hypersensitivity have been proposed as contributory immunologic mechanisms.

Cutaneous basophil hypersensitivity is a poorly understood type of delayed hypersensitivity with predominantly basophil infiltration that occurs transiently within 24 hours after cutaneous rechallenge with sensitizing antigen. Cutaneous basophil hypersensitivity is a protective response in tick bite reactions. Antigen-specific IgE molecules bind to the receptors on the surface of basophils. These basophils are attracted to the site of a tick bite and when the basophil comes in contact with the salivary antigens, the basophil degranulates. The primary effector substance released from the basophil is histamine, which mediates the death of the tick.

In a study on cutaneous basophil hypersensitivity in canine flea allergy, the number of basophils at the site of an intradermal injection of flea antigen increased from 4–18 hours after the injection (Halliwell and Schemmer, 1987). The peak occurred at 12 hours and the number had substantially fallen by 48 hours. Mononuclear cells increased after 18 hours while the percentage of eosinophils was fairly constant. These data support the contention that cutaneous basophil hypersensitivity may play a role in the immunopathogenesis of flea bite hypersensitivity.

Since fleas do not usually stay attached to the skin for long periods of time, cutaneous basophil hypersensitivity may be more detrimental than protective in flea allergy. Some degree of protection is suggested by the fact that flea hypersensitive dogs have fewer female fleas on their bodies than other dogs. Female fleas spend more time feeding than male fleas and are therefore more likely to be killed by the cutaneous basophil hypersensitivity. The poultry flea (*E. gallinacea*) and the sand flea (*T. penetrans*) are burrowing fleas and would be more susceptible to the effects of basophil hypersensitivity. The detrimental effect of cutaneous basophil hypersensitivity revolves around the persistence of the antigen at the site of the flea bite. The basophil will degranulate and release its vasoactive substances, which will cause inflammation of the skin without killing the flea since it has already gone.

Clinical features

Worldwide, there is no apparent breed or sex predilection for flea bite hypersensitivity. In some areas where genetic concentration has occurred due to line breeding, certain breeds may be predisposed. In atopic dogs, the incidence of positive skin tests to flea antigen has been reported to be as high as 80% as compared to a 40% or lower incidence in the general population (Scott *et al.*, 1995). This suggests that the atopic state favors the development or maintenance of the flea allergic state. Accordingly, the atopic breeds are more prone to develop flea bite hypersensitivity.

As with all other allergic disorders, clinical disease occurs only after a period of clinically insignificant sensitization. Animals with a genetic predisposition to develop allergies would be expected to be sensitized sooner then those with no such predisposition. When a nonpredisposed animal lives in an area where flea exposure is not overwhelming and is limited to three or four months of the year, sensitization often takes three or more years. With differing flea exposure, the sensitization period can be shortened or lengthened. With an allergic predisposition, the sensitization period can be very short and clinical disease can be seen during the first flea season. One author (WHM) cautions owners of very young animals (e.g. 6–18 months of age) with flea bite hypersensitivity that their pet is likely to show signs of other allergic disorders.

In areas where there is a distinct climatic difference between spring, summer, fall, and winter, flea bite hypersensitivity is a seasonal disorder. In many areas, the peak incidence is seen during the early–late summer and early fall. Chronically allergic animals will start to itch earlier and will show signs into winter. Provided that the house is not infested, the signs should resolve in the winter. In continually warm areas or where the house is infested, flea allergy can be a nonseasonal problem with seasonal variations.

The signs of flea bite hypersensitivity are similar to those seen in nonallergic flea bite dermatitis, but are much more profound. The intensity of the signs does not correlate with the number of fleas found. The primary lesion in both the dog and cat is a papule, which may develop an appreciable surrounding area of erythema. The papules usually become crusted. Lesions will be found anywhere the flea feeds. In the dog, the lower back (Figure 9.5), tail, posterior and medial thighs, and ventrum are affected, while the cat often has additional lesions between the shoulder blades (Figure 9.6). Because of the allergic nature of this condition, the primary lesions are often masked or confused by signs of self trauma. In the dog, acute moist dermatitis, secondary superficial bacterial folliculitis, alopecia, and secondary seborrhea are common findings. In the cat, severe excoriations, eosinophilic plaques, and eosinophilic granulomas can be superimposed on the underlying miliary dermatitis. Some cats have no primary lesions and present with widespread symmetrical self-induced hair loss.

In severely allergic animals, a generalized cutaneous reaction can occur. Some

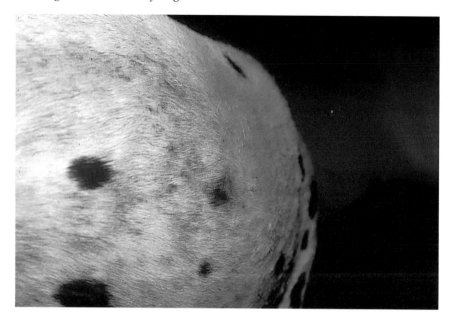

Figure 9.5   *An erythematous papular rash with traumatic hair loss over the rump.*

severely flea hypersensitive dogs resemble cases of sarcoptic mange clinically. In some cases, the owners will complain of facial and pedal pruritus, which coexist with the rump itching. This atopic-type pruritus can be explained by flea bites in those areas, concurrent atopy or food allergy, or a generalized IgE-mediated flea hypersensitivity.

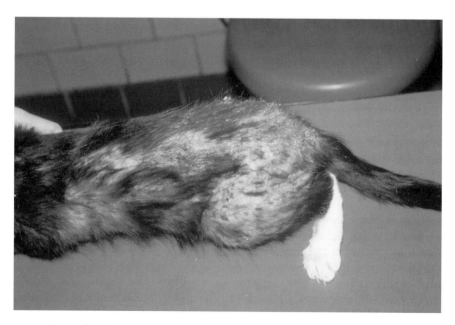

Figure 9.6   *Severe flea bite hypersensitivity in a cat.*

Diagnosis

A diagnosis of flea bite hypersensitivity can be proposed based on the physical find-ings. Demonstration of fleas or flea excreta supports the diagnosis, but does not con-firm it as the fleas may be a coincidental finding, or alternatively flea hypersensitivity can exist without direct evidence of fleas at one visit. Elimination of the clinical signs with eradication of the flea supports the diagnosis, but does not prove the hypersensi-tivity since immunologic abnormalities have not been documented.

In the dog and cat, the differential diagnosis includes atopy, food hypersensitiv-ity, superficial bacterial folliculitis, drug hypersensitivity, and intestinal parasite hypersensitivity. In the cat, the most common cause of miliary dermatitis is flea allergy, but all other causes of this syndrome such as *Cheyletiella* infestation, food allergy, and dermatophytosis must also be considered.

In most cases, the combination of compatible clinical signs and observed fleas is sufficient to render a tentative diagnosis of flea bite hypersensitivity. Although the clinician may find fleas on the animal, the owner often cannot. A flea comb is an excellent clinical aid as the fleas or flea excreta (Figure 9.7) can be removed from the animal and shown to the owner. The owner should be shown how to identify flea excreta as this may be the only sign of the presence of fleas once flea control is started. A moistened white paper towel will turn reddish-brown around the specks of dirt if the material is flea excreta (Plate 7). Street dirt will not cause the color change, but bloody crusts from skin wounds will. Bloody crusts are larger than flea excreta and the color change takes longer.

Skin biopsies can show a superficial perivascular dermatitis, which is typical of allergic disease. If eosinophils are the prominent dermal cell type or if eosinophilic intraepidermal microabscesses are seen, flea bite hypersensitivity is strongly sug-gested, but these features may not be seen. Hemograms may or may not show a peripheral eosinophilia.

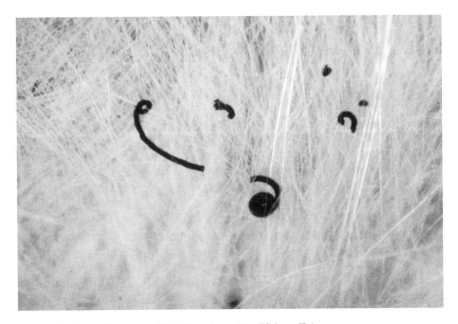

Figure 9.7   *Flea feces. (Courtesy of Vet-Kem Corp., Des Plaines, IL.)*

Intradermal skin testing with flea antigen is advocated as the diagnostic test for flea bite hypersensitivity. However, the results of the skin test are not foolproof. Negative reactions do not exclude the diagnosis while true positive results indicate a sensitivity, which may or may not be the cause of the animal's current problem. Figures indicating the sensitivity and specificity of flea antigen skin testing vary greatly (Van Winkle, 1981; Halliwell, 1984; Slacek and Opdebeech, 1993; Stolper and Opdebeech, 1994; Scott *et al.*, 1995; Willemse, 1996). Studies have shown that reactivity to commercial flea extracts differs from that seen with membrane or solubilized antigens (Slacek and Opdebeech, 1993; Stolper and Opdebeech, 1994). Using a commercial extract, Halliwell found that approximately 80% of skin test-positive dogs showed an immediate reaction while 10% showed only a delayed reaction. The remainder showed both reactions. Flea skin tests should be read immediately (15–30 minutes), at 4–8 hours (cutaneous basophil hypersensitivity), and at 24 and 48 hours (delayed hypersensitivity reaction). Often it is impractical for the veterinarian to read the results other than the immediate test results. The owners are therefore asked to read the sites for the delayed reactions, but these reports can be erroneous.

Presently, intradermal skin testing with flea antigen should be considered as a very highly supportive, but not absolutely diagnostic, test. Aqueous nonglycerinated extracts should be used at a concentration of no greater than 1:1000 (W/V) or 1000 Noon units/ml and should be injected with appropriate positive and negative controls. The test should be read at the times previously mentioned. Animals who show delayed reactions usually will react at 24 hours rather than at 48 hours and the reaction will often be an erythematous papule or plaque rather than the classic wheal.

Companies that provide serologic allergy tests typically include flea antigen in their test panel. To the authors' knowledge, there are no reports on the sensitivity and specificity of serologic testing for flea bite hypersensitivity. Since there are reports that allergic dogs have significant IgE antibody titers to insect and arachnid antigens (Griffin *et al.*, 1993) and that there probably is some cross-reactivity between the various insect allergens (Grier *et al.*, 1994; Pucheu-Haston *et al.*, 1995), serologic testing for flea bite hypersensitivity is probably no more reliable for diagnosis then is intradermal testing.

Clinical management
In general, flea bite hypersensitivity is a progressive disease provided the flea has not been eradicated (Scott *et al.*, 1995). Each year, clinical signs begin earlier in the season, are more severe, and persist longer. Accordingly, clinical management becomes more difficult. The cure for this disorder is complete eradication of the flea from the patient and its environment. Unfortunately, this is extremely difficult if not impossible in some areas.

With the whole flea extracts currently available, the results of immunotherapy for flea bite hypersensitivity have been disappointing. Flea bite hypersensitivity is therefore best treated by eradication of the flea. Since flea control measures take weeks to be maximally effective and most infested animals have inflamed skin, intercurrent medical treatments will be necessary when the animal is first presented. Early on, the pruritus of flea bite hypersensitivity will disappear entirely with the administration of appropriate doses of a glucocorticoid. Depending on the chronicity of the problem before diagnosis, a 5–10-day course of treatment should be sufficient to relieve the animal's discomfort. Very severe or chronic cases may require up to 21 days of steroid treatment. If effective flea control measures are started with the corticosteroid, the animal's flea burden should be sufficiently reduced by the time the steroid is withdrawn so that its pruritus does not return to any significant degree when the pills are stopped. If the flea control measures are haphazard or ignored entirely, the pruritus will return. Since administration of pills is far easier than flea control measures, this is a common scenario. Symptomatic treatment of flea bite hypersensitivity without concurrent flea control measures must be discouraged. With advancing time, the animal's steroid requirement will increase to dangerous levels. Eventually, the steroids will no longer be effective.

Depending upon the animal's environment and lifestyle, intense flea control measures may not be 100% effective in reducing the animal's pruritus to an acceptable level. Here, chronic medical management will then be necessary. Before the animal is doomed to a life of alternate-day steroids, the various nonsteroidal agents should be tried (see Chapter 6). As these agents seem to be most effective in the treatment of Type I hypersensitivity disorders and flea bite hypersensitivity has a complex immunopathogenesis, nonsteroidal agents may not be completely effective in any individual animal. If any particular drug reduces the animal's pruritus by 25% or more, it should be considered beneficial. The concurrent administration of the drug with the corticosteroid should allow a reduction in the steroid dosage.

Flea control.   The control of fleas requires a well-organized comprehensive program, which the client must understand (MacDonald, 1995; Scott et al., 1995). The owner must understand the hypersensitivity phenomenon and the nature of the flea and its life cycle. Most clients cannot absorb all of the necessary information in one short office visit and lapses in control can be expected. A client handout is an excellent management tool. The handout should explain the life cycle and lifestyle of the flea and describe in general terms the methods of flea control for the pet, other household pets, and the environment. A separate sheet should be attached that gives the specific instructions for the products to be used by this client. The client can read and absorb the information at his or her leisure and refer back to the document as needed since flea control is an ongoing battle.

In areas where there is a flea season, every effort should be made to eradicate the fleas from the environment during the winter. Once this is done, the animal should be disease-free until the next flea season. An owner with a flea allergic pet should start flea control in the early spring even if the animal's problem historically does not start until summer. The institution of early treatment will stress the necessity of good flea control and will usually prevent or minimize infestation of the pet's environment. If environmental infestation can be prevented, the management of the pet's hypersensitivity will be much easier and more rewarding.

An individual flea is easy to kill. Control is far more difficult because it involves the eradication of fleas from the pet in question, all contact animals, and the environment. If the pet in question is hypersensitive to fleas, the problem is further complicated because all fleas, not just most, must be eliminated. An effective control program must focus on all point sources of infestation. Environmental management is the key to success and has always been the weak link in most control programs because of its labor intensity and expense. The recent release of on- or in-animal products designed to prevent egg hatching or larval development provides the veterinarian and client with a simpler method of environmental control.

Treatment of the affected animal.   Unfortunately, dietary supplements of for example Brewer's yeast, garlic, and elemental sulfur and electronic flea collars are ineffective in the control of fleas (MacDonald, 1995; Scott *et al.*, 1995). These remedies may lessen the flea burden, but do not eradicate fleas. Insecticides must be used. Commonly used classic insecticides include the botanic products (pyrethrins, rotenone, and d-limonene) (Nicholson, 1995), synthetic pyrethroids, organophosphates, and carbamates. New agents are appearing and include fipronil, an insecticide from the phenylpyazole family (Postal *et al.*, 1995), and imidacloprid, a nitroguanidine compound. Some popular on-animal treatments contain organophosphates or carbamates, but their use appears to be declining because of concerns for animal toxicity and environmental pollution. Today, pyrethrin- or pyrethroid-containing products or the new generation of insecticides are most commonly used. These insecticides are combined with various repellents and potentiators to increase their efficacy and prolong their residual effects. Insecticides come in a myriad of formulations and can be applied via a flea collar, shampoo, aerosol spray, pump spray, foam, dust, dip, or spot application. One organophosphate, cythioate, is licensed for oral administration.

The most important aspect of flea control on animals is not the quick kill of the flea, but rather the residual effect of the product(s). Many product brochures claim a residual time that is not substantiated in the clinical situation (MacDonald, 1995). Poor owner application, animal factors such as swimming or grooming, and environmental infestation could explain this discrepancy. An effective well-applied standard flea dip appears to be effective for only 12–24 hours if the animal's environment is heavily infested. Present technologic advances have increased the residual effect of flea products and include the development of the synthetic pyrethroids and microencapsulation technology. Fipronil appears to have residual clinical activity for approximately 60 days (Postal *et al.*, 1995).

Selection of the insecticide depends on the local resistance of the flea population, the species and age of the animal being treated, the nature of the coat of the animal, and the wishes of the owner. Some owners will not use 'toxic' chemicals on their pets and are therefore restricted to the use of the botanic products. Fleas can become resistant to insecticides and this local resistance must be considered. In most instances, perceived 'resistance' is not true biochemical resistance but suboptimal performance due to poor application or a poor control program. Most insecticides will kill fleas, but environmental infestation or the short residual effect of the applied product can mean that fleas will quickly re-infest the animal.

In many countries, pesticide use is carefully controlled. The use of a pesticide in a manner inconsistent with its labeling is illegal. Veterinarians have been fined for extra-label use of a pesticide even when 'standard practice' indicates that extra-label use is safe and more effective. Accordingly, one should select products that are most flexible in their labeling. Products labeled for use no more frequently than once every 2–3 weeks give the veterinarian very little flexibility. In the clinical situation, few insecticides will be fully effective for three weeks. More frequent application of these potent products can be toxic, is an extra-label use of the product, and is illegal. The best products to use are those that are labeled without interval restrictions or can be modified by the direction of the veterinarian. With these products, the insecticide can be used legally as often as needed with little concern for toxicity. If the product used is licensed for dogs, puppies, cats, and kittens, the veterinarian can design a very effective control program with very few products.

The key to a successful flea control program is routine and regular use of an effective product. The frequency of application depends on the product used and the environmental flea burden. The best product in the world does no good if the owner cannot or will not use it. In the past, owners have been reluctant to repeatedly apply toxic chemicals to their animals. Today, the regular use of botanic products or the pyrethroids has lessened owners' fears. However, the substitution of these less potent products necessitates more frequent application and can make some control programs too labor intense for some owners. No one product or control program is best for all households. Product selection depends on the animal(s) being treated, the animal's lifestyle, and the owner's expectations and physical abilities. Pump spray insecticides are of little or no use for dogs with dense undercoats such as the chow chow. Dogs who swim daily must be treated differently than dogs who do not. Households with multiple dogs and cats, some or all of whom are allowed to run freely in the neighborhood, are most challenging. Any flea control program is destined to failure unless it is individualized for the household in question.

Flea combs.   The flea comb is an excellent nonchemical method of flea control, especially when the animal is not continually exposed to new fleas. A battery-powered comb that claims to electrocute fleas has just been marketed. No clinical data are available on its safety and efficacy. Obviously, the owner must have the time and desire to comb the animal thoroughly once or twice daily. Flea combing works best on short- to medium-coated small dogs and cats who spend most of their time inside. Regular flea combing is also a beneficial part of an insecticidal program. In most control programs, fleas disappear from the owner's sight long before they can be considered eradicated. Once or twice weekly flea combing of the animal with careful inspection of the hairball for fleas or flea feces helps the owner monitor the success of the program.

Flea collars.   The early veterinary literature is replete with reports on the efficacy of insecticidal flea collars. No such reports exist for the collars marketed and purchased today. As a sole agent, insecticidal flea collars are worthless in any serious flea control program. They will kill or repel some fleas, but nowhere near enough for a flea allergic animal. Their suboptimal efficacy does not exclude their use in all situations. Flea collars can be used in conjunction with other products provided the insecticides are compatible to increase the overall efficacy of the program. Flea collars are better then nothing when the owner will do no more.

Insect growth regulators, the backbone of environmental control programs, have some efficacy when they are applied to the animal. Collars containing these products are marketed and more will be released (Miller and Blagburn, 1996). Pre-release data on these collars show prolonged efficacy in killing flea eggs laid on the dog or cat, but no published controlled clinical studies on the collars' efficacy are available.

Flea shampoos and cream rinses.   The vast majority of flea shampoos, and to the best of the authors' knowledge, all of the insecticidal cream rinses contain pyrethrins or pyrethroids. Flea shampoos are excellent cleaning products and cream rinses condition the animal's coat. Both will kill fleas while the product is being applied, provided the contact time is sufficient. To kill fleas, natural or synthetic pyrethrins require a 10–15-minute contact time (Dryden, 1993b). A shorter contact time will stun but not kill the flea. Shampoos have little or no residual effect once the product is rinsed off. Manufacturers' data sheets for cream rinses suggest residual efficacy for up to seven days, provided that the product is applied carefully and rinsed lightly. No clinical studies are available to support or refute those claims so the place of cream rinses in a serious flea control program is unknown.

Flea shampoos clean the coat and can remove the surface lipid layer of the skin. The cleaning is beneficial, but the removal of the lipid layer can dry the skin and may shorten the residual efficacy of sprays or dips. Flea shampoos can irritate some animals and are more expensive then noninsecticidal grooming products. These shortcomings, coupled with the probability that most owners will not lather their pet for the necessary 10–15 minutes makes the regular use of flea shampoos of questionable benefit.

Flea powders.   The vast majority of flea powders contain carbamates (5–12.5%) as their main ingredient. Their application is very messy and dust surrounds the animal and the applier. All powders use talc as their vehicle and some also contain silicas or diatomaceous earth. The inclusion of these latter ingredients must be seriously questioned because they can cause chronic lung disease (Smith, 1995). If applied properly to haired skin, flea powders can have a very protracted residual effect. The application to sparsely or non-haired skin is of little value as the powder easily falls off when the animal stands or shakes. The talc absorbs sebum and repeated use will dry the skin and hair. Since all dogs are sparsely haired on their ventrum and most flea infested or allergic pets have areas of traumatic hair loss, complete flea control is difficult to achieve with a flea powder. If a powder is to be used, it must be supplemented with a spray for the hairless regions. With all of these shortcomings, the use of flea powders has declined dramatically in recent years.

Flea dips, foams, and sprays. Dips, foams, and sprays are different methods of applying a liquid insecticide to an animal's skin. Depending upon the active ingredients and the thoroughness of application, these methods of flea control tend to be the most effective way to kill fleas. Repeated use without intervening bathing of some pyrethrin and pyrethroid products may provide some repellent activity as well. Owners with physical disabilities can find it difficult to use these products. With repeated use of these liquids, the animal's coat develops a buildup of product, necessitating occasional bathing.

Flea dips (rinses) are very economic and provide the quickest and most thorough method of applying an insecticide to an animal's skin. They are also the messiest and can leave densely coated animals wet for hours. Cats rarely tolerate repeated dipping. In warm weather, animals can be dipped outside where they dry quickly. During cold or rainy weather many owners are reluctant to dip their pets. Small- to medium-sized dogs can be dipped in a bath tub, but large dogs present a real problem for most owners. If application by a professional is out of the question, an alternate method of control must be selected.

Flea foams (mousses) are relatively new and can be considered as expensive flea sprays. They receive widest use in cats, and although they can be used as the sole method of control on dogs, their expense often precludes this use. Spot use in dogs in areas where owners are reluctant to apply sprays or dips (e.g. the face) is becoming increasingly more popular. The product leaves the can as a foam, which is rubbed into the coat. As the bubbles burst, the insecticide reaches the skin. In treating small pets, especially cats, the owners should follow the product's directions carefully. It can be easy to intoxicate the animal if the mousse is applied at a greater rate then suggested by the manufacturer.

Flea sprays are basically diluted flea dips that have been stabilized, made more elegant, and are sold in spray cans or pump bottles. Since aerosol sprays are noisy and leave the can cold, they have no place in the treatment of animals. With the pump spray, the owner is in essence lightly dipping the animal. In very short-coated animals, effective spraying is straightforward. As the coat length increases, the ease of use decreases. The free hand must be used to lift the coat from the skin so that the spray can be applied directly to the skin. For large long-coated dogs like the golden retriever, effective pump spraying is very labor intense and uses a significant amount of product. Effective spraying of a densely undercoated dog like the chow chow is virtually impossible. If an owner is spraying two or more large dogs, the cost of treatment can become prohibitive. The owner can then make his or her own spray from an appropriate flea dip provided that the product's label does not exclude such use. The owner should buy a pump bottle and dilute enough of the dip concentrate so that the solution fills the reservoir bottle. Unless the flea dip package states that the diluted product is stable after dilution, the unused portion of the spray should be discarded. After several treatments, the owner will know how much product is actually used and can make the correct amount.

Within the last few years, some flea sprays and dips have included insect growth regulators along with the insecticide. Before 1996, products containing methoprene and fenoxycarb were available. In 1996, products with pyriproxifen, a potent growth regulator with purported adulticidal effects (Smith, 1995) were released and fenoxycarb was withdrawn in the USA by its manufacturer. Depending on the product selected, the manufacturer indicates that the growth regulator will kill eggs or inhibit their development for 30 or more days. Aside from the flea egg-control collar, all on-animal growth regulators are combined with an insecticide, which needs to be applied at least weekly. This frequent application of insecticide replenishes the growth regulator, thus providing an effective on-animal environmental product.

Spot-application products. Before 1996, there were two different products that could theoretically protect the entire dog from fleas with application of the insecticide to a very localized area of the skin over the back. In 1996, another spot-application product containing imidacloprid was released. These products are very appealing, especially to people with physical handicaps, because their application takes little time and effort. All products are marketed as part (not all) of a flea control program. The first product is a 65% permethrin concentrate, which is applied from 1 ml pouches to the skin over the dog's back. According to the product information sheet, the permethrin migrates over the dog's entire skin surface within three days of application and kills and repels fleas for up to four weeks. Shampooing will remove the product, but episodic swimming is reported to have little effect on efficacy. Manufacturer's efficacy figures depend upon the dog's weight and time from application and vary from 92–100%. The package insert gives no specific time for readministration, but indicates that the product should not be used more often than once weekly. The product is highly toxic to cats. The package insert cautions owners about letting their cat lick or play with a recently treated dog as the cat can become intoxicated.

The second spot-application product contains the organophosphate fenthion. The product is available in different size pouches for dogs of differing weights. Depending upon the dog's weight, the product, as marketed in the USA, delivers approximately 4–8 mg/kg of fenthion, which is absorbed into the animal's body. After the product is absorbed transdermally, it cannot be removed by bathing or swimming. Fleas are killed when they feed on a treated animal and ingest the fenthion. Since the product does not repel or kill fleas before feeding, the treated pet can still develop a flea-induced dermatitis. Manufacturer's data show that peak efficacy is not reached for three days after administration and is greater in dogs receiving 8 mg/kg. Manufacturer's efficacy figures vary from 97– 100% for 24 days after administration. The product is not to be applied more frequently than once every two weeks.

The newest product contains imidacloprid, a nitroguanidine compound that is licensed for both dogs and cats, and is applied over the back. Like the 65% permethrin product, it migrates over the animal's body and envelops it with a coating of insecticide. According to the manufacturer's data, the product is safe, odorless, will kill 98–100% of contact fleas within 24 hours of application, and has residual effectivity for up to four weeks on cats and for at least that period on dogs. Its features, especially the ability to use it on cats, are appealing, but its true place in flea control programs will not be known for some time.

These spot-application products are very appealing because of their ease of use. They are especially appealing for owners with swimming dogs, owners of a large number of dogs, or when the owner has a physical disability. Large controlled clinical studies on the efficacy of these spot-application products are not available. It is unlikely that they perform as well as their manufacturers indicate. Data generated in the 1970s when a 20% fenthion solution was used extensively at 20–30 mg/kg every 7–14 days suggest that the manufacturer's efficacy data for the commercial fenthion product are overly generous in the clinical setting. In those studies, doses of fenthion less then 20 mg/kg provided moderate control for approximately seven days (Mason *et al.*, 1984). For maximal efficacy, this product needs to be used with a compatible topical product or in an extra-label fashion. Anecdotal information suggests that the 65% permethrin product needs to be applied very frequently (e.g. weekly) for some dogs before the efficacy approaches that suggested by the manufacturer. At that frequency, the product becomes very expensive for owners of medium-sized or large dogs.

There is some concern that products using the enveloping technology might cause true biochemical resistance to the insecticide. As the insecticide envelops the animal's body, certain areas, especially the distal limbs, may not receive enough product to kill or repel fleas. Fleas can be observed on the feet of some dogs treated with the 65% permethrin product. It remains to be seen whether exposure to sublethal doses of insecticide will result in resistance.

Oral products. Three oral flea control products are currently marketed. Cythioate is an organophosphate administered orally ever hird day. Dogs are given 3 mg/kg while cats receive 1.5 mg/kg. In the USA, it is an FDA-controlled product and is not licensed for use in cats. The flea is killed if it feeds while the blood cythioate concentration is high enough. Manufacturer's efficacy figures vary from 90–95%. However, these figures are misleading since the cythioate blood concentration does not remain above the lethal level for the entire three days before the next administration. As licensed, cythioate appears to kill fleas for 24 hours or less.

The other two oral flea products are insect development inhibitors, which have ovicidal and larvicidal effects, but do not kill or repel adult fleas. These products are basically environmental treatments given to the animal. The most widely marketed product, lufenuron, is a benzyl–phenol urea compound that inhibits chitin synthesis in the developing flea (Hink *et al.*, 1994; Shipstone and Masson, 1995; Blagburn *et al.*, 1996; Smith *et al.*, 1996). It is given orally to dogs (10 mg/kg) or cats (30 mg/kg) once every 30 days. Fleas feeding during this time ingest the lufenuron, which results in death of the eggs or larvae. The second oral flea development inhibitor is cyromazine and is marketed for dogs only in combination with diethylcarbamazine (Shipstone and Masson, 1995). The drug is given daily at a dosage of 10 mg/kg. Cyromazine belongs to the triazine group. It does not inhibit chitin synthesis, but increases its stiffness so that the expansion needed for growth cannot occur. This increases the internal pressure in the larva and results in lethal body wall defects. Laboratory and clinical efficacy studies have shown a greater then 90% efficacy for both products (Hink *et al.*, 1994; Shipstone and Masson, 1995). Since mammals do not produce chitin, lufenuron and cyromazine both have a very wide margin of safety.

As the oral insect development inhibitors have no effect on adult fleas, clients must be warned that they will still be able to see adult fleas on their pets. These must be killed with an appropriate adulticide. Since there should be few or no fleas to replace those killed by the insecticide, the need for insecticides should be short-lived. If no adulticidal treatments are used, the number of adult fleas will decrease noticeably after 21 days of treatment and over 90% control will be seen after two months (Blagburn *et al.*, 1996; Smith *et al.*, 1996). Here, the decline in flea numbers is due to the natural or traumatic death of the feeding fleas.

Treatment of contact animals
Ideally, all contact dogs and cats should be treated with as much vigor as the flea hypersensitive pet. If the client owns many animals, especially cats, the cost and time commitment of this intense therapy may be prohibitive. Spot-application products and cythioate have their greatest application here. These products may not be efficacious enough for the allergic pet, but can help reduce the overall flea burden in a multiple animal household. Flea collars or cythioate, where licensed, will help decrease the flea population on cats when other products cannot be used.

Treatment of the environment
Environmental management is the most crucial part of any flea control program. None of the products used on animals is 100% effective so intense animal treatment is almost a waste of time and money if the heavily infested environment is ignored. Treatment of an infested household is expensive and time consuming. Prevention of infestation is the primary goal. In those areas where there is a flea season, every

effort should be made to eradicate the flea from the house, kennel, or barn during the winter. At the start of spring, flea control should be started on the animals and/or in the environment. The aim of this early treatment is to prevent infestation. If the pet's environment is nearly or entirely flea free, most of the battle has been won.

It makes little or no sense to treat an animal's environment intensively for fleas and then allow flea infested pets back into it. On the day(s) the environment is treated, all dogs and cats should be treated with the most effective topical agent available.

Indoor flea control.   In most cases, the fleas that an owner sees on his or her pets come from within the house. As discussed earlier, nonfed nonhosted adults are only a very small part of the indoor flea burden. The immature forms are most problematic and are concentrated in areas where the animal rests. However, fleas and their immature stages can be found everywhere the animal visits. If the animal does not enter certain rooms, these rooms should be flea free. All other areas should be treated. In large houses with one or more free-roaming pets, indoor flea treatment is time consuming and expensive. Halfhearted efforts are rewarded with little or no success. If the owner does not have the time or desire to treat his or her house correctly, a professional exterminator should be suggested. Since some exterminators suggest suboptimal control programs or may apply insecticides incompatible with those used on the animals, the exterminator's program should be reviewed before the house is treated.

Displaced or recently emerged adult fleas are easy to kill since they climb to the top of carpets to find a new host (Dryden, 1993a; Robinson, 1995). Eggs, larvae and pupae are more difficult to attack since they reside in areas that are hard to reach with chemicals. Accordingly, one household treatment is not likely to end the infestation. The owner should be warned of this in advance and control programs should be designed with a planned retreatment.

Cleaning is an essential part of flea control. Although the viability of eggs, larvae, and pupae is short in unprotected areas (e.g. window sills, seamless kitchen floors) these areas should be wiped or mopped with an appropriate cleaning solution. Items such as the pet's bedding and frequently slept-on throw rugs should be washed frequently. Carpeted areas and upholstered furniture are most problematic because the eggs, larvae, and pupae are deep in the material where they are protected from physical removal or contact with an insecticide sprayed on the surface. Vacuuming is the first line of defense in the cleaning process of most houses. Although vacuuming is not likely to remove larvae and pupae, it will remove eggs and the food necessary for larval development. The carpets, furniture cushions, areas under cushions, cracks in the floor, and the crevice along baseboards should be vacuumed carefully to remove as many of the immature forms and their food as is possible. With deep pile or shag carpets, high power vacuums are needed. Vacuuming may encourage pre-emerged adults to hatch so that they can be killed by the insecticide, which will be applied after the cleaning. The vacuum bag should be discarded after the cleaning is complete otherwise adult fleas can develop in and escape from the vacuum. Temperatures above 35°C (121°F) are lethal to larvae and pupae. Cleaning of carpets and furniture with a true steam cleaner is an excellent nonchemical method of flea control. Most rentable cleaners do not produce or maintain temperatures high enough to kill the hidden larvae so professional cleaning services must be used. Steam cleaning has the drawback that it increases the relative humidity in the fabric, which can accelerate the rate of egg development. Since cleaning is not likely to eradicate all fleas, a chemical must be applied to finish the job.

A wide variety of insecticides are available through veterinarians, hardware stores, and exterminators. All these products are carefully regulated and must be used according to label directions. Products vary in their potency and duration of action. Products with little residual effect (quick-kill) are inappropriate as the sole agent as the immature forms will repopulate the house very quickly. Products combining a quick-kill agent with an insect growth regulator or a residual insecticide are preferred.

Many clients and veterinarians are opposed to the idea of applying potent residual insecticide. Microencapsulation technology decreases these concerns. A thin chemical shell covers a minute amount of the insecticide. The shell protects the insecticide and allows a slow sustained release of a low, but insect-lethal, amount of the insecticide. Mammalian toxicity is greatly decreased. Household microencapsulated pyrethrins are reported to be effective for 30 days. Microencapsulated chlorpyrifos provides up to 90 days of control. Despite these improvements, many clients will not use these products.

Insect growth regulators interfere with the normal development of flea larvae (Dryden, 1993a; Palma *et al.*, 1993; MacDonald, 1995; Scott *et al.*, 1995; Smith, 1995). Classical growth regulators are juvenile hormone analogs, which mimic insect growth hormone. Growth hormone is necessary for early larval growth and development, but decreased levels are necessary to trigger larval metamorphosis. Sustained high levels of growth hormone, either natural or manmade, interrupts the maturation process, prevents pupation and, ultimately, results in larval death. This interruption in larval maturation is achieved when the adult female, egg, or larva is exposed to the compound. Adults are not killed by the compound, but will lay eggs, which will not develop. The efficacy of growth regulators applied to adults or eggs is the basis for their inclusion in on-animal products. Depending on the product selected, these compounds interfere with flea development for 30–52 weeks.

Thorough application of a residual insecticide or a quick-kill agent with a growth regulator will kill all displaced and recently emerged adults in the areas treated. If all flea infested areas are treated effectively, the house will be flea free on the day of treatment. However, owners will probably notice new fleas days to weeks later. The rate of appearance depends on the environmental conditions and the degree of infestation. These new fleas arise from the pupae. The pupal cocoon will absorb insecticides, resulting in the death of the pupa or pre-emerged adult. However, delivery of the insecticide to the cocoon is very difficult and it is unlikely that most pupae will be killed. If the house has been treated with a residual insecticide, these new fleas will be killed. When quick-kill and growth regulator products have been used, retreatment will be necessary because the adulticide will no longer be present. Although one could retreat the house with just a quick-kill insecticide, it is advisable to reuse the original product to guarantee an effective concentration of the growth regulator. In cool weather when pupal emergence can be prolonged, it may be necessary to treat the heavily infested house a third time.

The key to effective environmental treatment is the delivery system. The best insecticide is of little use if it is poorly applied. An incomplete understanding of the flea's habits and lifestyle coupled with misconceptions on how products work leads to much wasted effort on the client's part. The most poorly understood delivery system is the fogger or bomb. Foggers contain insecticides and/or growth regulators, which are aerosolized into droplets when the fogger is triggered. The droplets remain suspended in the air for some time and then fall to the ground by gravity where they dry on contact. The nozzle design and pressure system determines droplet size and consequently the dispersal of the insecticide. Large droplets fall to the ground relatively quickly while fine particles stay suspended longer and can travel further.

Foggers do not cover room corners well and do not penetrate under furniture cushions or furniture to any great extent. These undertreated areas tend to be where the flea infestation is heaviest. The droplets dry on contact and may not penetrate deeply into carpets or upholstery. The product information on many foggers indicates that large areas can be treated with each fogger. Owners typically buy the number of foggers necessary to treat the number of square meters of living space in their house. However, since areas such as doorways and corridors interfere with dispersal of the product, most houses need to be treated with many more foggers than used. For maximum effect, a separate fogger should be used in nearly every room. When the appropriate number of foggers is purchased for the initial treatment and the retreatment, this method of treatment is very expensive. Many individuals reserve foggers for the treatment of large unfurnished areas like basements.

The most efficient way to treat a house is to spray the product on to the area to be treated. Premise products are sold in standard aerosol cans, inverted aerosol cans, pump sprays, or as concentrates. Hand pump sprays are worthless for the treatment of large areas. The user's hand will quickly tire. Spray tanks with a pressurized reservoir are much more user friendly. Since most veterinary premise products do not come in a concentrate, the owner must purchase these products from an exterminator. Today, aerosolized products are receiving widest use. Standard aerosol cans often fail to deliver product if the can is tipped while spraying under furniture. The inverted aerosol can does not suffer from this problem. Whichever method of delivery is selected, the owner must apply the product at the delivery rate indicated by the manufacturer. Underapplication to save a few dollars of product is very likely to fail.

Many individuals are opposed to the use of any insecticide in their environment. This has led to the development of premise sprays containing just growth regulators or the use of environmental desiccants. Since these products do not kill adults, the pets and humans in the household may still be bothered by flea bites until all the adult fleas die of old age. However, since no new fleas should develop from the eggs, the environment will eventually be flea free provided no new fleas are brought in from outside. The premise sprays available contain the products discussed above. Electronic flea traps may be useful in this situation to reduce the adult flea burden.

Diatomaceous earth and borates have received widest use as noninsecticidal premise products (MacDonald, 1995). Diatomaceous earth works by disrupting the epicuticle of the flea and larvae, resulting in dehydration and death (Bowman, 1995; Smith, 1995). Chronic lung disease has been recognized in miners of this product

(Smith, 1995). Since the product is messy to use, of unproven efficacy, and inhalation is likely, diatomaceous earth should not be used.

Borates were originally thought to work solely by desiccation (MacDonald, 1995; Smith, 1995). Although desiccation is probably part of their mode of action, recent work indicates that the larvae are killed when they ingest the product. Borates are thought by many to be completely innocuous. As with any chemical, this is, however, not true and the US Borax company has issued a strong cautionary statement on the widespread use of borates in households (Smith, 1995). Any borate product not specifically licensed for household application should not be used. Sodium polyborate has an acute oral LD_{50} of 3.5 g/kg in laboratory animals. To the authors' knowledge, no animal illness or deaths have been attributed to sodium polyborate. However, the National Animal Poison Control Center has received multiple calls on supposed cases of animal toxicosis (Smith, 1995). Sales figures are not available to allow a calculation of the incidence of adverse reactions per households treated. The number is likely to be very low (MacDonald, 1995). Since the use of borates is relatively new, there are concerns about what effect chronic borate exposure will have on the humans and animals in the household. Until the long-term safety of the borates is known, potential users should be informed of the concerns that exist.

The most widely known borate product can be applied by company technicians or by the owner. Until recently, this product was applied only by the company's technicians. When applied by the company with special machines, the carpet would be packed with sodium polyborate crystals and would be guaranteed flea free for one year (MacDonald, 1995). Vacuuming does not decrease the efficacy, but shampooing will. Treated carpets will suppress flea development for over 18 months. The number of satisfied users, including veterinary dermatologists, is very high. This company, as well as others, also markets borate products for client application. No studies are available to show whether one of these self-applied products is superior to the others. As with any self-applied product, the potential for misapplication with increased toxicity must be considered. Clients interested in this approach to environmental flea control must be told to follow the manufacturer's directions carefully. With careful application, these self-applied products should be equally or nearly as effective as the technician-applied product.

Kennel control.   Fleas are easy to control in a modern well-designed kennel. These kennels have seamless fiberglass or stainless steel cages, separate ward areas, and paved outdoor runs. Little more than routine and regular use of a high-pressure hose is needed to keep the environment flea free. At the other end of the spectrum is the equivalent of a dog slum. All outdoor areas are dirt covered and animals are housed either alone or in groups in wood houses bedded with straw, hay, or wood shavings. Sanitary efforts are typically nonexistent and the owner will refuse to make any significant effort to improve them. It is hopeless to treat this type of kennel and only repeated use of residual insecticides will have any effect on reducing the flea burden for the dogs.

Some concerned owners have one or several dogs kept in dog houses surrounded by a dirt run. These kennels can be effectively treated provided a well-designed plan is followed. Firstly, all bedding and organic debris in the run area must be removed. Dog houses on or near ground level should be moved so that the ground beneath can be cleaned. Ideally, the dog houses should be reinstalled on blocks or posts so that the area can be cleaned regularly and air can circulate beneath. If ground contact cannot be avoided, the area should be treated with an externally approved residual insecticide (e.g. carbamate powder) or quick-kill/growth regulator product. The dog house should be sprayed with a quick-kill/growth regulator product and clean bedding should be provided. Spraying and rebedding should be scheduled every fourteenth day for at least one month. The dirt run area should be addressed as discussed below.

Outdoor flea control.   In most instances, the pet confined to his or her own property picks up no more than 5% of its flea burden from the outside environment. Untreated, flea infested neighborhood cohorts are a much greater source for most pets. Free-roaming suburban or rural dogs and cats are exposed to fleas from their untreated friends, the dens or burrows of infested wild animals, and from frequently used resting spots, which they and their friends have infested. Obviously, little can be done to prevent outside infestation of the free-roaming pet and this source of fleas can be eliminated only by confinement.

Products containing an outdoor-approved insecticide or growth regulator are available. Application of these products to an entire yard is unnecessary in many cases, will be marginally effective in rainy areas, and can be environmentally unsound if an insecticide is used. Although eggs can fall from an animal's body anywhere as it runs through the yard, only the areas where the animal rests or is confined by a chain or a fence are likely to be significantly infested. In the typical yard, most of the grass is kept cut short, is free of organic debris, and is not shaded from the sun. Under these conditions, the soil rapidly dries and reaches very high temperatures. The probability of an egg developing to an adult flea under these harsh conditions is very remote. Soil conditions for flea development are ideal in shaded areas and where the vegetation is tall. Flower gardens, uncut fields, and areas under large-shade trees are natural trouble spots. Manmade trouble spots include areas under decks, porches, and dog houses and shaded runs with a crushed stone or dirt floor. By mowing uncut areas, pruning to decrease shade coverage, or appropriate fencing, the number of trouble spots that might need insecticidal attention can be greatly decreased.

Animals forced to spend long hours outside must be provided shade. If the ground in these areas is paved, flea development is unlikely and can be terminated by frequently hosing the area. When the flooring is dirt, sand, crushed stone, or board on or just above the ground surface, environmental conditions for flea development are likely to be ideal. Licensed yard and kennel products should be used as they have been formulated for maximum residual effect in all weather conditions and the manufacturer's instructions must be followed carefully. If insecticidal products are used, all the insecticides used to treat the animal and the house should be reviewed carefully so that the animal is not intoxicated by cumulative absorption from all sources. If the yard and kennel sprays contains an organophosphate or carbamate, similar agents should not be used in the house or on the animal.

The use of biologic weapons in outdoor flea control is receiving increasing attention. A nematode, *Steinernema carpocapsae*, is marketed as one such weapon (Henderson *et al.*, 1995). Once the nematodes are established in sufficient numbers in moist soil, they seek flea larvae and pupae and kill them. The nematodes need to be replenished periodically and will die off when the flea larvae have gone. To remain viable, the surface soil moisture must be about 20%, and these is therefore usually a need for frequent watering. This watering requirement can be unacceptable if the treated area drains poorly and the animal has to rest in mud. Laboratory data show high efficacy, especially in gravel, but no clinical studies have been published on its efficacy in the clinical situation (Henderson *et al.*, 1995).

Immunotherapy
The efficacy of immunotherapy for flea bite hypersensitivity is extremely controversial. Some early clinical reports extol its virtue, but controlled studies do not substantiate these findings. Two double-blinded studies run at the University of Florida concluded that presently available flea antigen injections cannot be recommended for therapy (Halliwell, 1981; Kunkle and Milcarsky, 1985). Halliwell studied the response of flea allergic dogs to six weekly intradermal injections of various commercial flea antigens while Kunkle studied the response of cats to 20 weekly intradermal or subcutaneous injections of one particular antigen. Kunkle found that two of her 18 treated cats responded markedly while one additional cat showed a moderate improvement. One of the cats who responded markedly received intradermal injections while the other cat received subcutaneous injections. The other responder also received subcutaneous injections. In Halliwell's study, some improvement was noted in some of the dogs, but the overall assessment was that his protocol was probably not helpful.

The apparent ineffectiveness of flea immunotherapy in animals is in agreement with studies in humans with insect hypersensitivity when whole insect extracts have been used for immunotherapy (Wilson *et al.*, 1993). In man, it has been shown that immunotherapy with specific insect venoms is much more efficacious than when whole insect extracts are used. A better flea antigen would probably increase the efficacy of immunotherapy in pets.

Presently, immunotherapy for flea allergy cannot be recommended except as a last ditch effort before euthanasia or chronic high-dose glucocorticoid administration. If immunotherapy is attempted, it should be used in conjunction with the best flea control program attainable. Weekly subcutaneous injections of 0.5–1.0 ml of a commercial flea antigen should be given. Since at least 15 of the antigens found in flea saliva are complete antigens rather than haptens (Halliwell, 1984; Scott *et al.*, 1995), the previously recommended intradermal route of administration is probably not necessary. If a response is seen, the vaccine should be given on an 'as needed' basis during flea season. If no response is seen after six months of treatment, it is unlikely that continued immunotherapy will be helpful.

Mosquito bite hypersensitivity

This is an apparently uncommon condition that has only been documented in the cat (Mason and Evans, 1991; Ihrke and Gross, 1994), but it is probably more common than recognized. Since some dogs have clinical histories and lesions comparable with those seen in the cat, the condition probably occurs in dogs (Scott *et al.*, 1995). Positive intradermal skin test reactions to mosquito antigen are reported in both species (Mason and Evans, 1991; Willis and Kunkle, 1996).

Pathogenesis
Affected cats show an immediate intradermal reaction to mosquito antigen, indicating a Type I hypersensitivity disorder. In some cats, skin biopsies show eosinophilic granulomas with collagen degeneration without a significant diffuse eosinophilic dermatitis. This suggests that the pathogenesis may be more complicated than a simple Type I hypersensitivity reaction.

Clinical features
No age, breed, or sex predilection has been recognized. Affected animals are not reported to be allergic to other allergens. All cases have involved outdoor or indoor–outdoor cats living in areas where mosquitos are prevalent. Indoor cats kept in unscreened rooms may be equally susceptible. The onset of signs is during warm weather. The first episode may occur anytime during the spring or summer. Subsequent episodes in later years would be expected to occur sooner since the cat is already sensitized.

Mosquitos feed in non- or sparsely-haired areas. In the cat, this includes the nasal planum, the bridge of the nose adjacent to the nasal planum, the pinnae, and the footpads. Other areas of skin exposed by clipping or the cat's excessive grooming can also be involved. Most affected cats have a facial dermatitis, which is variably pruritic. The earliest lesion is an inflammatory papule or nodule, which is typically eroded and crusted. If the cat is very pruritic or has been bitten by many mosquitos, individual lesions can be hard to identify. Advanced cases have an ulcerative crusted dermatitis of the bridge of the nose (Plate 8) and ears. Some cats only develop papular–nodular lesions on the edge of the pinnae (Figure 9.8). These

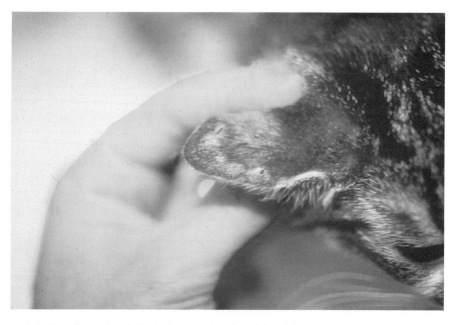

Figure 9.8 *Papular and nodular lesions on the edge of the right pinna in a cat with mosquito bite hypersensitivity.*

lesions tend to be minimally symptomatic. Restriction of lesions to the footpads is rare. If involved, they usually accompany facial disease and are swollen and hyper-keratotic.

Diagnosis
The ease of diagnosis depends on the chronicity of the problem and the severity of the cat's pruritus. In early cases where there are nontraumatized papular–nodular lesions in appropriate areas, the tentative diagnosis is straightforward. Differential diagnoses include all other causes of folliculitis or furunculosis. In mosquito bite hypersensitivity, aspiration cytology of a papule shows a heavy eosinophilic infil-trate. In chronic pruritic cases, the major differentials include pemphigus foliaceus or erythematosus, feline scabies, atopy, and food hypersensitivity. Skin biopsy shows perivascular–diffuse eosinophilic dermatitis with or without collagen degen-eration and excludes all differentials except atopy or food hypersensitivity. If signifi-cant lesions preceded the cat's pruritus, atopy and food hypersensitivity are unlikely. Intradermal testing with mosquito antigen (1000 protein nitrogen units) (PNU) should be positive in affected animals. The specificity of this testing is unknown since to the best of the authors' knowledge this testing has not been validated in large numbers of normal cats.

Treatment
Isolation from mosquitos is essential to treat and prevent this condition. Once removed from mosquitos, mild cases will resolve spontaneously within 7–10 days. Corticosteroids can hasten the healing and will be required in advanced cases. Oral or injectable drugs can be used, depending upon the course of treatment needed. Oral prednisolone (2.2 mg/kg q. 24 h) or injectable methylprednisolone acetate are most commonly used (see Chapter 6). Prevention is of paramount importance as the next exposure will result in more severe lesions. Ideally, the cat should be kept inside in a screened room from dusk to dawn, the peak feeding period for mosquitos. If restrictive housing is impossible, the frequent application of flea products with repellent activity may be helpful. Flea foams receive wide use in affected cats. Only the sparsely-haired areas need treatment.

Canine facial eosinophilic furunculosis

This is a fairly common condition with an acute onset of papular–nodular facial lesions. In most cases, the muzzle or the bridge of the nose is involved, but lesions can be seen anywhere.

Pathogenesis
The pathogenesis is purely speculative (Holtz, 1990; Gross, 1993; Scott *et al.*, 1995). The sudden onset of the lesions coupled with the pronounced eosinophilic infil-trate has led investigators to believe that it represents a Type I hypersensitivity reaction to biting or stinging insects. Bees, wasps, black flies, and horseflies have been implicated (Griffin, 1993; Gross, 1993). Since the reaction is seen in some dogs

in the middle of winter, spiders, other arachnids, or household insects may also be involved (Scott *et al.*, 1995).

Clinical features
Dogs of any age, breed or sex can be affected, but most cases involve medium- to large-sized dogs who spend a great deal of time outside. The typical history indicates that the dog was perfectly normal when it went outside, but returned with striking lesions hours later. The lesions develop to their full extent within 24 hours. They are tender, but are not usually pruritic.

The earliest lesions are erythematous or hemorrhagic blisters or papules and they are usually multiple (Plate 9). These lesions progress to papules and nodules, which are often ulcerated and crusted. The most common area of involvement is the skin surrounding the nasal planum, either on the muzzle or bridge of the nose. Lesions can also be seen in the periocular region, on the pinnae, and elsewhere. Provided the dog has no further exposure and does not traumatize the lesions, no new lesions will develop after the first 24 hours and those that are present start to regress slowly.

Diagnosis
The sudden onset of tender facial furuncular lesions that do not progress in size or number after 24 hours is characteristic of this disorder. If the animal is presented within the first 24 hours, other causes of furunculosis, especially staphylococci and dermatophytes, must be considered. Aspiration cytology of an intact papule or nodule in this condition will show an intense eosinophilic infiltration. Signs of secondary staphylococcal infection may be seen in ulcerated or chronic lesions.

Skin testing with insect or arachnid antigens may be beneficial in determining the cause of the disorder.

Treatment
With isolation from further insect bites or stings, the lesions will resolve spontaneously. However, healing is slow and can lead to permanent scarring. The response to glucocorticoids is rapid and dramatic. Most cases are treated with oral prednisolone (1–2 mg/kg q. 24 h) for 3–14 days. Some dogs cannot tolerate these high doses of prednisolone and have been treated successfully with potent topical steroids or other oral corticosteroids.

It is rare for a dog to have more than one episode of disease. If relapses are seen, the dog should be skin tested to identify the offending parasite. Effective preventive measures depend upon the life cycle of the insect involved.

Miscellaneous disorders

Approximately 10% of classically atopic dogs have negative intradermal or serologic allergy tests to pollens, molds, house dust and house dust mite, fleas, and other environmental allergens and do not improve with restrictive dietary testing for food hypersensitivity (Griffin, 1993; Griffin *et al.*, 1993). Figures for the cat are unknown, but are probably lower. This has led to the testing of allergic suspects with various insect antigens. There are hundreds of stinging, biting, and nonparasitic insects that could be problematic for dogs or cats. Unfortunately, antigens for most are not commercially available so their role in the allergies of pets may never be known.

Investigators are currently skin testing dogs for the following biting insects: fire ant (100 PNU/ml), black fly (1000 PNU/ml), deer fly (1000 PNU/ml), horse fly (1000 PNU/ml), mosquito (1000 PNU/ml), and *Culicoides* gnat (1:1000 W/V) (Griffin, 1993; Koch and Peters, 1994; Buerger, 1995; Scott *et al.*, 1995; Rothstein *et al.*, 1996; Willis and Kunkle, 1996). The appropriate skin test dilutions are shown in the trailing parentheses and are based on the work of Willis and Kunkle (1996). These investigators tested various dilutions of insect allergens in 26 normal dogs and found these concentrations to be nonirritating. They and others have found that allergic dogs commonly react to one or more of these insect allergens, either as their sole reaction or in addition to reactions to fleas or other classical antigens. The percentage of dogs reacting positively varies with the study and the insect used, but figures range from 2–32% (Griffin, 1993; Buerger, 1995; Willis and Kunkle, 1996).

Serologic testing for insect and arachnid allergens is being carried out on an experimental basis. Dogs frequently show positive reactions to one or more allergens (Griffin *et al.*, 1993; Grier *et al.*, 1994; Pucheu-Haston *et al.*, 1995). Reciprocal inhibition studies have shown *in vitro* cross-reactivity between flea, black ant, black fly, and cockroach extracts (Pucheu-Haston *et al.*, 1995).

Willis and Kunkle found no statistical difference between the skin test reactivity of normal and allergic dogs to insect antigens (Willis and Kunkle, 1996). The meaning of positive test results is therefore open to question. Clearly, the reaction indicates that the insect or one that closely cross-reacts is in the dog's environment, has bitten the dog, and has induced an IgE or IgGd response. What remains to be proven is the clinical significance of the antibody.

Rothstein *et al.* (1996) studied the responsiveness of two groups of dogs to immunotherapy. The first group of 31 dogs had insect allergens in their immunotherapy prescription mixture while the second group of 13 had standard environmental allergens only. There was no statistical difference in the response rate to immunotherapy between the two groups. These preliminary data suggest that clinical insect hypersensitivity other than to fleas is uncommon in dogs. Serologic and intradermal testing of larger numbers of dogs will hopefully clarify the issue. Until these data are available, immunotherapy cannot be recommended. Skin testing results should be used to design an insect avoidance or repellent program.

The allergenicity of house dust and other storage mites is well known (see Chapter 3). These arachnids leave their body parts and excreta in the environment where dogs or cats can inhale, ingest, or transdermally absorb them. A very common household insect, the cockroach, is an important allergen in people via the same mechanism. Reports on skin test reactivity of allergic dogs to cockroach antigen vary from 0–60% (Nesbitt, 1978; Griffin, 1993; Buerger, 1995; Willis and Kunkle, 1996). These data have led to the testing of dogs with multiple environmental insect allergens. Currently, housefly (100 PNU/ml), black ant (100 PNU/ml), caddis fly (1000 PNU/ml), moth (100 PNU/ml), and cockroach (1000 PNU/ml) are being studied. Again, Willis and Kunkle could not differentiate normal from allergic dogs based on their reactivity to these insects. Until the significance of 'inhaled' insect allergens is known, the authors do not recommend immunotherapy with insect allergens. An exception might be where the animal reacts only to these nonbiting insects. Since the immunotherapy prescription mixture would only contain these allergens, efficacy could be determined fairly simply.

Arachnid hypersensitivity disorders

The role of arachnids in hypersensitivity disorders of dogs and cats is well known. Aside from the widespread problems associated with house dust and other environmental mites, the remainder of the disorders discussed here are far less common.

Tick bite hypersensitivity

Depending on the environmental conditions, ticks can be plentiful and are a major health concern for dogs and cats because they suck blood, are vectors for various infectious diseases, and damage the skin. The skin damage depends upon the number of attached ticks and the location of attachment (Scott *et al.*, 1995). With large numbers attached, the animal can lick or chew at the area to dislodge the ticks. In the vast majority of cases, the individual lesions are small erythematous puncture wounds with no hint of hypersensitivity. Rarely, the dog or cat will develop a large ulcerated nodule or focal area of necrosis at the site of tick attachment. Skin biopsy can show changes typical of either a Type III or Type IV hypersensitivity reaction. Treatment involves removal of the tick, prevention of reinfection with topical products or the amitraz tick collar, and symptomatic treatment of the lesion with either topical or oral glucocorticoids.

Ear mite hypersensitivity

Otoacariasis caused by *Otodectes cynotis* is common in the dog and cat. Otic symptomatology is very variable and ranges from none (asymptomatic) to an intensely pruritic otic disease with or without exudation. Some animals will also traumatize other areas of their bodies.

O. *cynotis* is a nonburrowing psoroptid mite that feeds on host lymph and whole blood. During feeding, the host is exposed to mite antigens and can mount an immune response to these allergens. Powell *et al.* (1980) showed the presence of IgE-like reagin in cats experimentally-infected with *O. cynotis*. These cats showed immediate but not delayed skin test reactions when tested with mite extracts. After 35 days of exposure, two-hour skin test reactions occurred with the histologic features of an Arthus (Type III) reaction. Serum precipitating antibodies occurred by day 45.

These data show that cats and probably dogs can become hypersensitive to the ear mite. Asymptomatic animals are probably not allergic while severely pruritic animals are hypersensitive.

Scabies hypersensitivity

Scabies mites are burrowing arachnids and are exposed to the host's immune system. Hypersensitivity to scabies mites is well known in humans (Wilson *et al.*, 1993). Once infected with scabies mites, the individual typically remains symptom free for approximately four weeks and then the lesions and pruritus begin. Symptoms can persist for 1–2 weeks after the mites are eradicated. When these treated patients are reinfected, only 40% develop clinical disease and the signs can occur within 24 hours of exposure. Humans will show an immediate skin test reaction to scabies extract if they have had the disease within one year of testing. Delayed hypersensitivity skin test reactions can also be seen. These results coupled with the ability to demonstrate circulating immune complexes and altered immunoglobulin levels support the presence of an allergic component in this disease.

Dogs with sarcoptic mange typically itch well out of proportion to the number of mites present, have a significant peripheral lymphadenopathy, and respond poorly to glucocorticoid therapy (Scott *et al.*, 1995). Asymptomatic carriers can also be identified. These findings combined with the ability to demonstrate an eosinophilia, proteinuria, or immune complex glomerulonephritis in some dogs strongly support the theory that dogs can also become allergic to scabies mites (Baker and Stannard, 1974). Recent work in dogs has shown the presence of scabies-specific antibodies in infected dogs (Bornstein and Zakrisson, 1993; Thoday, 1993). These antibodies disappear after treatment. In light of the hypersensitivity, which will not disappear the moment the mites are killed, owners of dogs with scabies should be warned that their animal's pruritus might persist for 2–5 weeks after treatment has been started.

Miscellaneous disorders

Hypersensitivity to the *Cheyletiella* or *Notoedres* mite has not been studied. Since the range of symptoms seen in infected animals varies from none (asymptomatic carrier) to intense pruritus, hypersensitivity no doubt plays a role in the severity of the clinical disease. An exaggerated response could also be expected in some animals transiently infested with straw mites, fowl mites, or some other mite.

References

Baker BB, Stannard AA. A look at canine scabies. *J. Am. Anim. Hosp. Assoc.* **10:** 513, 1974.

Blagburn BL, Hendrix CM, Vaughan JL, *et al.* Efficacy of lufenuron against developmental stages of fleas (*Ctenocephalides felis felis*) in dogs housed in simulated home environments. *Am. J. Vet. Res.* **56:** 464, 1996.

Bornstein S, Zakrisson G. Humoral antibody response to experimental *Sarcoptes scabiei* var *vulpes* infection in the dog. *Vet. Dermatol.* **4:** 107, 1993.

Bowman DD. *Georgis' Parasitology for Veterinarians*, 6th edition. W.B. Saunders, Philadelphia, p.2, 1995.

Buerger RG. Insect and arachnid hypersensitivity disorders of dogs and cats. In Bonagura JD (ed.) *Kirk's Current Veterinary Therapy XII.* W.B. Saunders, Philadephia, p. 631, 1995.

Dryden MW. Biology of fleas of dogs and cats. *Comp. Cont. Ed.* **15:** 569, 1993a.

Dryden MW. Biology of fleas on dogs and cats. *Proc. Am. Acad. Vet. Dermatol. Am. Coll. Vet. Dermatol.* **9:** 75, 1993b.

Greene WK, Carnegie RL, Shaw SE, *et al.* Characterization of allergens of the cat flea, *Ctenocephalides felis*: Detection and frequency of IgE antibody in canine sera. *Parasit. Immunol.* **15:** 69, 1993a.

Greene WK, Penhale WJ, Thompson RCA. Isolation and *in vitro* translation of messenger RNA encoding allergens of the cat flea, *Ctenocephalides felis. Vet. Immunol. Immunopath.* **37:** 15, 1993b.

Grier TJ, Willis EL, Esch RE, *et al.* Canine insect hypersensitivity: immunochemical evidence for common or cross-reactive antigens. *Proc. Am. Acad. Vet. Dermatol. Am. Coll. Vet. Dermatol.* **10**: 21, 1994.

Griffin CE. Insect and arachnid hypersensitivity. In: Griffin CE, Kwochka KW, McDonald JM (eds) *Current Veterinary Dermatology.* St. Louis: Mosby Year Book, p. 133, 1993.

Griffin CE, Rosenkrantz WS, Alaba S. Detection of insect/arachnid specific IgE in dogs: comparison of two techniques utilizing western blots as the standard. In Ihrke PJ, Mason IS, White SD (eds). *Advances in Veterinary Dermatology* – Volume 2. Oxford: Pergamon Press, p. 263, 1993.

Gross TL. Canine eosinophilic furunculosis of the face. In Ihrke PJ, Mason IS, White SD (eds) *Advances in Veterinary Dermatology* Volume 2. Pergamon Press, Oxford, p. 239, 1993.

Halliwell REW. Hyposensitization in the treatment of flea bite hypersensitivity: Results of a double-blinded study. *J. Am. Anim. Hosp. Assoc.* **17**: 249, 1981.

Halliwell REW. Factors in the development of flea-bite allergy. *Vet. Med.* **79**: 1273, 1984.

Halliwell REW, Schemmer KR. The role of basophils in the immunopathogenesis of hypersensitivity to fleas (*Ctenocephalides felis*) in dogs. *Vet. Immunol. Immunopathol.* **15**: 203, 1987.

Halliwell REW, Longino SJ. IgE and IgG antibodies to flea antigen in differing dog populations. *Vet Immunol. Immunopathol.* **8**: 215, 1985.

Henderson G, Manweiler SA, Laurence WJ, *et al.* The effects of *Steinernema carpocapsea* (Weiser) application to different life stages on adult emergence of the cat flea *Ctenocephalides felis* (Bouche). *Vet. Dermatol.* **6**: 159, 1995.

Hink WF, Zakson M, Barnett S. Evaluation of a single oral dose of lufenuron to control flea infestations in dogs. *Am. J. Vet. Res.* **55**: 822, 1994.

Holtz CS. Eosinophilic dermatitis in a Siberian Husky. *Calif. Vet.* **44**: 11, 1990.

Ihrke PJ, Gross TL. Conference in dermatology – No. 2. *Vet. Dermatol.* **5**: 33, 1994.

Koch HJ, Peters S. 207 intrakutantests bei hunden mit verdacht auf atopische dermatitis. *Kleintierpraxis* **39**: 25, 1994.

Kunkle GA, Milcarsky J. Double-blind flea hyposensitization in cats. *J. Am. Vet. Med. Assoc.* **186**: 677, 1985.

MacDonald JM. Flea control: An overview of treatment concepts for North America. *Vet. Dermatol.* **6**: 121, 1995.

Mason KV, Evans AG. Mosquito bite caused eosinophilic dermatitis in cats. *J. Am. Vet. Med. Assoc.* **198**: 2086, 1991.

Mason KV, Ring J, Duggan J. Fenthione for flea control on dogs under field conditions: Dose response efficacy studies and effect on cholinesterase activity. *J. Am. Anim. Hosp. Assoc.* **20**: 591, 1984.

McKeon SE, Opdebeech JP. IgG and IgE antibodies against antigens of the cat flea, *Ctenocephalides felis felis*, in sera of allergic and non-allergic dogs. *Int. J. Parasitol.* **24**: 259, 1994.

Miller TA, Blagburn BL. Ovisterilant efficacy of pyriproxyfen collars on dogs and cats. *Proc. Am. Acad. Vet. Dermatol. Am. Coll. Vet. Dermatol.* **12**: 63, 1996.

Nesbitt GH. Canine allergic inhalant dermatitis: A review of 230 cases. *J. Am. Vet. Med. Assoc.* **172**: 55, 1978.

Nicholson SS. Toxicity of insecticides and skin care products of botanical origin. *Vet. Dermatol.* **6**: 139, 1995.

Palma KG, Meola SM, Meola RW. Mode of action of pyriproxifen and methoprene on eggs of *Ctenocephalides felis* (Siphonaptera: Pulicidae). *J. Med. Entomol.* **30**: 421, 1993.

Postal JR, Jeamin PC, Consalvi P. Field efficacy of a mechanical pump spray formulation containing 0.25% fipronil in the treatment and control of flea infestation and associated dermatological signs in dogs and cats. *Vet. Dermatol.* **6**: 153, 1995.

Powell MB, Weisbroth SH, Roth L, *et al*. Reaginic hypersensitivity in *Otodectes cynotis* infection of cats and mode of mite feeding. *Am. J. Vet. Res.* **41**: 877, 1980.

Pucheu-Haston CM, Grier TJ, Esch R, *et al*. Allergenic cross-reactivity in flea reactive canine sera. *Proc. Am. Acad. Vet. Dermatol. Am. Coll. Vet. Dermatol.* **11**: 26, 1995.

Robinson WH. Distribution of cat flea larvae in the carpeted household environment. *Vet. Dermatol.* **6**: 145, 1995.

Rothstein E, Miller WH Jr, Scott DW, *et al*. Investigation of insect hypersensitivity and response to immunotherapy in allergic dogs. *Vet. Dermatol.* (Submitted 1996)

Scott DW, Miller WH Jr, Griffin CE. *Muller and Kirk's Small Animal Dermatology*, 5th edition. W.B. Saunders, Philadelphia, 1995.

Slacek B, Opdebeech JP. Reactivity of dogs and cats to feeding fleas and to flea antigens injected intradermally. *Aust. Vet. J.* **70**: 313, 1993.

Shipstone MA, Masson KV. The use of insect development inhibitors as an oral medication for control of the fleas *Ctenocephalides felis, Ct. canis* in the dog and cat. *Vet. Dermatol.* **6**: 131, 1995.

Smith CA. Current concepts: Searching for safe methods of flea control. *J. Am. Vet. Med. Assoc.* **206**: 1137, 1995.

Smith RD, Paul AJ, Kitron UD, *et al*. Impact of an orally administered insect growth regulator (lufenuron) on flea infestations of dogs in a controlled simulated home environment. *Am. J. Vet. Res.* **57**: 502, 1996.

Soulsby EJL. *Helminths, Arthropods, and Protozoa of Domesticated Animals*. Lea & Febiger, Philadelphia, 1982, p. 357.

Stolper R, Opdebeech JP. Flea allergy dermatitis in dogs diagnosed by intradermal skin test. *Res. Vet. Sci.* **57**: 21, 1994.

Thoday KL. Serum immunoglobulin concentrations in canine scabies. In: Ihrke PJ, *et al*, (eds). *Advances in Veterinary Dermatology* – Volume 2. Oxford, Pergamon Press, 1993, p. 211.

Trudeau WL, Fernandez-Callas E, Fox RW, *et al*. Allergenicity of the cat flea (*Ctenocephalides felis felis*). *Clin. Exp. Allergy* **23**: 377, 1993.

Van Winkle KA. An evaluation of flea antigens used in intradermal skin testing for flea allergy in the canine. *J. Am. Anim. Hosp. Assoc.* **17**: 343, 1981.

Wilson DC, Levna WH, King LE Jr. Arthropod bites and stings. In: Fitzpatrick TB. Eisen AZ, Wolff K, *et al*. (eds): *Dermatology in General Medicine* 4th edition. New York: McGraw Hill Book Company, 1993, p.2810.

Willemse T. The diagnostic value of whole-body flea extract in dogs with clinical flea bite hypersensitivity. *Proc. World. Cong. Vet. Dermatol.* **3**: 11, 1996.

Willis CE, Kunkle GA. Intradermal reactivity to various insect and arachnid allergens in dogs from the southeastern United States. *J. Am. Vet. Med. Assoc.* **209**: 1431, 1996.

—————10—————
Miscellaneous Allergic Disorders

Bacterial Hypersensitivity

Although the term bacterial hypersensitivity has been used since the late 1960s to describe an intensely pruritic disorder associated with staphylococcal infection, the appropriateness of this term to describe the condition was and continues to be a point of debate. Although some clinical and immunologic data support the concept of bacterial hypersensitivity, irrefutable proof for its existence is absent. Until the disorder is completely described, the authors have elected to continue with the term bacterial hypersensitivity.

Staphylococcal skin infections are common in the dog and usually has an underlying dermatologic disorder predisposing it to infection (Scott *et al.*, 1995). Most dogs with bacterial pyoderma have some pruritus and this should stop with appropriate antibiotic therapy. Pathologic pruritus is triggered by a variety of mediators, which include histamine, proteolytic enzymes, kallikrein, and bradykinin. In staphylococcal skin infections, antibody production for opsonization and neutrophil phagocytosis and killing are important to eliminate the organisms. Proteolytic enzymes released from the neutrophils or other modulators generated through the humoral amplification system cause the infected skin to itch. In some animals, staphylococcal antigens may result in the degranulation of skin mast cells, resulting in pruritus well out of proportion to the severity of the clinical lesions (Mason and Lloyd, 1989).

Although Walton first introduced the concept of clinical bacterial allergy in dogs in 1966, Baker (1974) was the first investigator to describe staphylococcal allergy in dogs. Baker stated that dogs with a bacterial allergy could present with a recurrent bacterial infection or as a classically allergic dog with or without an obvious infection. The dogs with the allergic presentation showed secondary seborrheic changes and hair loss. Some dogs also had a blepharitis and iritis. The history from these animals often indicated that the dog had had a previous staphylococcal infection, which presumably sensitized the dog. Baker proposed that inapparent staphylococcal infections of the tonsils, anal sacs, or internal organs acted as sources of antigen release in those dogs with no obvious skin infection. Colonization of normal skin must also be considered (Mason and Lloyd, 1989).

Pathogenesis

The initial theories on bacterial hypersensitivity were developed from the data generated by skin testing suspect dogs with staphylococcal antigens and the results of skin biopsies (Baker, 1974; Scott *et al.*, 1978). Skin testing was carried out with a staphylococcal cell wall antigen and toxoid mixture. All dogs showed immediate reactions (i.e. within 15 to 30 minutes) characterized by erythematous wheals varying from 14–20 mm in diameter. In normal dogs, the lesion faded slowly and an indurated, occasionally erythematous nodule, 5–9 mm in diameter, remained at the late readings at 24–48 hours. In hypersensitive dogs, the delayed reactions were very inflammatory and varied in size from 9 to 75 mm. The lesions were not wheals but rather erythematous, indurated, oozing, and variably necrotic nodules. Biopsies of skin test reactions and clinical lesions typically showed signs of a vasculitis. These data indicated that staphylococcal hypersensitivity most closely approximated a Type III hypersensitivity disorder.

More recent work has focused on antistaphylococcal IgG and IgE antibody titers and the effects of staphylococcal antigens on mast cell degranulation (Mason and Lloyds, 1989; Morales *et al.*, 1994). Dogs with recurrent infections have higher antistaphylococcal IgG and IgE antibody titers than healthy dogs (Morales *et al.*, 1994). Dogs with non-recurrent pyoderma, recurrent pyoderma secondary to atopic disease, and idiopathic recurrent pyoderma all have elevated titers of antistaphylococcal IgG, the highest of which is seen in dogs with deep pyoderma. IgE titers are highest in dogs with recurrent idiopathic superficial pyoderma or recurrent pyoderma secondary to atopy. Staphylococcal protein A, a cell wall antigen found in many strains of *Staphylococcus intermedius*, can bind nonspecifically to mast cell-bound IgE and cause mast cell degranulation (Mason and Lloyd, 1989). Mast cell degranulation increases the permeability of the epidermis to staphylococcal antigens, increasing the likelihood of further mast cell degranulation in dogs with antistaphylococcal IgE titers. Coupling this information with the high frequency of recurrent, pruritic, superficial folliculitis in allergic dogs suggests that bacterial hypersensitivity may be more common than recognized and may not be strictly a Type III hypersensitivity disorder.

Clinical features

The work of Baker, Breen, and Scott has led to the description of the clinical lesions associated with staphylococcal hypersensitivity, namely the erythematous pustule, the hemorrhagic vesicle or bulla, or the patch of seborrheic dermatitis (Baker, 1974; Breen, 1976; Scott *et al.*, 1978). All forms result in pruritus, which disappears with the administration of appropriate antibiotics. The erythematous pustule is a follicular papule or pustule with a large erythematous halo. The hemorrhagic bulla (Plate 10) also has a ring of peripheral erythema. The seborrheic patch varies in its appearance. Small lesions are annular areas of hair loss and erythema that expand peripherally with a zone of inflammation and peeling (epidermal collarette) at the leading edge (Figure 10.1). The epidermal collarette indicates that a pustule, vesicle, or bulla was present, but ruptured recently. As the lesion ages, its size increases and the central erythema fades and often becomes hyperpigmented. Lesions can coalesce and form large areas of hair loss, which look inactive centrally (Figure 10.2). Examination of the leading edge of the hair loss will indicate active inflammation. Rarely, one will see a glucocorticoid unresponsive 'allergic' dog with no visible pyoderma or one whose pruritus is triggered by an obvious infection, but the pruritus is intense and well out of proportion to the severity of the infection (Miller, 1991). Baker proposed that the site of antigen

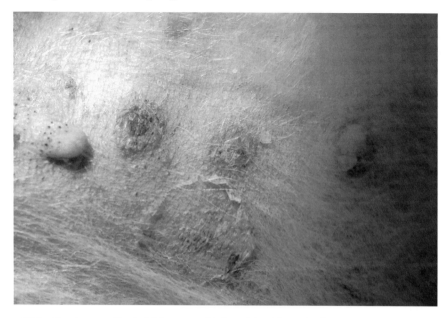

Figure 10.1   *Focal areas of bacterial hypersensitivity with epidermal collarettes.*

release in dogs with nonlesional pruritus was from an inapparent infection of the tonsils, anal sacs, or internal organs. The newer information on the effects of transepidermal protein A indicates that a hidden nidus of infection may not be necessary.

None of the lesions associated with staphylococcal hypersensitivity are pathognomonic for this condition. The erythematous pustule and seborrheic patch are often

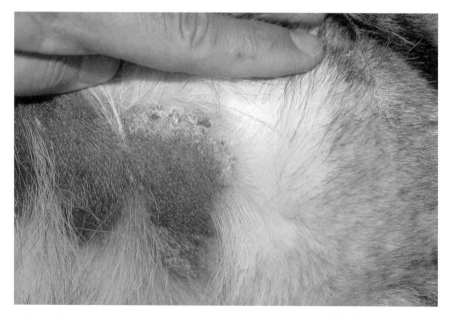

Figure 10.2   *Coalescence of individual lesions into a larger area.*

seen in dogs with pyodermas without staphylococcal hypersensitivity. The hemor-rhagic bulla is much more suggestive of staphylococcal hypersensitivity, but can also be seen in dogs with vasculitis. The animal's history will support the tentative diagnosis of a bacterial allergy. The animal's pruritus is not lessened with appropri-ate glucocorticoid therapy, but stops with prolonged antibiotic therapy. As dis-cussed before, routine infections can also be pruritic, so a response to antibacterial therapy is not diagnostic. The dog with a staphylococcal hypersensitivity should remain normal for some period of time after the antibiotics are discontinued, but should spontaneously develop new lesions in normal skin or start to itch at normal skin. Signs typically recur within 30–60 days. Dogs who develop new lesions in areas of diseased skin may have a staphylococcal hypersensitivity superimposed on another condition or may simply be experiencing a recurrent pyoderma secondary to another problem. Dogs with nonlesion pruritus who stop itching with antibiotic therapy and start itching again when the drug is discontinued are strong candidates for a bacterial allergy.

Diagnosis

The history and physical findings can strongly support the tentative diagnosis of staphylococcal hypersensitivity, but confirmation of the diagnosis requires skin biopsies and/or skin testing. The cell wall antigen used by Baker and others to docu-ment staphylococcal hypersensitivity is no longer manufactured. In the US there is only one licensed staphylococcal antigen for use in dogs (Scott et al., 1995). This product is a phage lysate of S. aureus and has been used extensively in the treatment of dogs with recurrent pyoderma (De Boer et al., 1990; Scott et al., 1995). According to the manufacturer, full-strength antigen (0.05–0.1 ml) is used for skin testing. One author (LMR) regularly uses this product at a 1:10 dilution and feels that it can be irritating at this dilution. Although various investigators verbally suggest that test-ing this product is as accurate as that done with the staphyloccal toxoid, the authors have been unable to find any reports comparing the reactivity of this product in healthy dogs and dogs with nonrecurrent pyoderma, recurrent pyoderma without bacterial hypersensitivity, and recurrent pyoderma with presumed hypersensitivity. Because of its potential irritation, one author (LMR) interprets positive reactions cautiously. Until detailed data with this product are available, the results of skin testing are uncertain.

Mason and Lloyd skin-tested a small number of normal dogs with various dilu-tions of staphylococcal protein A and specially prepared extracts of S. aureus and S. intermedius (Mason and Lloyd, 1995). The dogs showed greater reactivity to the S. intermedius extract than to the S. aureus extract at the same dilution. Protein A extracts were more reactive than either of the staphylococcal products. No diseased dogs were tested. Since S. intermedius is the primary cutaneous pathogen in dogs, results of testing diseased dogs are eagerly awaited.

The biopsy results vary with the nature of the clinical lesion and the vascular changes are of critical importance. The erythematous pustules and hemorrhagic bullae show signs of vascular inflammation with extravasation of red blood cells or dermal hemorrhage (Scott et al., 1978, 1995). These findings are not typical of non-allergic pyodermas. The seborrheic lesions tend to show more vascular dilatation and neutrophilic infiltration, but can be indistinguishable from other seborrheic lesions.

Treatment

The diagnosis of staphylococcal hypersensitivity does not necessarily mean that the dog will need specific therapy. Diseased skin is easily infected and recurrent infections can sensitize the animal. If the dog has an underlying disease that can be identified and treated, resolution of the disorder coupled with prolonged (i.e. 4–8-week) antibiotic therapy may 'cure' the dog. Scott reported that 45% of his 31 cases fell into this category (Scott *et al.*, 1978). The hypersensitivity in these animals would persist for some time, but the normalization of the skin would eliminate or minimize the animal's exposure to the antigen.

Dogs who have a staphylococcal hypersensitivity for no apparent reason or who do not 'self-cure' with resolution of the underlying disease will require long-term, presumably lifelong, therapy. Therapy can consist of antibiotics or immunotherapy. The ideal method of treatment is immunotherapy. Animals who do not respond to the immunotherapy may be controlled with long-term antibiotic therapy.

Immunotherapy appears to be safe and is relatively inexpensive. Since the products used are immunostimulants, they are also used in the treatment of recurrent pyodermas secondary to immunodeficiencies. All the various bacterial antigens used for immunotherapy are probably antigenically different and are used in different ways in different dogs to treat different diseases. It is therefore difficult, if not impossible, to state an accurate success rate of therapy for staphylococcal hypersensitivity.

Baker described a protocol where 0.1 ml was given intradermally and larger volumes were given either subcutaneously or half intramuscularly and half subcutaneously (Baker, 1974). He reported that this therapy was uniformly effective and that one course of therapy was usually effective, but some dogs need periodic booster injections. Scott followed Baker's protocol and successfully treated six of nine dogs (Scott *et al.*, 1978). All these dogs needed booster injections every 1–3 months. Pukay (1985) used a very similar protocol and noted an excellent response in 14 of his 16 cases. Of the dogs who responded 44% required a booster injection within 30 days while the remainder required an injection within two months. Thus the reported success rate with Baker's protocol varies from 67–88%.

Bacterial antigens are used to treat dogs with recurrent idiopathic pyodermas (Becker *et al.*, 1989; De Boer *et al.*, 1990; Scott *et al.*, 1995). Autogenous bacterins, lysates of staphyloccal cells, and a *Propionibacterium acnes* suspension appear to receive widest use. Detailed reports on the efficacy of the latter two products are available (Becker *et al.*, 1989; De Boer *et al.*, 1990), but it is unclear whether the patients were staphylococcal hypersensitive or developed recurrent pyodermas for other reasons. Because of study design and method of reporting, a critical review of the investigators' data is difficult. Both products showed some efficacy, but the figures given in the reports can be interpreted as being overly generous.

Because the *Propionibacterium* must be given by intravenous injection and staphyloccal cell lysates or autogenous bacterins are administered by subcutaneous injections, the latter two products receive widest use (De Boer *et al.*, 1990; Scott *et al.*, 1995). There are no reports comparing the efficacy of the different biologicals in the same group of patients. Until such data are available, it might be prudent to try a different product if the first treatment protocol is ineffective. The authors are unaware of any protocols including an intradermal fraction as proposed by Baker. The bacterial antigens are given weekly with gradually increasing doses of 0.1 or 0.25 ml until the maintenance dose of either 0.5 or 1.0 ml is reached. For very large dogs, doses up to 2.0 ml have been used. One author (WHM) gives incremental doses of 0.1 or 0.2 ml every other day until the final dose is reached and has not seen any adverse reactions to this accelerated schedule. Maintenance injections are given once weekly. Animals who do not respond after three months of maintenance therapy are not likely to do so. The addition of a 0.1 ml intradermal fraction might increase the efficacy in dogs who do not respond to sub-cutaneous administration. Dogs who respond to the weekly injections may be able to be maintained with less frequent injections.

Animals with staphylococcal hypersensitivity or idiopathic recurrent pyoderma who fail to respond to immunotherapy can be treated successfully with long-term antibiotics. These treatments involve either the periodic use of full-dose therapy or a maintenance protocol. If the animal's episodes of disease are separated by months of normalcy, each episode should be treated until the infection is completely resolved and then the drug should be discontinued. This pattern is unusual. Most animals with staphylococcal hypersensitivity remain infection free for only a relatively short period. With frequent relapses, the dog should be treated on a maintenance basis to prevent relapses. Maintenance antibiotic treatments will not resolve a preexisting infection. Accordingly, the animal must be treated with an appropriate full-dose course of antibiotics before maintenance treatment is started. Currently, three protocols for maintenance antibiotic administration are used with no published data to indicate which might be safest and most effective (Scott *et al.*, 1995). For discussion sake, let us say that the full therapeutic dose of the drug to be used is 500 mg, given twice daily. The oldest maintenance protocol reduces the dose to 500 mg, given once daily. If this procedure keeps the animal infection free for 60 days or longer, some investigators would reduce the dose to 500 mg every other day or 250 mg daily. The other two maintenance protocols involve the administration of the full therapeutic dose (e.g. 500 mg q. 12 h), but not on a continuous basis. In one protocol, 500 mg q. 12 h is given every other day while it is given in a pulsatile fashion in the other. In the pulse proto-col, the drug is given at 500 mg q. 12 h daily for seven days and then is withdrawn for seven days. If no relapses are seen within 60 days in either protocol, further reduc-tions are made, either by giving the drug every third day or by separating the week of drug administration by 10 or 14 days. It is unlikely that further reductions would be possible. Chronic maintenance antibiotic protocols are very effective and remarkably safe, but should not be instituted until all other avenues of treatment have been exhausted. Chronic antibiotic therapy is expensive and could lead to a variety of prob-lems, including bacterial resistance, chronic intoxication, altered bowel function, and drug reactions. Before maintenance treatment is undertaken, the animal should have a complete and thorough workup, including an intradermal or serologic allergy test for atopy and restrictive dietary trial for food hypersensitivity.

Drug Hypersensitivity

Drugs are low molecular weight compounds that can produce side effects of an expected or an unexpected nature (Van Arsdel, 1988; Blacker *et al.*, 1993; Scott *et al.*,

1995). Although expected drug reactions can be undesirable (e.g. hair loss associated with the use of some chemotherapeutic agents) they can be explained by the pharmacologic or physiologic effect of the drug. Unexpected reactions that affect the skin are called drug eruptions and they can have an immunologic or a nonimmunologic basis. In man, it is estimated that drug eruptions will occur in 2–3% of medical inpatients (Blacker *et al.*, 1993). Reports of drug eruptions in animals are infrequent, but are probably more common than the literature indicates (Affolter and von Tscharner, 1993; Noli *et al.*, 1995; Scott *et al.*, 1995).

Pathogenesis

Drug eruptions can be caused by the drug, impurities in the drug, drug metabolites, binding agents such as starches and stearates, and flavoring agents. Molecules of increased size and complexity are more immunogenic and drugs that contain proteins can be more allergenic. Since most drugs are haptens, they must bind to host proteins before they become allergenic. Drugs that bind easily to proteins are more likely to cause drug eruptions.

Aside from the nature of the drug, other factors influencing the frequency of drug eruptions in man include the dose, route of administration, previous administration of the drug, and previous drug allergies. The possibility of a drug eruption is increased by the simultaneous local and systemic administration of the same drug, intermittent use of the drug, or by using a repositol form of the drug. Other risk factors include the genetic background of the patient, the nature of the disease being treated, concomitant drug therapy, and intercurrent infections. Most of these predisposing factors have not been evaluated in animals.

Immunologic drug eruptions do not occur at the first administration of the drug. Sensitization must occur first and usually takes at least one week. Reactions that occur in many patients and occur at the first administration are not immunologically mediated. Drug eruptions can be caused by Type I, II, III, or IV hypersensitivity reactions and although certain drugs typically cause one type of reaction, there is no specific reaction pattern for any one drug. In man, maculopapular rashes and urticarial reactions are the most common manifestations of a drug eruption. Less common reaction patterns include fixed drug eruptions, contact dermatitis, erythema multiforme, toxic epidermal necrolysis, pemphigus-like eruptions, lupus-like eruptions, vasculitis, and photosensitization. Except for the fixed drug eruption, these reactive patterns have a sudden onset and are symmetric and widespread.

The list of drugs known to cause drug eruptions in people is extensive (van Ansdel, 1988; Blacker *et al.*, 1993). Drugs from these lists that are frequently used in companion animal medicine are the penicillins*, cephalosporins*, chloramphenicol*, sulfa drugs*, tetracyclines*, griseofulvin*, ketoconazole*, barbiturates*, cimetidine*, phenytoins*, phenylbutazone, aspirin, furosemide, neomycin*, retinoids*, and topical anesthetics*. Less commonly used drugs include phenothiazine drugs*, propylthiouracil*, gold salts*, female sex hormones*, dapsone*, quinidine*, thiabendazole*, and nystatin. The drugs marked by the asterisk have been reported to cause eruptions in companion animals (Scott *et al.*, 1995). Other drugs reported to cause reactions in dogs and cats include 5-fluorocytosine, diethylcarbamazine, thiacetarsamide, levamisole, prednisolone, thyroid extract, gentamicin, ivermectin, a variety of topical products, and a variety of biologicals (blood transfusions, vaccines, bacterins, and antisera) (Scott *et al.*, 1995). It is very likely that every commonly used drug in veterinary medicine has caused a drug reaction in some animal. Which drugs have the highest incidence of adverse reactions in companion animals? Detailed sales data on each drug are needed to answer this question accurately, and all veterinarians would have to report the reactions seen in their practice to a central processing office. Obviously, these data are not available. In the authors' experience, reactions to sulfa-type antibiotics are most common.

Clinical features

Drug hypersensitivities can be manifested by systemic signs (e.g. anorexia, fever of unknown origin, lameness), systemic illnesses (e.g. hemolytic anemia, immune-mediated thrombocytopenia), dermatologic disease only, or a combination of these (Plate 11) (Noli *et al.*, 1995). If the sensitized animal receives the drug again, the reaction seen at each administration can be the same or can change. Typically, drug hypersensitivities are progressive in their severity.

The cutaneous manifestations of drug hypersensitivity in animals are usually lesional. The reaction induces exfoliation, papules, vesicles, ulcers, and a variety of other lesions. These preexisting lesions can be painful or pruritic. Noneruptive pruritus mimicking atopy, food hypersensitivity, and the various other allergic disorders discussed in this text is rare. Since this type of reaction probably involves a Type I hypersensitivity, the animal's pruritus should intensify shortly after the drug is given and should lessen as the drug is cleared from the body. Drugs with very long half-lives will not show this variation. Unless the drug history of the 'allergic' patient is carefully examined, drug hypersensitivity is often overlooked in these patients.

The lesions of a drug eruption can mimic any known dermatosis and can be urticarial, angioedematous, papular (Figure 10.3), exfoliative (Figure 10.4), vesiculo-bullous (Figure 10.5), erythrodermatous, purpuric (Plate 12), or ulcerative. Draining nodular lesions, focal or diffuse alopecic conditions, fixed drug eruptions, and pseudolymphomatous changes can also be seen (Affolter and von Tscharner, 1993; Scott *et al.*, 1995). Depending upon the nature and distribution of the lesions, the patient can look like he or she has something as simple as a folliculitis or something as bizarre as pemphigus, discoid lupus erythematosus, erythema multiforme (Figure 10.6), toxic epidermal necrolysis (Plate 13), or cutaneous lymphoma. If the cutaneous signs are accompanied by systemic signs of illness, systemic lupus erythematosus, various systemic infectious diseases, necrolytic migratory erythema, and other serious disease must be investigated.

Diagnosis

To diagnose a drug eruption, one must have an index of suspicion since these reactions can mimic many skin conditions. A careful history about all medications and nutritional supplements is critical. After the initial sensitization period, drug eruptions can occur at any time during administration and may even occur a few days after the drug is discontinued. If an animal has a drug history, a drug hypersensitivity may be

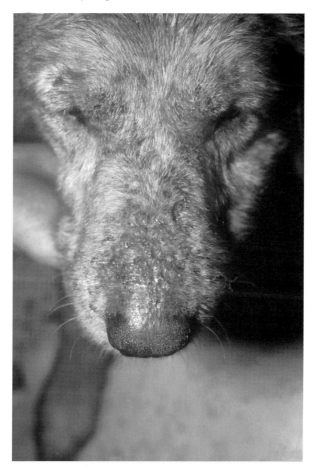

Figure 10.3   *Multiple crusted and ulcerated papular lesions due to a trimethoprim–sulfadiazine drug reaction.*

present. The presumptive diagnosis of drug hypersensitivity is easiest when the drug is given for a nondermatologic condition and the animal develops compatible skin lesions somewhere during the course of treatment. Animals being treated for a dermatologic condition can be more problematic. If the owner reports that the condition initially responded to the medication and then stopped improving or worsened, a drug eruption may be superimposed upon the original condition. Alternatively, the medication may have lost its effectiveness and the progression might be due to ineffective treatment. If the client returns the animal to the veterinarian who first examined it, a thorough examination, paying particular attention to the distribution and nature of the new lesion should indicate whether the skin disease is the same or different. A different pattern of lesions should suggest a drug reaction. If the client seeks a second opinion from a veterinarian who has never seen the dog before, the diagnosis of drug reaction will probably be delayed.

Presently, there are no commercially available, reliable, specific tests to document a drug hypersensitivity in animals. Spontaneous resolution of the eruption with drug withdrawal implicates the drug as a causative factor, but does not prove the

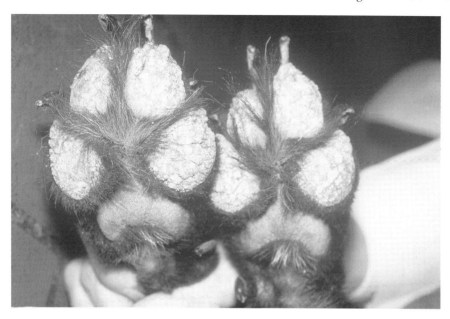

Figure 10.4 *Digital hyperkeratosis and exfoliation due to an oxacillin drug reaction.*

immunologic basis. Drug challenge would strengthen the definitive diagnosis, but is not advised as the next reaction can be much more severe.

Skin biopsies are very helpful in the diagnosis of drug reaction in that they may define a specific cause for the animal's lesions, will help eliminate some diseases from consideration, and can strongly support the diagnosis of drug eruption. In a

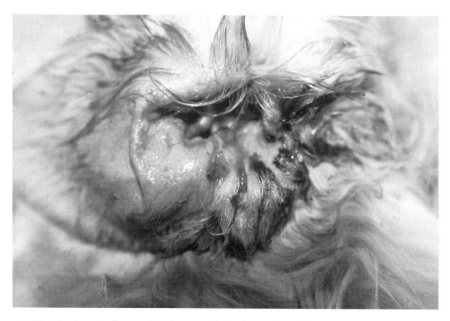

Figure 10.5 *Acute vesicular reaction due to topical miconazole solution.*

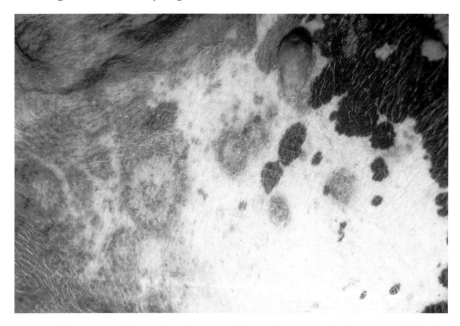

Figure 10.6 *Donut-type lesions of erythema multiforme due to a trimethoprim–sulfadiazine drug reaction.*

histologic study of 67 cases with a widespread drug reaction, 40% had a lichenoid interface dermatitis, 37% had erythema multiforme, 9% had vasculitis, 9% had toxic epidermal necrolysis, and 6% had a pemphigus-like reactions (Affolter and von Tscharner, 1993). Each of these histologic reaction patterns can be seen in a variety of conditions, including drug reaction. Although a histologic reaction pattern may not be pathognomonic for drug reaction, the knowledge that drug reaction can cause this eruption should prompt a careful review of the patient's drug history.

Treatment

If a drug eruption is suspected, the drug should be discontinued. If the animal is receiving multiple drugs, they should all be discontinued, but if this is not possible the last drug added would be most suspect. With drug withdrawal, most drug eruptions stop progressing and start to heal spontaneously in 7–14 days. Depending upon the severity of the skin lesions, complete healing can take weeks to months. Eruptions due to repositol or body-stored (e.g. gold salts) agents continue for long periods and are very problematic.

Beyond drug withdrawal, there are no uniformly required treatments for animals with a drug reaction. Mild cases resolve spontaneously and various symptomatic measures (e.g. bathing) are evaluated on a case-to-case basis. Animals with serious reactions such as toxic epidermal necrolysis require intensive supportive care and may die despite heroic efforts. One author's (TW) success in the management of cases with toxic epidermal necrolysis has been increased by severely limiting the amount of manipulation the animal receives. The animal is not clipped or bathed.

For animals with a documented drug eruption, prophylaxis is of utmost importance. Readministration of the drug or a similar one could cause a much more serious reaction. It is important that the owner is told of their animal's sensitivity to the drug so that they can take this information with them if they travel. Patients allergic to penicillin should not be treated with any other drug of the penicillin family and cephalosporins should be used cautiously as these drugs contain the β-lactam ring found in penicillin.

Fungal Hypersensitivity

Although fungal infections are relatively common in animals and the immunologic reaction to the organism can be complex, hypersensitivity seems to play a minimal role in most cutaneous fungal disorders (Lehmann, 1985). Some cases of dermatophytosis and *Malassezia* dermatitis can be exceptions.

Dermatophytosis

In most dogs and cats, the inflammation and pruritus associated with a *Microsporum canis* infection is minimal. Typically any pruritus associated *M. canis* infection occurs only after the clinical lesions are well established. When the infecting organism is a *Trichophyton* spp., a geophilic organism like *Microsporum gypseum*, or some other very unusual organism, the inflammation and pruritus induced can be significant and pruritus can be the presenting complaint. The clinical presentation, coupled with a disproportionate inflammatory response suggests hypersensitivity (Lehmann, 1985; Scott *et al.*, 1995).

Clinical features
Focal inoculation of the skin with a dermatophyte, especially an atypical one like *M. gypseum*, can cause a kerion reaction. The kerion reaction is a well-circumscribed, nodular lesion with a fairly acute onset and is very inflamed (Figure 10.7). Close inspection, especially after the lesion has been squeezed, demonstrates multiple draining tracts. Secondary staphylococcal infection is common. Typically, species of dermatophytes not well adapted to the host in question (e.g. *Trichophyton mentagrophytes* in a dog) are isolated. Skin biopsies show a very inflammatory furunculosis with few fungal elements.

With regionalized or generalized infection with an unusual dermatophyte, especially *Trichophyton* spp., the involved skin is erythematous, hairless, scaly, and pruritic. Most owners will comment that pruritus was the first sign that the animal had a skin problem. If the region involved is one with an allergic predilection (e.g., the facial area), it is easy to attribute the changes seen to atopic pruritus. Administration of corticosteroids has minimal impact on the pruritus and can worsen the infection. Careful inspection of the junction between the haired and hairless skin is necessary. Pruritic dermatophytic lesions have sharply demarcated, well-circumscribed borders (Plate 14) while the borders of lesions created by the animal scratching itself are ill-defined with a gradual transition from haired to hairless skin. Diagnosis is via trichrography or fungal culture.

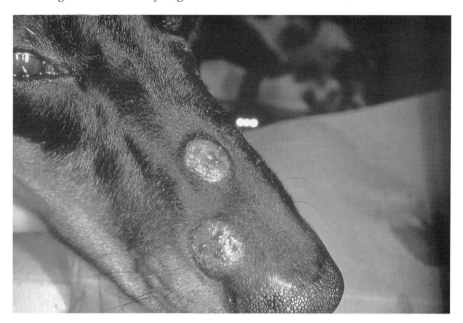

Figure 10.7   *Two kerion reactions on the bridge of the nose. The serosanguinous discharge overlies the draining tracts.*

Treatment

For kerion reactions, the lesion should be evaluated for a secondary staphylococcal infection and if one is documented the animal needs to receive an appropriate oral antibiotic for 2–4 weeks. The lesion is best treated with a topical product containing an antifungal agent and a corticosteroid. Systemic antifungal agents are rarely required. With more widespread disease, topical antifungal shampoos and dips (rinses) are indicated. To hasten the animal's response, systemic antifungal agents are usually used.

Malassezia dermatitis

Although *Malassezia pachydermatis* was recognized as a cause of skin disease in dogs years ago (Dufait, 1983), *Malassezia* dermatitis has become an increasingly more common finding in the dog (Mason and Evans, 1991; Scott *et al.*, 1995). It has been reported in the cat, but is rare in this species (Bond *et al.*, 1995; Scott *et al.*, 1995). It is not uncommon for the busy dermatology clinic to see one or more cases in the dog each week. This increased frequency is partly due to the knowledge that the disease exists and that patients must be evaluated for it. However, this does not explain the high incidence seen today. Predisposing causes of secondary *Malassezia* dermatitis include breed, the long-term administration of glucocorticoids or antibiotics, bacterial skin disease, and an underlying allergic or seborrheic skin disease (Plant *et al.*, 1992). Since most of the predisposing factors have been problems in dermatology for years, other unidentified causes may also be important.

Pathogenesis

M. pachydermatis is a nonmycelial lipophilic yeast and is part of the normal cutaneous flora of the dog (Plant *et al.*, 1992; Scott *et al.*, 1995). In the normal animal, the number of organisms per cm^2 of skin is very small. Proliferation is encouraged by the buildup of sebum or by excessive moisture. In excessive numbers, the organisms alter the surface lipid layer and produce seborrheic changes, which may or may not be pruritic. Although some dogs with *Malassezia* dermatitis have a flaky dermatitis, most lesions are greasy and malodorous. The dog's level of pruritus is variable and ranges from very little to a maniacal, steroid-nonresponsive, intense itching. Since yeast lipases liberate inflammatory fatty acids from sebum, a low level pruritus can be attributed to chemical irritation. An alternative mechanism is necessary to explain the intensely pruritic animal, especially since the number of organisms found in some of these dogs is low. Hypersensitivity to cell wall components or a metabolic byproduct of the yeast is likely and is supported by some preliminary data.

To date, no studies comparing the histologic and clinical features of *Malassezia* dermatitis in large numbers of dogs have been published. Histologic data that are available suggest that yeast hypersensitivity exists. Dogs with a pruritic *Malassezia* dermatitis or West Highland white terriers with epidermal dysplasia show a superficial, predominantly lymphohistiocytic, perivascular–interstitial dermatitis with prominent exocytosis of lymphocytes into the epidermis and follicular epithelium (Scott and Miller, 1989; Scott *et al.*, 1995). West Highland white terriers also show a subepidermal and perifollicular band of mast cells (Scott and Miller, 1989). With resolution of the yeast infection, these inflammatory changes disappear. These findings suggest that some dogs develop a Type I and/or IV hypersensitivity to the yeast.

Human atopic patients commonly show immediate and delayed skin test reactions to *Malassezia* extracts (Kieffer *et al.*, 1990). This testing is just underway in dogs. Morris skin tested normal dogs, atopic dogs without a *Malassezia* dermatitis, and atopic dogs with *Malassezia* dermatitis with various dilutions of a *Malassezia* extract and eight chromatographic fractions of it (Morris and Rosser, 1995). At a 1:10 dilution of most fractions, there was a clear difference in immediate skin test reactivity between the dogs. Atopic dogs with *Malassezia* dermatitis typically showed the greatest reactivity while normal dogs showed little reactivity. Atopics without *Malassezia* dermatitis showed intermediate reactivity. Nagata developed his own *Malassezia* antigen and compared the skin test reactivity of normal dogs with that of dogs with seborrheic dermatitis (Nagata and Ishida, 1995). Normal dogs showed no immediate or delayed reactivity while 30% and 7% of the seborrheic dogs showed immediate or delayed reactivity, respectively. Over 90% of the dogs with negative skin test reactions responded to shampoo treatments while 67% of the skin test-positive dogs required systemic antifungal therapy to resolve their dermatitis. As more investigators study the immunology of *Malassezia* dermatitis, these preliminary findings will, no doubt, be supported.

Clinical features

The current veterinary literature lists various breeds predisposed to *Malassezia* dermatitis. Most are those with pronounced body folds (e.g., Basset hound), an allergic predisposition (e.g. Jack Russell terrier), a seborrheic predisposition (e.g. Cocker spaniel) or a combination of these (e.g. West Highland white terrier) (Scott *et al.*, 1995). Probably all dogs with an allergic or seborrheic predisposition are prone to the problem. Unless the dog is exquisitely sensitive to the yeast from previous episodes of disease, the initial clinical signs will be that of the underlying disease. When the hypersensitivity to the yeast develops, the clinical history can change markedly. A common example is that seen in many atopic dogs when their gluco-corticoid-responsive seasonal pruritus suddenly escalates, responds poorly to ever increasing doses of glucocorticoids, and becomes nonseasonal.

Dogs with *Malassezia* hypersensitivity have a regionalized or generalized pruritic seborrheic dermatitis. Pruritus is variable, but is often intense and responds poorly to corticosteroid treatment. Body folds and intertriginous regions (Figure 10.8), especially those on the feet, are often severely involved. Affected areas are variably haired, erythematous, scaly, crusty, greasy, and very malodorous. Depending upon the severity of the dog's pruritus and the chronicity of the disease, the dog's whole body can be bald, red–hyperpigmented, and greasy (Plate 15) with very pronounced skin folds. The differential diagnosis depends on the clinical presentation. When the animal has a generalized steroid-nonresponsive condition the list of differential diagnoses should include food hypersensitivity, scabies, staphylococcal infection, and *Malassezia* dermatitis.

Malassezia dermatitis is rare in the cat. Beyond feline immunodeficiency virus infection, no predisposing causes have been established. Clinical findings include ceruminous otitis externa mimicking ear mite disease, feline acne, and a generalized seborrheic condition.

Diagnosis

Although *M. pachydermatis* is part of the normal cutaneous flora, it is difficult to demonstrate in normal dogs (Plant, 1992; Scott *et al.*, 1995). The organism can be identified by culture or exfoliative cytology. In diseased animals, exfoliative cytology is most commonly used. Surface debris is collected by scraping or rubbing the affected area with a moistened cotton swab or a scalpel blade, by direct exfoliation with cellophane tape, or by pressing a clean glass slide on to the lesion. Cellophane collected samples are usually examined with new methylene blue stain while the other samples are heat fixed, stained with a conventional differential stain, and examined (Figure 10.9). Usually the confirmation or negation of the tentative diagnosis is straightforward. Yeast are either numerous or nonexistent. In some cases, an occasional yeast (0–1/cm^2) is seen on each of multiple slides. With such small numbers it can be difficult to make a firm diagnosis of *Malassezia* dermatitis. The significance of these yeast is proven by skin biopsy and/or response to treatment.

A common complaint is that exfoliative cytology shows no yeast. An obvious answer is that the animal does not have a *Malassezia* dermatitis but rather a seborrheic condition with a different cause. Dogs with a staphylococcal seborrheic dermatitis can look and smell like those with a *Malassezia* dermatitis, but will not respond to anti-yeast treatments. If the cytologic preparation is not examined with the 40× objective, the staphylococci will be missed. Other explanations for negative cytology in dogs with *Malassezia* dermatitis include poor site selection, poor sample collection, and the nature of hypersensitivity. The yeast replicate in the surface keratin layer and if this layer is removed for example by the animal's scratching, bathing, or clipping, the yeast population will be drastically reduced. With hypersensitivity, the few remaining yeast in the hair follicle infundibulum or elsewhere on the body can maintain the dermatitis. When the clinical presentation strongly

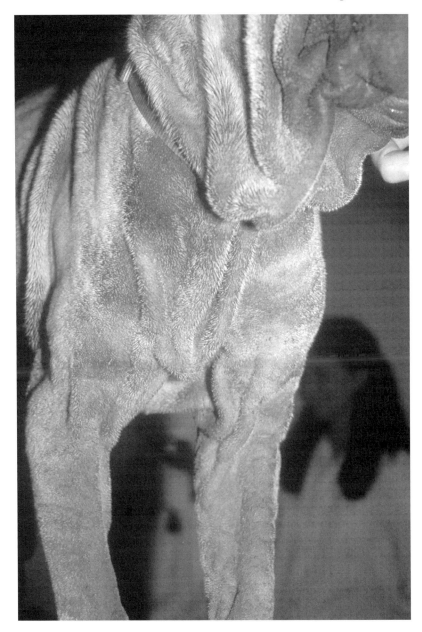

Figure 10.8 *Alopecia, hyperpigmentation, and greasiness of the folds in a Chinese shar pei.*

suggests a *Malassezia* dermatitis but the initial round of cytology is negative, more cytologic samples should be evaluated or skin biopsies should be taken.

Skin biopsy is useful in the diagnosis of *Malassezia* dermatitis and can be helpful in defining the underlying disease provided that the inflammation associated with the yeast dermatitis does not overwhelm the histologic features of the underlying condition. If secondary yeast hypersensitivity is strongly suspected, skin biopsies to characterize the underlying disease should be postponed until the yeast dermatitis

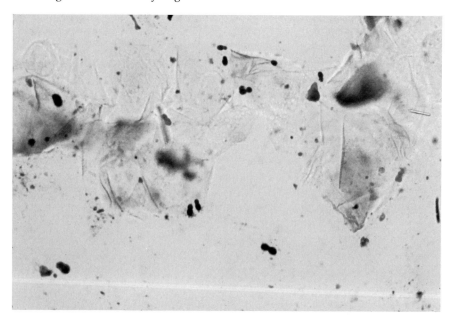

Figure 10.9 *Multiple* Malassezia *organisms from a cat with a generalized seborrheic dermatitis. (Diff Quik 100X)*

has resolved. Since the organisms live in the surface keratin layer, it is imperative that the biopsy sites are selected and collected carefully. Excoriated areas should be avoided and lesions with visible scale, crust, or grease should be selected. Multiple biopsies should be taken, especially if cytology shows no or only a few yeast. The biopsy sites should not be clipped closely or cleaned with scrubs of any kind. Close clipping, as is done for most skin biopsies, and routine surface preparation will remove the keratin layer and the yeast.

Treatment

Although some dogs have an idiopathic nonrecurrent *Malassezia* dermatitis, most have some allergic or seborrheic disorder that predisposes to yeast overgrowth. Successful treatment of the animal involves resolution of both the *Malasseziai* dermatitis and the underlying disease. If the underlying disease is overlooked, the yeast infection will recur and the second and subsequent episodes will be more severe.

If the surface and follicular keratin layers are removed with antiseborrheic shampoos, the yeast will also be removed. Since it is difficult to remove all the surface and follicular keratin and therefore the yeast by bathing, shampooing alone may be inadequate in dogs with *Malassezia* hypersensitivity. This was demonstrated nicely by Nagata when he needed to treat 67% of his skin test-positive dogs with oral antifungal agents (Nagata and Ishida, 1995).

Since the two most widely used antifungal agents, ketoconazole (5–10 mg/kg q. 12 h) and itraconazole (5 mg/kg q. 24 h), are expensive and adverse reactions are associated with their use, topical treatments are usually dispensed before systemic antifungals are used (Scott *et al.*, 1995). Densely-coated dogs will probably not respond to topical treatments unless the coat is cut short to allow adequate bathing of the skin. Shampoo selection depends upon the greasiness of the skin. When the skin is fairly dry, shampoos containing ketoconazole, miconazole, chlorhexidine, or a combination of these can be effective. Sulfur or selenium sulfide products receive widest use for greasy dogs. The bathing is done daily to twice weekly, depending upon the severity of the dog's condition. Afterbath rinses with a 2% lime sulfur solution or enilconazole provide residual activity and may prolong the interval between baths. The ears and localized areas on the skin can be spot-treated with a variety of topical products containing nystatin, miconazole, ketoconazole, or other effective antifungals.

When bathing is ineffective by itself or cannot be done, oral antifungals are necessary. The medication is given for 7–10 days after the skin lesion has resolved. Typical courses of treatment are 30–45 days. The dog with idiopathic *Malassezia* hypersensitivity or sensitivity due to an unresolvable underlying problem will require lifelong treatment. Although topical treatments can be effective for a period of time, the response will be lost eventually and oral treatments will be needed. Since ketoconazole and itraconazole are so expensive, very few cases are treated on a maintenance basis. In the authors' limited experience, the administration of ketoconazole every second or third day can be effective in preventing or postponing relapses.

Helminth Hypersensitivity Disorders

With rare exception, the helminths that affect dogs and cats live within the animal's body. During the parasites' development, their cuticular antigens are exposed to the host's immune system. IgE is thought of as the antiparasitic and antiallergen antibody. Its production in response to ascarids and other parasites is a well-known phenomenon. Halliwell (1975) demonstrated that anti-ascarid IgE molecules bind to skin and other mast cells. Hirshman *et al.* (1981) have shown an airway hypersensitivity in dogs to ascarid antigen. Butler *et al.* (1983) reported that dogs naturally or experimentally sensitized to ascarid antigen would develop both respiratory and cutaneous allergic reactions when challenged with antigen. Accordingly, parasitized animals may show signs of cutaneous allergy.

Intestinal parasite hypersensitivity

Hypersensitivity with cutaneous manifestations to intestinal parasites is rare and has been reported in dogs and cats (Miller, 1978; Scott *et al.*, 1995). Ascarids, hookworms, tapeworms, and whipworms have all been implicated. Since roundworms and hookworms migrate through the host's tissues during their development, these parasites should be more allergenic.

Clinical features
Cutaneous manifestations of hypersensitivity to internal parasites include:

■ persistent or recurrent urticaria;
■ a widespread, pruritic papulocrustous dermatitis;

- nonlesional pruritus in the distribution of atopy or food hypersensitivity (Figure 10.10).
- Animals sensitized to hookworms may develop pruritic erythematous papular–nodular lesions at the site of larval penetration of the skin.

Diagnosis

Due to its rarity, the index of suspicion for intestinal parasite hypersensitivity will be low unless the patient has concurrent gastrointestinal signs. A fecal sample from all 'allergic' animals should therefore be examined before considering allergy testing. A diagnosis of parasite hypersensitivity should be entertained when the fecal sample is positive. Resolution of the cutaneous signs with the administration of the appropriate anthelminthic supports the diagnosis but does not prove its allergic basis.

Endoparasitized dogs have high IgE titers, which can cause false-positive serologic allergy test results (Scott *et al.*, 1995). If the 'allergic' animal has intestinal parasites but worming does not change the animal's skin condition, further allergy testing will be necessary. It is advisable to postpone the testing to allow the antiparasite serum IgE levels to drop. With antigen withdrawal, the duration of a reaginic antibody response in atopic dogs has been estimated to be 60 days (Schultz and Halliwell, 1985). This figure may not apply to antiparasitic antibodies, but it would seem appropriate to delay serologic allergy testing for this period.

Filarial hypersensitivity

Dirofilaria immitis and *D. repens* are the most common species of filarial nematodes that can cause skin disease in pets (Scott *et al.*, 1995). The frequency of infection

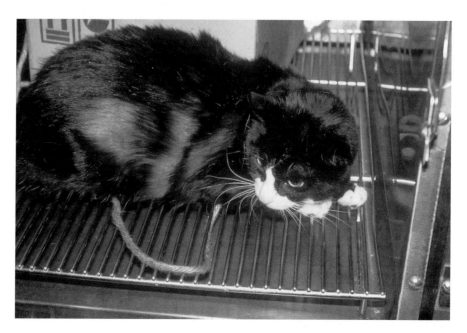

Figure 10.10   *Traumatic hair loss in a cat with a roundworm hypersensitivity.*

varies greatly with geographic location. Various other filarial nematodes exist worldwide, but are of uncertain significance in the skin. Although skin lesions have been seen in association with both *D. immitis* and *D. repens* infection, hypersensitivity apparently only plays a role in the lesions seen in some heartworm infected dogs.

Clinical features
Skin lesions are rare in dogs with heartworm disease. Most of the affected dogs have demonstrable microfilariae in the blood, but about 20% have occult dirofilariasis. The most commonly reported cutaneous manifestation of *D. immitis* infection is a pruritic nodular skin disease of the head and limbs (Figure 10.11) (Scott, 1979, 1987). Lesions may be seen elsewhere and the animal's pruritus responds poorly to the administration of corticosteroids. Other presentations include:

- an intensely pruritic papulocrustous dermatitis mimicking canine scabies;
- a pruritic ulcerative disease of the head and limbs;
- alopecia of the chest and limbs;
- seborrheic skin disease (Mozos *et al.*, 1992; Scott *et al.*, 1995).

Heartworm disease is documented in the cat and is probably more common than recognized. Since most affected cats are lightly infected, they are usually neither microfilaremic or antigenemic, making diagnosis difficult (Knight, 1995). Currently, the antibody serologic test is considered to be more sensitive in the cat. One author (WHM) has seen one, and possibly two, cat(s) with a presumed heartworm-associated dermatitis. Both cats had an allergic-like generalized pruritic skin disease, a persistent high peripheral eosinophilia, and signs of respiratory disease. During the evaluation of their respiratory system, heartworm disease was found. One cat was treated for heartworms and its skin disease disappeared. The other cat was not treated.

Diagnosis
All of the clinical presentations other than the nodular lesions on the head and limbs mimic reaction patterns seen in atopy, food hypersensitivity, scabies, and a variety of other dermatoses. Unless the skin is biopsied and the microfilariae are seen within the tissues, the index of suspicion for filarial hypersensitivity will be low. Accordingly, all 'allergic' dogs who live in or have visited a heartworm endemic area should be checked for heartworms before allergy testing is undertaken. The same may be true for cats. Since approximately 20% of infected dogs will test negative for microfilariae while less than 1% of microfilaremic dogs test negative for heartworm antigen, the serologic heartworm tests, especially the antigen test, are preferred (Knight, 1995). If a Knott's test-negative dog or cat has a persistent peripheral eosinophilia and/or basophilia, it should be tested for heartworms using the appropriate serologic test. If the testing is positive, the animal must be treated.

Treatment
Dogs with heartworm hypersensitivity will stop itching and their lesions will heal

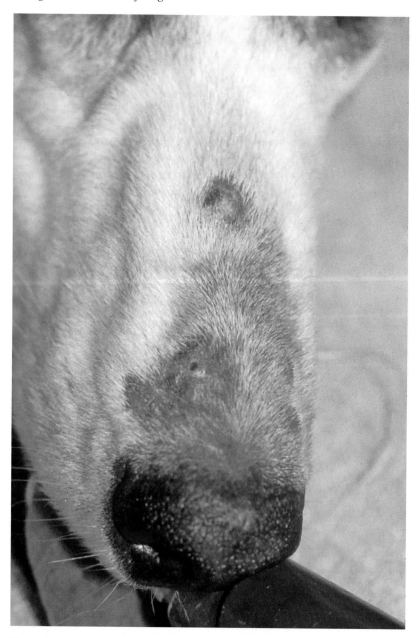

Figure 10.11 *Pruritic papular lesions on the bridge of the nose in a dog with heartworm hypersensitivity. (Courtesy of DW Scott.)*

spontaneously with the administration of an appropriate adulticide and microfilaricide (Scott, 1979; Scott and Vaughan 1987; Mozos *et al.*, 1992). Pruritus disappears in about two weeks and lesional healing is complete in another 3–6 weeks. Because of its rarity, most pruritic dogs with heartworm disease will continue to itch after the heartworm disease has resolved, indicating that the heartworm disease was a coincidental finding.

Hormonal Hypersensitivity

Hormonal hypersensitivity is a rare allergic condition where an animal presumably becomes hypersensitive to its own endogenous sex hormones (Chamberlain, 1974; Scott and Miller, 1992; Scott *et al.*, 1995). It occurs in both males and females, but because of the cyclic variation in serum sex hormone levels in the bitch, it is most commonly recognized in the female dog. To the authors' knowledge, the disorder only occurs in intact animals. If an affected animal is neutered after years of disease, some residual pruritus may persist from the adrenal sex hormones.

Clinical features

As in other allergic conditions, pruritus is the clinical sign of this disorder. Initially, there is nonlesional pruritus of the lower back, perineum, and posteromedial thighs (Figure 10.12 and Plate 16). As the itching usually is fairly intense, secondary changes are common. In females, the signs start around a heat period or an overt pseudocyesis and stop when this reproductive event is over. Typical of allergic disorders, the next exposure produces more intense signs, which last longer. Some bitches will become so sensitive that the signs will be nonseasonal although estral exacerbations can be recognized. Males show nonseasonal signs, which intensify with time (Scot and Miller, 1992). Chronically affected animals will traumatize their face, feet, and axillary regions as well as the posterior parts of their body. Even early in the course of the disease, the response to adequate doses of corticosteroids is poor.

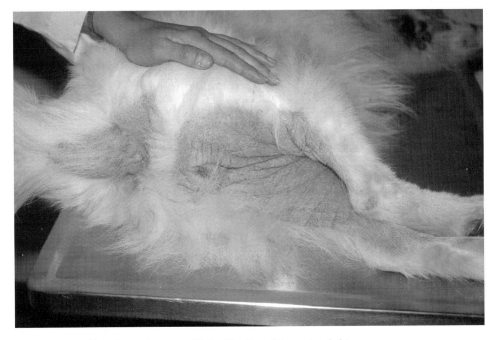

Figure 10.12 *Alopecia, erythema, and lichenification of the perineal skin.*

Diagnosis

Early on, these animals are most easily confused with dogs who are food or flea hypersensitive. As the signs progress, atopic disease must also be considered. Helpful diagnostic clues for hormonal hypersensitivity include the onset or worsening of clinical signs around a reproductive event and resistance to glucocorticoid. Unless complicated by a secondary bacterial or *Malassezia* infection, the pruritus of atopy, some cases of food hypersensitivity, or early flea bite hypersensitivity typically stops when adequate doses of a glucocorticoid are administered, but in over 60% of the cases of food hypersensitivity and all cases of hormonal hypersensitivity, the response to glucocorticoids is poor. The pruritus either does not lessen at all or decreases, but not to the level expected. Since food hypersensitivity is not typically cyclic, this differential can be dismissed in bitches who have gone through one or more episodes of disease. If the patient is a male or a bitch presented in her first episode, food hypersensitivity can not be dismissed without testing. If dietary restriction testing is done on the bitch whose pruritus is still focused around her estral period, it is likely that she will be nonpruritic by the time the 4- to 10-weeks of dietary testing have been completed. If the bitch is not challenged with her old food as she should be, an erroneous diagnosis of food hypersensitivity will be made.

Currently, the definitive documentation of a hormonal hypersensitivity is impossible. In the past, skin testing with aqueous solutions of estrogen, progesterone, and testosterone was used to substantiate the diagnosis. These hormones are expensive and difficult to obtain so testing is not routine. The diagnosis is supported by the elimination of all the appropriate differential diagnoses and by the animal's response to neutering. After surgery, most dogs show a significant improvement within two weeks. If a female dog is a breeding bitch or the owners are reluctant to neuter the dog without an absolute diagnosis, oral or repositol testosterone should be administered at a dose of 0.5–1.0 mg/kg to a maximum total dose of 30 mg (Scott et al., 1995). The bitch with hormonal hypersensitivity should stop scratching with this drug and the signs should recur when the drug is withdrawn. In males, diethylstilbestrol (0.1–0.5 mg total dose) is the hormone used to 'prove' hormonal hypersensitivity (Scott and Miller, 1992). Progestational compounds can also be used; but because they have some anti-inflammatory properties and can decrease pruritus in some animals, response is difficult to interpret. Testosterone administration is likely to intensify the pruritus.

Treatment

Although medical management with testosterone or estrogen is appealing to some owners, these drugs should only be used as a presurgical diagnostic test. Treatment consists of neutering the animal.

References

Affolter VK, von Tscharner C. Cutaneous drug reactions: A retrospective study of histopathologic changes and their correlation with clinical disease. *Vet. Dermatol.* **4:** 79, 1993.

Baker E. Staphylococcal disease. *Vet. Clin. N. Am.* **4:** 107, 1974.

Blacker KI, Stern RS, Wintroub BU. Cutaneous reactions to drugs. In Fitzpatrick TB, *et al.* (eds) *Dermatology in General Medicine*, 4th edition. McGraw Hill, New York, p. 1783, 1993.

Becker AM, Jamik TA, Smith EK, *et al. Propionibacterium acnes* immunotherapy in chronic recurrent canine pyoderma. *J. Vet. Intern. Med.* **3:** 26, 1989.

Bond R, Dodd AM, Lloyd DH. Isolation of *Malassezia sympodialis* from feline skin and mucosa. *Proc. ESVD,* **12:** 220, 1995.

Breen PT. Secondary bacterial hypersensitivity reactions in canine skin. *Proc. Am. Anim. Hosp. Assoc.* **43:** 134, 1976.

Butler JM, Peters JE, Hirshman CA, *et al.* Pruritic dermatitis in asthmatic Basenji-Greyhound dogs: A model for human atopic dermatitis. *J. Am. Acad. Dermatol.* **8:** 33, 1983.

Chamberlain KW. Hormonal hypersensitivity in canines. *Canine Pract.* **1:** 18, 1974.

DeBoer DJ, Moriello KA, Thomas CB, *et al.* Evaluation of commercial staphylococcal bacterin for management of idiopathic recurrent superficial pyoderma in dogs. *Am. J. Vet. Res.* **51:** 636, 1990.

Dufait R. *Pityrosporum canis* as the cause of canine chronic dermatitis. *Vet. Med. Sm. Anim. Clin.* **78:** 1055, 1983.

Halliwell REW. The site of production and localization of IgE in canine tissues. *Ann. N. Y. Acad. Sci.* **254:** 476, 1975.

Hirshman CA, Downes H, Leon DA, *et al.* Basenji-Greyhound dog model of asthma. Pulmonary responses after β-adrenergic blockage. *J. Appl. Physiol.* **51:** 1423, 1981.

Kieffer M, Bergbrant IM, Faergemann J. Immunologic reactions to *Pityrosporum ovale* in adult patients with atopic and seborrheic dermatitis. *J. Am. Acad. Dermatol.* **22:** 739, 1990.

Knight DH. Guidelines for diagnosis and management of heartworm (*Dirofilaria immitis*) infection. In Bonagura, JD (ed.) *Kirk's Current Veterinary Therapy XII.* W.B. Saunders, Philadelphia, p. 879, 1995.

Lehmann PF. Immunology of fungal infections in animals. *Vet. Immunol. Immunopathol.* **10:** 33, 1985.

Mason IS, Lloyd DH. The role of allergy in the development of canine pyoderma. *J. Sm. Anim. Pract.* **30:** 216, 1989.

Mason IS, Lloyd DW. The macroscopic and microscopic effects of intradermal injection of crude and purified staphylococcal extracts on canine skin. *Vet. Dermatol.* **6:** 197, 1995.

Mason KV, Evans AG. Dermatitis associated with *Malassezia pachydermatis* in 11 dogs. *J. Am. Anim. Hosp. Assoc.* **27:** 13, 1991.

Miller TA. Immunology in intestinal parasitism. *Vet. Clin. N. Am.* **8:** 707, 1978.

Miller WH Jr, Antibiotic-responsive generalized nonlesional pruritis in a dog. *Cornell Vet.* **81:** 389, 1991.

Morales CA, Schultz KT, DeBoer DJ. Antistaphylococcal antibodies in dogs with recurrent staphylococcal pyoderma. *Vet. Immunol. Immunopathol.* **42:** 137, 1994.

Morris DO, Rosser EJ. Immunologic aspects of *Malassezia* dermatitis in patients with canine atopic dermatitis. *Proc. Annu. Memb. Meet. Am. Acad. Vet. Dermatol. Am. Coll. Vet. Dermatol.* **11:** 16, 1995.

Mozos E, Ginel JS, Lopez R, *et al.* Cutaneous lesions associated with canine heartworm infection. *Vet. Dermatol.* **3:** 191, 1992.

Nagata M, Ishida T. Cutaneous reactivity to *Malassezia pachydermatis* in dogs with seborrheic dermatitis. *Proc. Annu. Memb. Meet. Am. Acad. Vet. Dermatol. Am. Coll. Vet. Dermatol.* **11:** 11, 1995.

Noli C, Koeman JP, Willemse T. A retrospective evaluation of adverse reactions to trimethoprim–sulphonamide combinations in dogs and cats. *Vet. Quart.* **17:** 123, 1995.

Plant JD, Rosenkrantz WS, Griffin CE. Factors associated with and prevalence of high *Malassezia pachydermatis* numbers on dog skin. *J. Am. Vet. Med. Assoc.* **210:** 879, 1992.

Pukay BP. Treatment of canine bacterial hypersensitivity by hyposensitization with *Staphylococcus aureus* bacterin-toxoid. *J. Am. Anim. Hosp. Assoc.* **21:** 479, 1985.

Schultz KT, Halliwell REW. The induction and kinetics of an anti-DNP IgE response in dogs. *Vet. Immunol. Immunopathol.* **10:** 205, 1985.

Scott DW. Nodular skin disease associated with *Dirofilaria immitis* infection in the dog. *Cornell Vet.* **59:** 233, 1979.

Scott DW, MacDonald JM, Schultz RD. Staphylococcal hypersensitivity in the dog. *J. Am. Anim. Hosp. Assoc.* **13:** 766, 1978.

Scott DW, Miller WH Jr, Griffin CE. *Muller and Kirk's Small Animal Dermatology*, 5th edition. W.B. Saunders, Philadelphia, 1995.

Scott DW, Miller WH Jr. Epidermal dysplasia and *Malassezia pachydermatis* infection in West Highland White terriers. *Vet. Dermatol.* **1:** 25, 1989.

Scott DW, Miller WH Jr. Probable hormonal hypersensitivity in two male dogs. *Canine Pract.* **17:** 14, 1992.

Scott DW, Vaughn TC. Papulonodular dermatitis in a dog with occult filariasis. *Comp. Anim. Pract.* **1:** 31, 1987.

Van Arsdel PP Jr. Drug hypersensitivity. In Bierman CW, Pearlman DS (eds) *Allergic Diseases from Infancy to Adulthood*, 2nd edition. W.B. Saunders, Philadelphia, p. 684, 1988.

Walton GS. Symposium on allergic and endocrine dermatoses in the dog and cat. I. Allergic dermatoses of the dog and cat. *J. Sm. Anim. Pract.* **7:** 749, 1966.

Index

Numbers in *italics* refer to illustrations

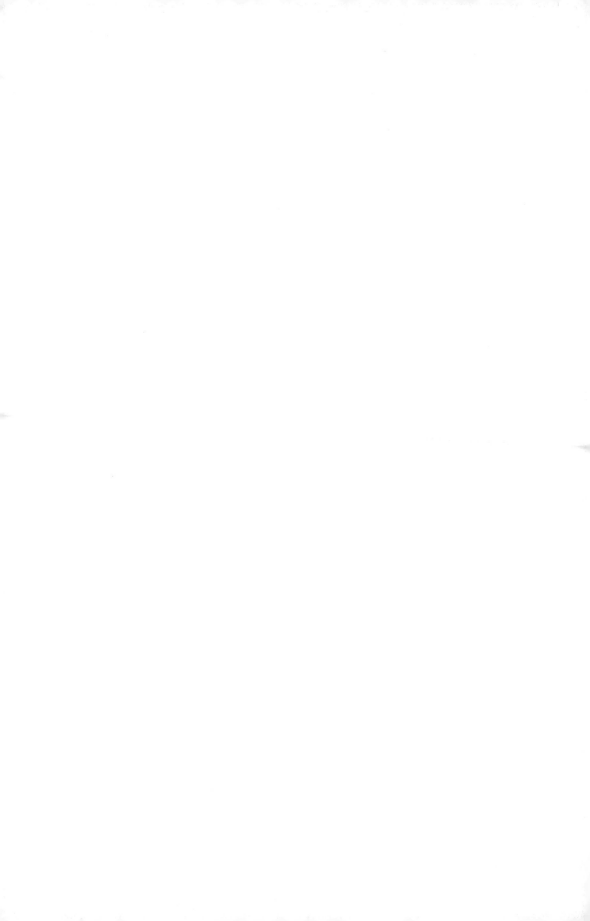